PANDEMIC OBJECTS

CONTENTS

00		FOREWORD	5
		INTRODUCTION	6
01	COMMUNICATE	HOMEMADE SIGNS	12
		RAINBOWS	18
		COSTUMES	26
		THE GROUND	32
		KEFFIYEH MASKS	38
		JAPANESE MEASLES PRINTS	46
		HIV/AIDS POSTERS	52
02	DOCUMENT	LISTS	60
		DRONES	66
		FAMILY PORTRAITS	72
		BARRICADES	82
		POSTCARDS	88
		THE SEA	98
03	SELF-CARE	FLOUR AND YEAST	108
		GARDENS	114
		POTTED PLANTS	120
		DOGS	124
		ANIMAL CROSSING	130
		TIKTOK	136
		STREAMING SERVICES	142
		WINDOWS	148
		CEMETERIES	154
04	ABSTAIN	CASH	160
		CLOTHING SHOPS	166
		HANDBAGS	172
		HAIR SALONS	176
		MUSIC VENUES	180
		PUBS	186
		THE UNDERGROUND	190
05	PIVOT	DATING APPS	198
		ROSES	204
		AL FRESCO	210
		PUBLIC PARKS	214
		STUDENT HOUSING	220
		BEDS	228

06	REAPPROPRIATE	CONVENTION CENTRES	236
		DISABLED PARKING SPACES	242
		GOVERNMENT LETTERS	248
		TOTE BAGS	252
		GOOGLE STREET VIEW	256
		CHAIRS	262
07	REVIVE	SOAP	270
		SEWING MACHINES	276
		MILK	282
		HOPSCOTCH	286
		RADIATORS	292
		RADIO	298
08	SCALING UP	TOILET ROLL	306
		LAPTOPS	312
		DOOR HANDLES	318
		COPPER	322
		CARDBOARD BOXES	326
		TESTING KITS	332
09	APPENDIX	HANDS	338
		STREET TREES	
		DIGITAL ARCHIVES	
		BEARDS	
		COCKTAIL GLASSES	
		FINGER OXIMETERS	
		HAND SANITISER	
		MOURNING RINGS	
		ICONS	
		PLAYGROUNDS	
		SPREADSHEETS	
		BARRIER TAPE	
		BALCONIES	
		SKIPPING ROPE	
		CARAVANS	
10		EPILOGUE	348
		ACKNOWLEDGEMENTS	350

Foreword

Ingrid Schroder

In the spring of 2020, the rhythms of daily life and the patterns of the year fell, one after another. As we retreated home, there was a startling awareness of being part of something immense and uncertain. We were not the first generation to have experienced a sudden shift of perspective but the isolation that characterised the sequence of lockdowns gave us little opportunity to share this moment of crisis or to come together to overcome it.

So many of the objects contained in this book reflect the closing-in experienced as a result of the pandemic and the highly individualised nature of self-protection, fear and adaptation. Most of us witnessed from afar the relentless race to keep people alive in overstretched hospitals and to find cures, vaccines and anti-dotes in the labs; meanwhile we stayed home, baking and pickling, schooling children who would have long and lasting gaps in their social maturity.

These were months of extremes that threw so many constants up in the air. Amid the distressing absurdity of global political leadership, its shifts and uncertainties, we became acutely aware of the grave effects of policies, the rigidity of borders and the precarious nature of freedom. But just as the impact of such a rapidly spreading virus felt enormous, our immediate communities became exponentially richer. For many, the restrictions of movement gave way to so much more time, and an intensity of mutual care among the few people we could interact closely with.

The strict limitations and the abiding fear that accompanied so much of everyday life in 2020 also gave depth and intimacy to our relationships. The objects and people around us were made more tangible through their extreme familiarity. The examples that follow reflect this unique preciousness, not through hasty appeals to nostalgia, but through their distillation of the new habits and rituals that we reached for in a moment of crisis to persevere and provide care and support to one another.

Introduction

Brendan Cormier

In normal times, the swirling constellation of objects that mediate daily life – by the very nature of their ordinariness – tends to slip into the background, to become invisible. Amid the disruption of a pandemic, however, the camouflage surrounding these things is lifted, allowing for new perspectives and revelations. *Pandemic Objects* began as an editorial project at the Victoria and Albert Museum, starting in April 2020 and running for roughly a year and a half, through the most tumultuous and harrowing moments of the Covid-19 pandemic. The premise of the blog was based on a simple observation: during a global crisis, everyday objects change in their function and develop new meanings.

For a museum devoted to design and material culture, this felt urgent to capture. What the pandemic made clear was how modern life relies on the interworking of a vast network of objects and material flows, without which things fall apart fast. It also demonstrated the incredible elasticity and adaptability of objects as they are hacked, transformed and redeployed for other purposes – with the aid of a little human (and non-human) ingenuity. In both cases, it reaffirmed the V&A's mission, both to promote the significance of objects and design and to support critical thinking around their impact on our present and future worlds.

Many museums shared this drive to document the pandemic. Though hampered by lockdowns and furloughs, several institutions started 'rapid response' collecting initiatives to acquire objects that would stand material witness to the grim milestones of Covid-19. Curiously, the term 'rapid response collecting' had already been coined in 2013 at the V&A, by Kieran Long and his division of contemporary design and architecture curators, as a provocation to think more responsively about what can be acquired into a collection. It borrowed the language of emergency, in recognition that if certain cultural phenomena weren't collected quickly, they risked being lost forever. Seven years later, when the world faced a real existential emergency, it was appropriate that the term found widespread adoption among many museums as their flagship pandemic initiative.

This wasn't the case everywhere. Many institutions made a conscious decision not to address the pandemic at all. Some expressed doubt about what contribution a cultural space could make to a crisis that was largely dominated by challenges better left to scientists, doctors and public health professionals. There was also an understandable wariness of being seen as exploitative or attention-seeking, when the real focus should be on solving the pandemic itself. In May 2020, the design critic Kate Wagner wrote a scathing piece of criticism regarding the output from websites like *Dezeen*, *ArchDaily* and *designboom*, which for the first few months of lockdown were promoting precisely this – poorly-conceived attention-seeking designs which were meant less as earnest attempts to address the crisis, and more to generate clicks to the website.

On the other hand, a predominant narrative in design over the last several decades has been its unique ability to solve problems. This kind of problem-solving design felt absent from the pandemic story. This may have been about scale: any product designed to be delivered to millions of people usually goes through a multi-year development phase – a timeline which was impossible during the pandemic, where situations changed daily. Rather than focus on bold new innovations, *Pandemic Objects* considered the adaptive uses and past lives of the things we already had. The real design stars of the pandemic were sewing machines, cardboard boxes, hand sanitiser, and on and on: objects invented decades if not centuries ago, whose adaptability, longevity and resilience spoke to a deeper kind of design intelligence than most products on the market today.

If so much of the pandemic could be characterised by making do with what was on hand, then so too was the experience of putting together the *Pandemic Objects* project. I proposed the idea in early April 2020, before furloughs had begun. There had been a flurry of discussion at the V&A about how to transition to a digital museum, but it was clear that elaborate visions of virtual walk-throughs and online interactive exhibitions would take months or even years to develop. A project that consisted mostly of writing, which could sit on a pre-existing piece of digital infrastructure – our blog – seemed a straightforward and expeditious way to begin. As a brief, I gave a simple prompt to colleagues working across the museum: choose an object that has changed in either meaning or function over the course of the pandemic and talk about what that reveals.

Pandemic Objects highlighted the power of writing as a key output of museum work. I described it as 'an editorial project', yet this still confounded a number of journalists and the general public, who assumed that the blog was an online component to a larger exhibition or collection project. Yet many of the things discussed on the blog were uncollectable because they were so generic: collecting and exhibiting a roll of toilet paper to reflect a moment of panic-buying seemed odd. More important was to document, in writing, what significance toilet roll gained in 2020, and what that said about our emotional attachment to things. The blog was a way to collect an observation, rather than collecting a thing in itself.

A curious side effect of this approach was how the project provided a new lens for understanding the V&A collection. Historically, the way our objects have been written about and interpreted has been dominated by art historical categorisations and imperatives. In our cataloguing systems, labels and publications far more has been written about the evolution of styles, techniques, decorative motifs and biographical accounts of individual artists than about the meaning of objects in everyday life or the world-changing events in which they were implicated. The blog provides a good example of how the viewing of a collection from a lateral angle can provoke a new slate of interpretations for objects.

While posts were published fast and furious in the first few months of lockdown, they settled into a leisurely pace by the autumn, and then a trickle by the middle of 2021. As people returned to work and the museum opened up again, the focus shifted to getting visitors back and catching up on the backlog of work stalled by the pandemic. People had less time to write, but there was also a shift towards not wanting to dwell on Covid-19 any longer, to put it in the past. The last post, which was published on 22 September 2021, was never meant to be the conclusion; it just happened that way.

A new project then emerged: finding a way to archive *Pandemic Objects*, to make sure it would be available as a record for future generations to discover. Since the outbreak, it has been remarkable to see how quickly collective forgetting could sink in. Grand premonitions about the end of the automobile, the end of air flight, the end of the office and so on seemed to vanish into thin air. Utopian thinking about the reorganisation of cities, neighbourhoods, work structures and the economy dried up. We were back to business as usual, which created urgency to find a permanent and more polished format for *Pandemic Objects*. And although internet archiving has improved recently, there is still nothing better than a book for the preservation and dissemination of information. The volume you are reading now is the realisation of that goal, a fruitful collaboration with the Architectural Association – to which I am eternally grateful – to edit and revise *Pandemic Objects* into both a document about a moment in time, but hopefully also a sourcebook of insight about the nature of objects.

01

COMMUNICATE

The first thing to do in a crisis is to get your story straight. Covid-19 complicated this aim through a series of unknowns: a novel virus, an unprecedented global spread and a generation of people who had never experienced the challenges of a pandemic before. Governments struggled to sort out their messaging, and social media fanned the flames of uncertainty, doubt and hysteria.

In this informational lacuna, improvisation kicked in and, along with it, a series of bottom-up interventions that often used makeshift and at-hand objects for the simplest and most urgent of communication: hand-written signs on shopfronts, rainbow drawings facing the street from household windows, spray-painted ground markings delineating social distancing, pots and pans for cheering on key workers. As the pandemic progressed, so too did the nuance of what was communicated and how. Playful costumes were deployed as both information campaigns and much-needed mood lighteners, while obligatory face masks became carriers of multiple political and social messages.

Each pandemic is marked by its own visual output. Japanese woodblock prints during a 19th-century outbreak of measles tell stories of inequality, fear and suspicion that spread as viciously as the virus. A worldwide series of poster campaigns during the HIV/AIDS crisis in the 1980s and 1990s underlined the pressure to disseminate informed methods of prevention. With Covid-19, the visual output has been so immense and informal that future historians will have difficulty unravelling the material, but recurrent across all that visual matter is the creativity with which people have used the simplest of objects and means to talk and be heard.

HOMEMADE SIGNS

How cities and neighbourhoods saw the rebirth of grassroots communication through homemade signs, and what it means for the public sphere

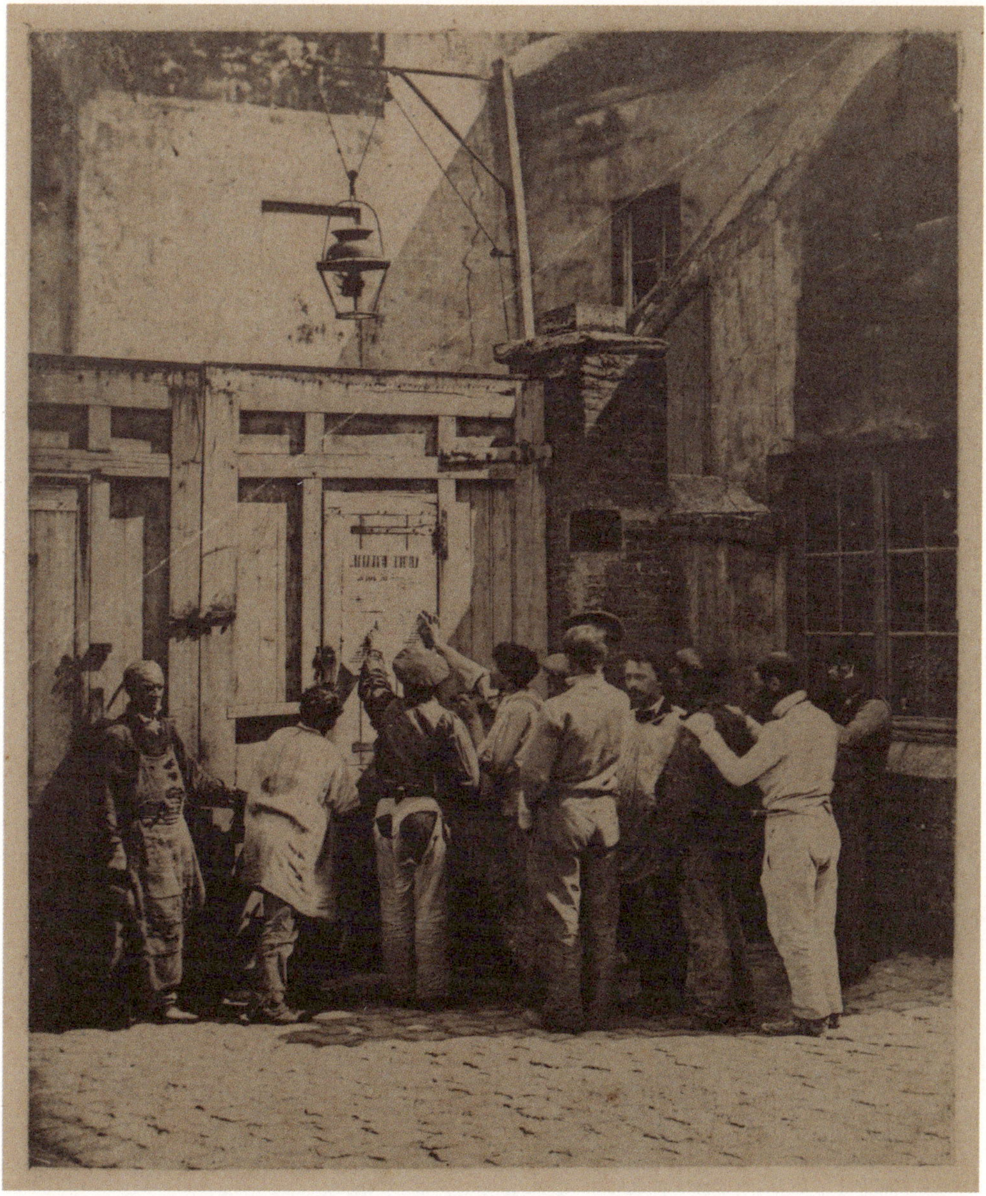

Camille Silvy,
Proclamation of the Army of July,
Paris, 1859.

'Due to Covid-19'. Those three words – the standard introduction to a homemade notice posted in a shop window – symbolised a stunning shift in the way public life was experienced during the pandemic. Written, scribbled and typed millions of times in the first weeks of the pandemic, most often on stock A4 paper and taped to windows and doors, these hastily put together signs provided an essential system for organising new social cues and protocols to deal with the crisis.

Not only did the proliferation of these homemade signs represent one of the most immediate and visible changes to public space during the lockdown, their ad-hoc nature also reflected the uncertainty, confusion and improvisational nature of the early days of the outbreak. These signs generated a strange intimacy between the maker and those reading them, and provided a guide for how to behave according to new needs and boundaries in a rapidly shifting situation. One moved through familiar spaces by reading instructions. While most wording was prosaic and perfunctory – 'we are closed', 'no cash', 'only two in the shop at a time', 'we now do takeaway' – various strange, humorous and touching informalities could also be found in typos, handwriting and local references.

Rather rapidly, these signs expanded to encompass more than just instruction. Children took to drawing rainbows (see Rainbows p18) and other positive messages, and posting them in front windows. The poster *Thank God for Immigrants* by artist Jeremy Deller and graphic designer Fraser Muggeridge quickly sold through its limited run and also appeared in windows around the UK. Chalk and spray paint were used to communicate messages of both hope and criticism (see Hopscotch p286 and The Ground p32), directly transforming the surfaces of the city.

The proliferation of homemade signs brought to the surface an aspect of the city that had fallen out of public discourse in recent years. This could be referred to as the editorial layer of a city – all the words, messages and images that are broadcast to us in public spaces through shop signage, parking regulations and bus shelter advertisements. This layer not only helps with day-to-day navigation – knowing where to go, what a shop sells, or where and when you can park – but also produces the character of a city and its power relations, determined by those who are granted the right to broadcast messages and those who are not.

The power dynamics wrapped up in the regulation of these rights have historically been subject to a much fiercer debate than as seen in recent years. In the early 2000s, for instance, spurred on by publications like *Adbusters* and Naomi Klein's *No Logo*, significant critique emerged about the loss of a democratic voice in public space. While beautification policies in municipalities around the world had explicitly banned certain forms of individual and community expression (graffiti, flyposting, etc), corporations were allowed to cover public space in advertising. Impassioned activists rallied to protect the right of communities and individuals to find a voice on the street and aimed to curb the presence of corporate messaging in public space.

These debates eventually faded into the background. Mass communication technologies were becoming far more readily available, and the rising popularity of internet forums and social media in the latter half of the 2000s replaced much of the need for community postering. A parallel and fast-developing world of online communication caused many of the messages that had previously adorned signposts, billboards and building façades to shift location and be consumed through what was rapidly becoming a ubiquitous handheld device: the mobile phone. Meanwhile, the editorial layer of the city could quietly be reformatted, cleaned up and regulated from above.

The re-emergence of homemade signs – while imbued with the tragedy of the pandemic – has also rekindled the idea that cities and public spaces can, and should, be physical expressions of the communities that inhabit them. This, along with the use of simple tools – a pad of paper, some tape and a pen – is all you need for your voice to be heard.

Text by Brendan Cormier

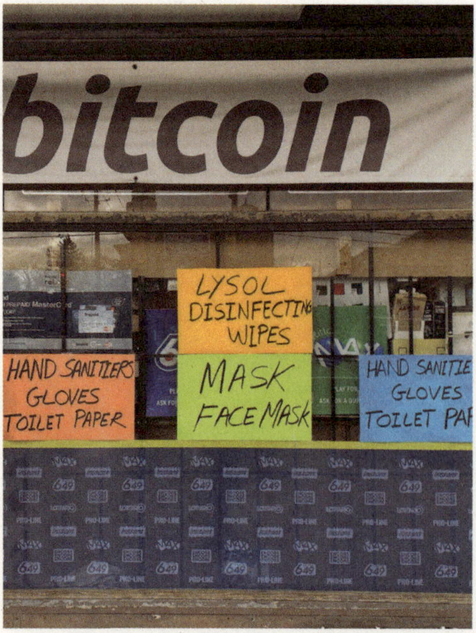

Signs advertising goods
for sale, Toronto, Canada.

Signs on a bottle shop
in Toronto, Canada.

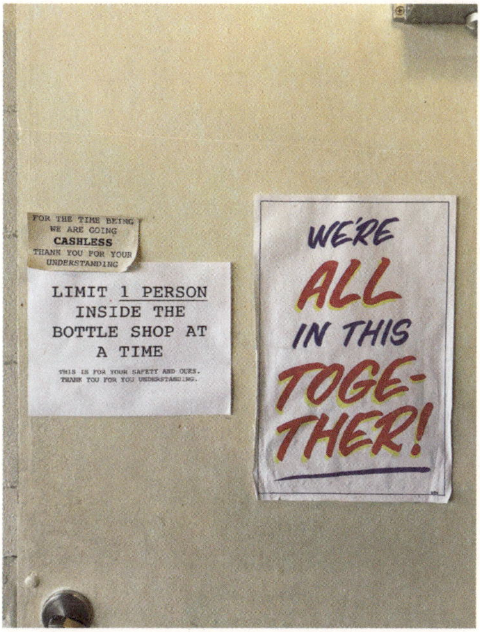

Signs on a shop
in Akashi, Japan.

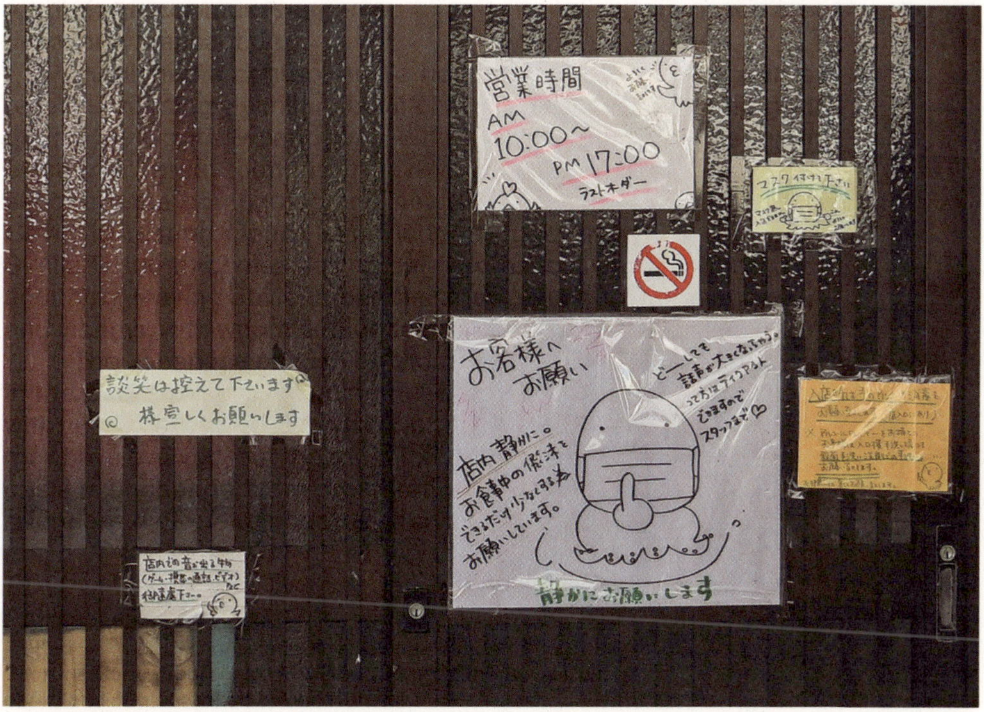
営業時間
AM
10:00~
PM 17:00
ラストオーダー
談笑は控えて下さいます
様宜しくお願いします
お客様へ
お願い
店内 静かに。
お食事中の飛沫を
できるだけ少なくする為
お願いしています。
静かにお願いします

RAINBOWS

Cheer Bear, manufactured
by Kenner Products, 1983.

How the pandemic spawned a worldwide phenomenon of rainbow drawings, showing the collective power of children's voices

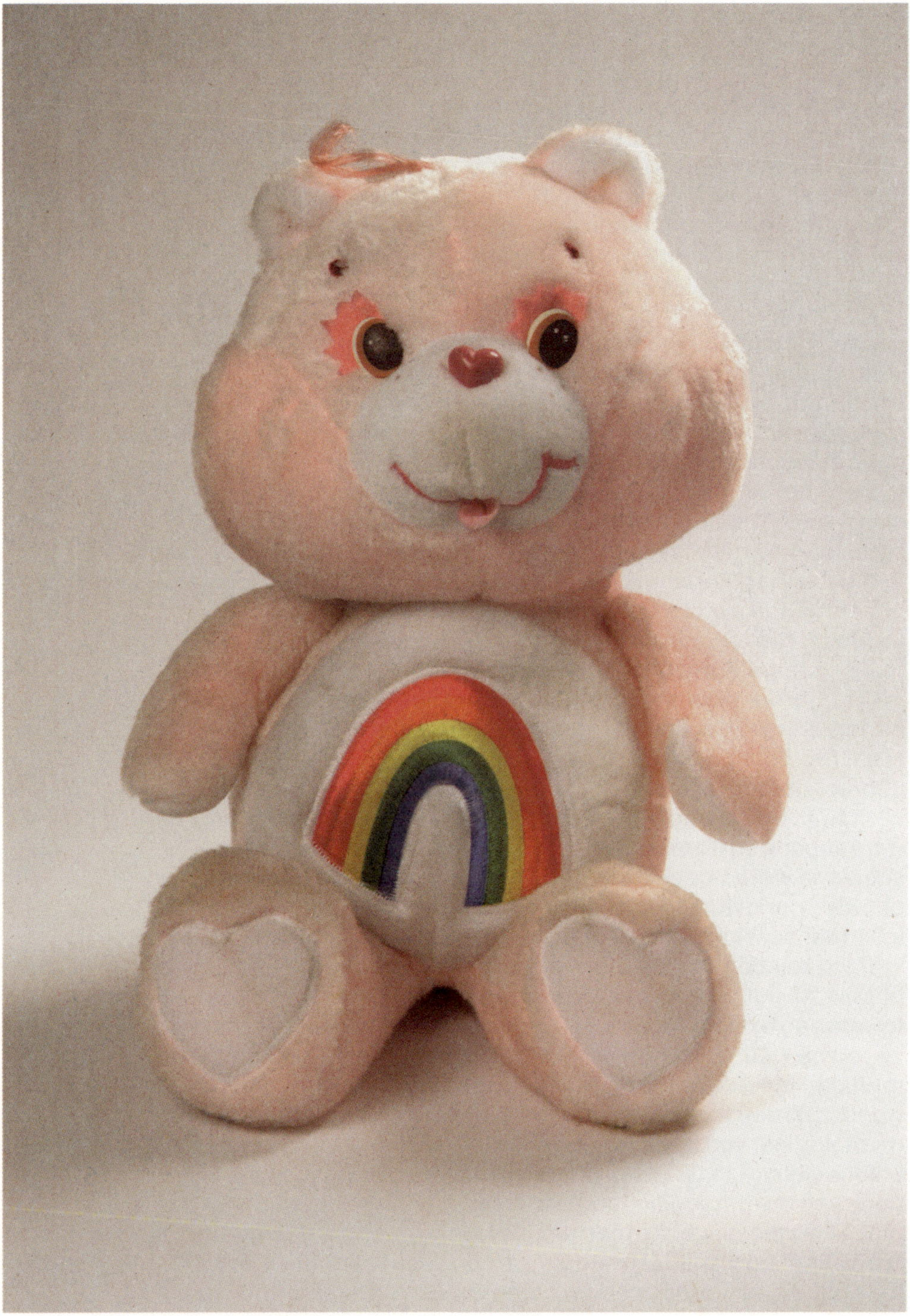

COMMUNICATE

In February 2020, Europe's first wave of Covid-19 infections hit northern Italy. News reports showed deserted Italian streets, with only a few people venturing out for indispensable supplies – giving a preview of what would soon come to pass around the world. Against this bleak backdrop, another phenomenon emerged, one which showcased the resilience and creativity of children and their families: homemade signs proclaiming 'Andrà tutto bene' (all will be well), accompanied by the hopeful image of a rainbow, hanging from balcony railings and windows in towns and cities throughout the country.

The phrase 'Andrà tutto bene' entered the country's consciousness in early March, when hand-written post-it notes with the phrase mysteriously began appearing on front doors in the Lombardy region – a clandestine act to brighten the spirits of troubled citizens. Soon after, a group of families in southern Italy encouraged their children to craft signs using the same phrase with added rainbows. When photos of these signs were shared online and in the news, the practice quickly became a national phenomenon before spreading to other countries, including the UK. What started as a modest activity to bring hope and cheer to those in need resulted in an international movement of incredible force: hundreds of thousands of signs made by children, representing an outpouring of empathy at an unprecedented scale.

John Constable, *Landscape with a Double Rainbow*, Great Britain, 1812.

In the UK, as lockdown inevitably materialised and children were separated from their friends and sequestered to their homes, solutions were needed for home schooling and to nourish their creative curiosities. By mid-March, encouraged by parents and in virtual sessions with teachers, children across the UK began crafting rainbow images to hang in their own windows. While the phrase 'All will be well' was used less in the UK, messages evolved towards an explicit focus on supporting the NHS and key workers.

The use of rainbows in these images was evocative on multiple levels. Rainbows have been symbols of hope and wonder throughout history, and are deeply embedded in various mythologies, with legends and beliefs created to explain their unique beauty. In Greek mythology, Iris was the messenger of the gods and the personification of the rainbow, travelling from Olympia to give messages to mortals. In Navajo tradition, the rainbow is the path of holy spirits, frequently depicted in sacred sand paintings, which are produced in ceremonies for healing purposes

and destroyed afterwards. The Old Testament's *Book of Genesis* describes a rainbow appearing at the moment that a great flood recedes, allowing an ark to finally dock with its cargo of people and animals. Irish legend has it that reaching the end of a rainbow will lead to a pot of gold guarded by a leprechaun.

Over the centuries these myths and legends percolated throughout culture. From the end of the 18th century and throughout the 19th century, western European art was dominated by landscape painting, with English Romantic artists such as John Constable and JMW Turner often exploring the magical light effects of rainbows in their works. More recently, the artist Ugo Rondinone has used rainbows in *Vocabulary of Solitude* and his *Rainbow Poems* series, which include enigmatic phrases about shared experience in public space. With these giant rainbow-coloured phrases, Rondinone, as a gay artist, was drawing on the more recent symbolic history of the rainbow as an LGBTQ+ emblem. Designed by artists and activists including Gilbert Baker, Lynn Segerblom and James McNamara in 1978, the rainbow flag became a symbol unifying LGBTQ+ people around the world.

In popular culture, the rainbow has featured heavily in film and television as a symbol of longing and of hope. Major moments in the history of film include Judy Garland singing 'Over the Rainbow' in *The Wizard of Oz* (1939) and Kermit the Frog's rendition of 'Rainbow Connection' 40 years later in *The Muppet Movie* (1979). In April 2020, Kermit would reprise this in a new version for social media, bringing new fans to a classic song that resonated with children's creative endeavours during lockdown.

In May 2020, recognising the cultural importance of the rainbow-drawing phenomenon under lockdown, the V&A Museum of Childhood (now Young V&A) launched an open call to collect examples of children's rainbow artwork from around the world. Thousands of emails were received, interpreting the rainbow motif in diverse ways using a wide variety of materials at hand. After whittling down the submissions to what was most easily collectible and preservable, the museum was able to officially acquire more than 100 works which are now in its permanent collection.

Aside from the reuse and reinterpretation of the rainbow symbol, these works point to another significance: that children can express themselves and be heard in the public sphere. Alongside their rainbow artworks, many children sent out a clear and powerful statement: that we must protect the institution of the NHS and its workers. This strong political point was bolstered by a shared graphic symbolism that echoed the online mechanics of memes, showing a collective endorsement of a healthcare system that is highly regarded around the world. The rainbow artwork phenomenon, and its backing of the NHS in the UK, offers an inspiring lesson in the power of creativity and how children can find a way to make themselves heard.

Text by Kristian Volsing

Handprint banner made by Molly and Merle from Somerset, featured in the V&A exhibition *All Will Be Well: Children's Rainbows from Lockdown* which opened in December 2020.

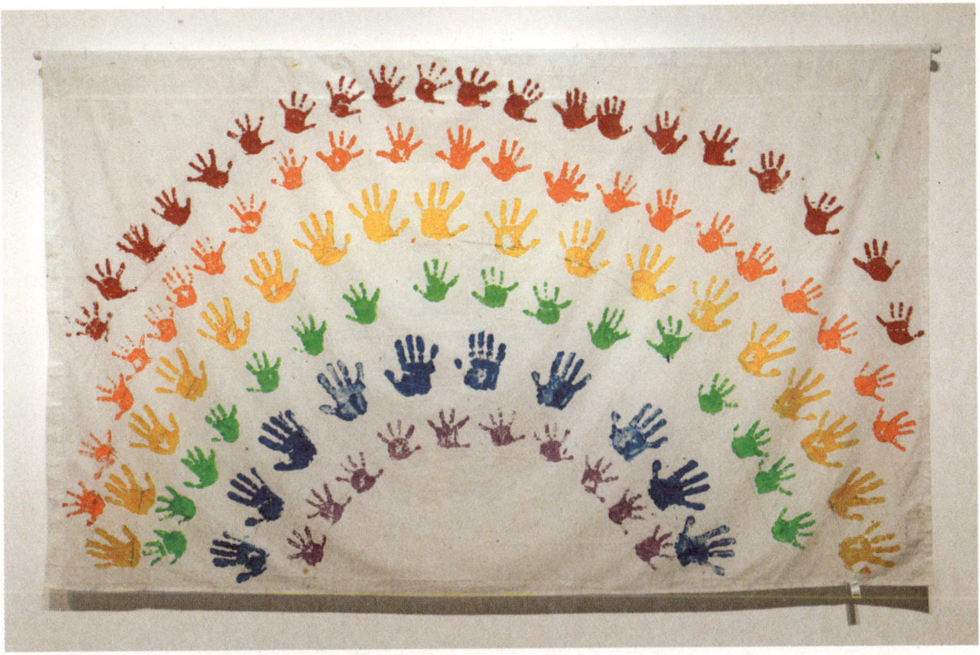

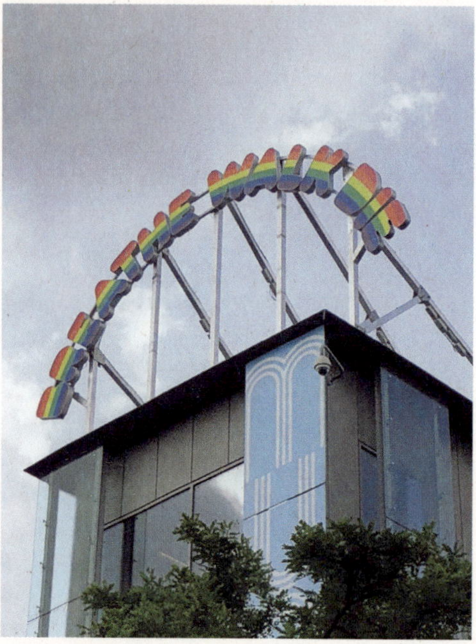

Ugo Rondinone's artwork *Breathe Walk Die* on the edge of the roof of Museum Boijmans Van Beuningen in Rotterdam, 2016.

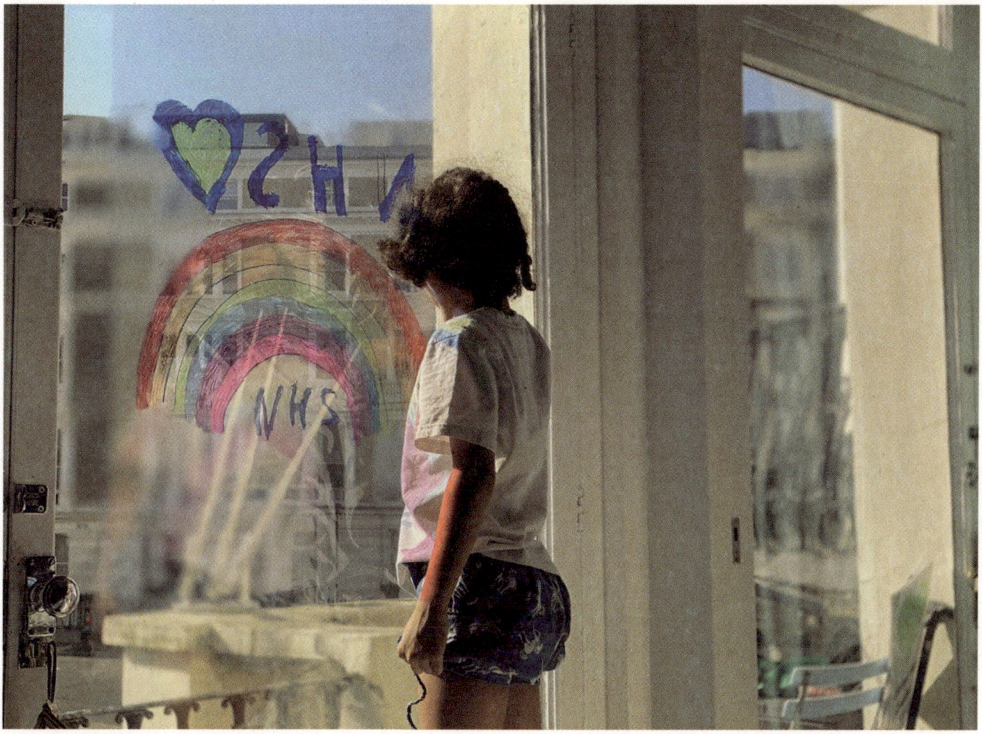

Eliza from Ladbroke Grove, London making a stained glass window effect rainbow.

COSTUMES

How costumes provided a productive form of escapism as well as a way of communicating with others

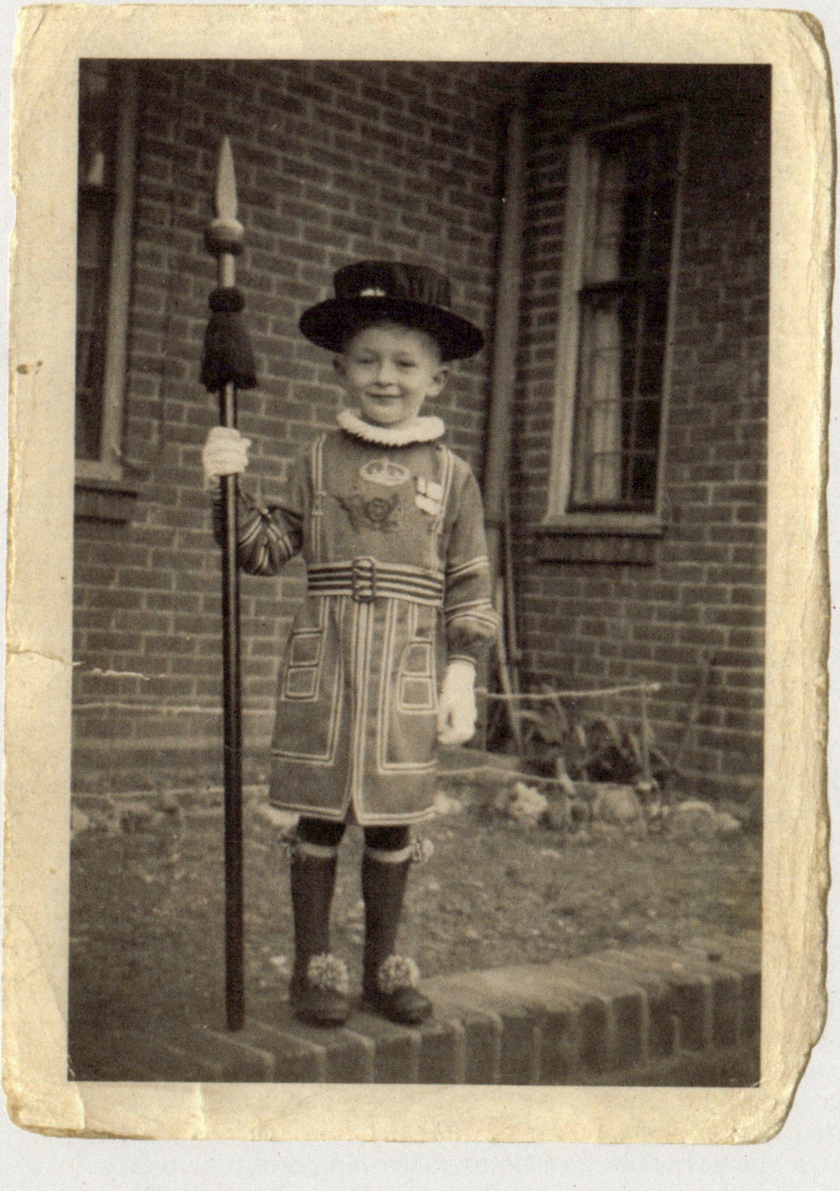

Michael Allnutt wearing a costume of a Beefeater's Tudor State Dress made by his parents in honour of the coronation of Queen Elizabeth II in 1953.

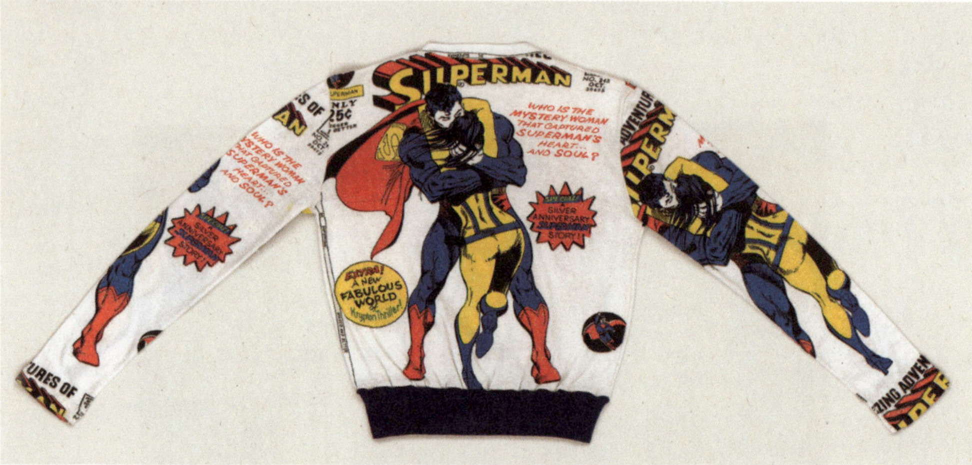

Superman T-Shirt designed by Marshall Lester, UK, 1973–74.

The trend of dressing up in costume – or fancy dress, as it is known in the UK – during the Covid-19 pandemic is evidence that an outfit is not just a statement, but also a psychological device. Whether as a form of public service – as seen in various communication campaigns about the virus – or a way to pass the time and entertain others, costumes of all kinds populated news feeds and social media streams, reinforcing the idea that dressing up can be a powerful and transformative act.

At the beginning of the pandemic, the psychological need to perforate the darkness of the news cycle saw children and adults alike using costumes as a way to cope. During lockdown, in Puertollano, Spain, three-year-old Mara and her father Jaime wore matching costumes as they carried out their rubbish bins to make being outside less frightening. Key workers around the world used costumes to send messages of cheer or for public service and information campaigns. During the first lockdown in the UK, Glen Walton, a postal worker from Nottinghamshire, dressed up as a wrestler, a robber, a princess and the Pokémon character Pikachu to amuse his district and normalise the scary situation. 'It's all been doom and gloom lately and I wanted to change it,' Walton said. 'It's been brilliant. People have been cheering and clapping, and kids have been in the windows waving.'

To inform commuters about the threat of Covid-19, and the need to wear masks, police officers in Chennai and New Delhi wore specially adapted helmets, bedecked with red spikes to look like the virus. The police officers' costumes illustrated the transmission of the disease from one person to another. 'The helmet is an attempt to do something different,' explained Rajesh Babu, an officer in Chennai. 'When I wear this, the thought of coronavirus comes into the minds of the commuters. Children react especially strongly after seeing this and want to be taken home.' Bolivian police took a similar approach. In La Paz, the virus was anthropomorphised into garish green and purple cartoon characters who roamed the streets reminding people to follow the health guidelines.

While it is considered culturally acceptable for children to wear costumes as a way to transform how they feel and are perceived, it is less common for adults to do so. Yet popular culture is littered with examples of adults using transformative costume – such as Jerrica Benton transforming into her alter ego Jem, lead singer of The Holograms, and Clark Kent emerging from the telephone box as Superman. It is not surprising that during the pandemic, many adults embraced the making and wearing of costumes as a transformative and creative act.

Costumes can provide a sense of both empowerment and liberation. Festivals like Halloween, which celebrate the ghoulish and creepy, might have seemed redundant or distasteful in the face of the pandemic, but actually provided a fun and safe way for people to face their fears, while empowering children and adults alike to explore creative ideas and providing an opportunity for some much-needed frivolity.

Text by Katy Canales

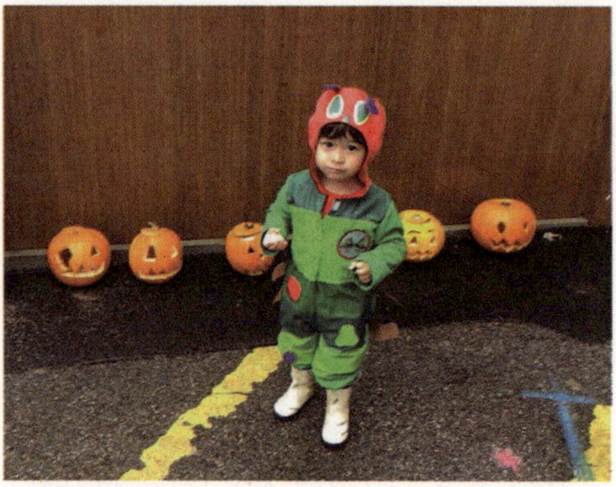

The author's son dressed up as The Hungry Caterpillar for his nursery's Halloween celebrations.

Father Jaime and daughter Mara dressed up for one of their trips to empty the household rubbish during lockdown.

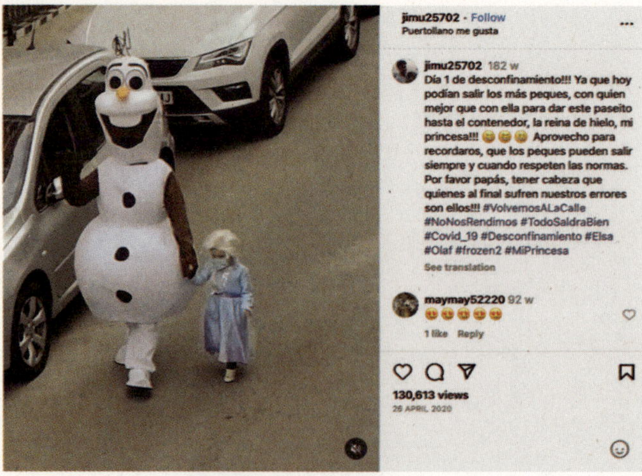
jimu25702 · Follow
Puertollano me gusta
jimu25702 182 w
Día 1 de desconfinamiento!!! Ya que hoy podían salir los más peques, con quien mejor que con ella para dar este paseito hasta el contenedor, la reina de hielo, mi princesa!!! 😄😄😄 Aprovecho para recordaros, que los peques pueden salir siempre y cuando respeten las normas. Por favor papás, tener cabeza que quienes al final sufren nuestros errores son ellos!!! #VolvemosALaCalle #NoNosRendimos #TodoSaldraBien #Covid_19 #Desconfinamiento #Elsa #Olaf #frozen2 #MiPrincesa
See translation
maymay52220 92 w
😍😍😍😍😍
1 like Reply
130,613 views
26 APRIL 2020

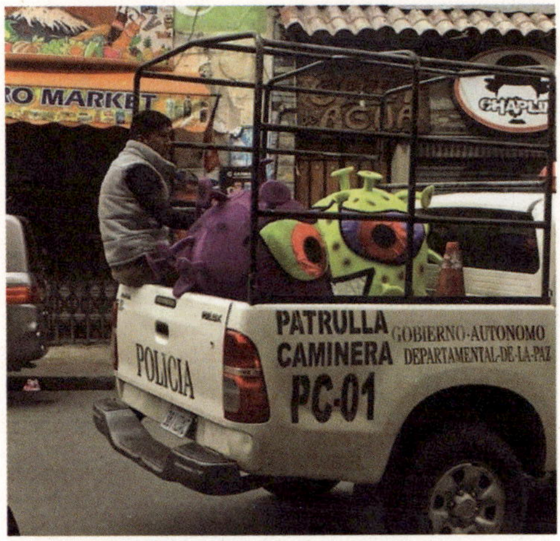

Coronavirus costumes as part of an information campaign in La Paz, Bolivia.

THE GROUND

How the ground became a canvas for multiple forms of expression

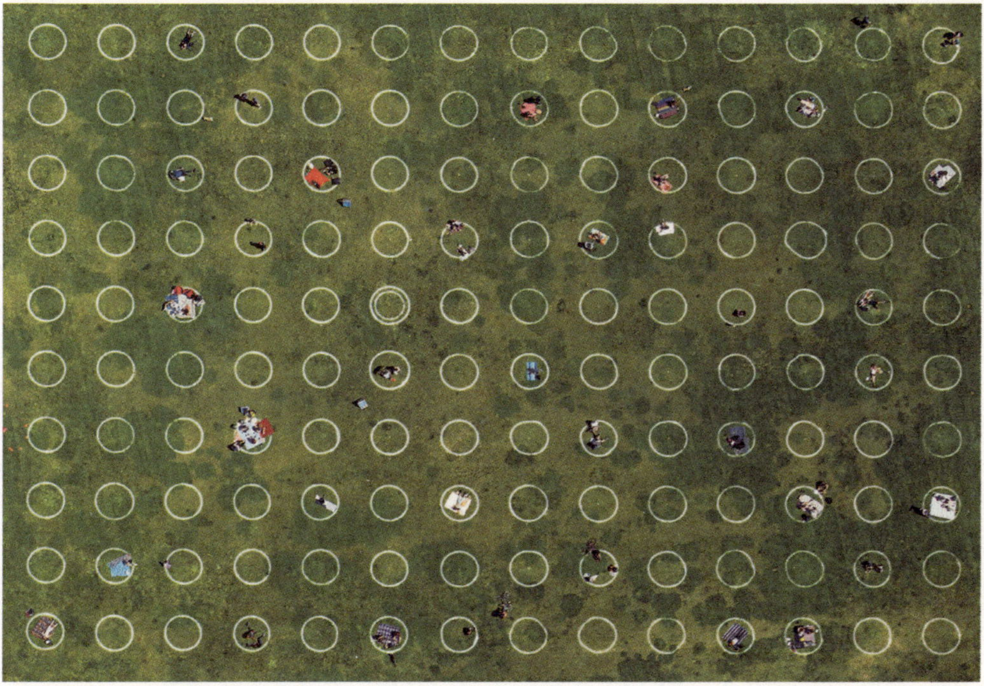

Circles in Mission Dolores Park, San Francisco.

The ground took on a new resonance during the pandemic. Despite its ubiquity in cities, the black asphalt and grey concrete of the ground generally fades into the backdrop. As a site of dirt and of the discarded, it was precisely this lack of preciousness which made the ground an ideal canvas for ad-hoc creativity.

As in many cities around the world, the pavements of London were decluttered to create more space for footfall, with new types of signage appearing on footpaths. During the first lockdown in 2020, stencilled directives cropped up on pavements across the city, bearing instructions such as 'KEEP YOUR DISTANCE', or in the form of symbols, such as pictograms of two people separated by a double-pronged arrow. These 2D graphics quickly faded from exposure to weather and the friction from thousands of shoes wearing away at the surfaces on a daily basis. Unlike most signs found in the public realm, the graphics on the ground were not intended to be permanent, and often drew on materials that were readily available. Indoors, these markings could be found in supermarkets, where people formed orderly queues with the aid of stickers bearing footprints. As more of the public sphere gradually reopened – schools, offices and pubs – the footprints started to appear everywhere.

The act of marking areas for us to stand, routes we are supposed to walk or spaces in which we can lounge within the public realm manifests an apparatus of power that constantly mediates our interactions with our surroundings. However, these floor markings, in their most appealing usage, provided more than just a mapping out of social distancing; they managed to embellish our experiences and instil a sense of levity at an unsettling time. Smiley faces on the playground of a primary school in France, for example, brought joy to the unnatural experience of being shuffled around. At the Coconut Beach club in Münster, Germany, 1.5m-spaced circles placed on the dance floor and markers showing where to queue at the bar enabled 100 revellers to find enjoyment while social distancing.

Parks around the world introduced painted circles that demarcated areas where people from the same household could group together. Domino Park in Brooklyn, New York City, for instance, arranged around 30 circles in rows, each 2.4m in diameter. Italian design studio Caret painted white squares onto the cobblestones of Piazza Giotto in Vicchio, near Florence, creating a gridded layout communicating how people should move around the space. Rather than being at odds with the Cinquecento architecture that encloses the piazza, the white squares formed a pattern that was visually complementary and allowed for a multiplicity of interactions with the space.

The proliferation of the virus brought to the fore the degree to which we are all interconnected. In an article responding to the pandemic, appearing in French publication *AOC* in March 2020, Bruno Latour discussed this idea: ‘Every entity on this same planet has its very own way of hooking up with each other and all the other elements that compose the collective at a given moment.’ Floor markings that brought us together in new, safer networks were a reminder that no one is a discrete or isolated entity. Through them, the ground took on new resonance, expressing the networks and interpersonal infrastructures that people rely on but rarely see.

Text by Priya Khanchandani

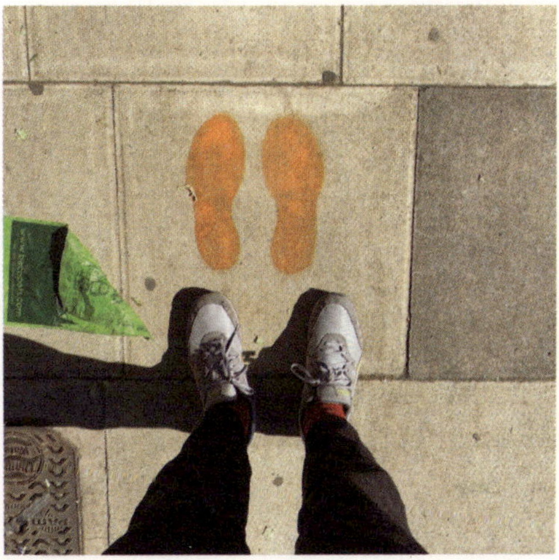

An indication of where to stand.

Social distance markers by a school in Canonbury, London.

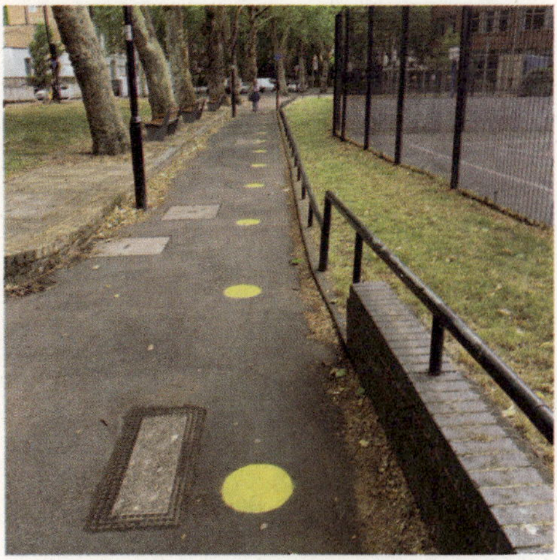

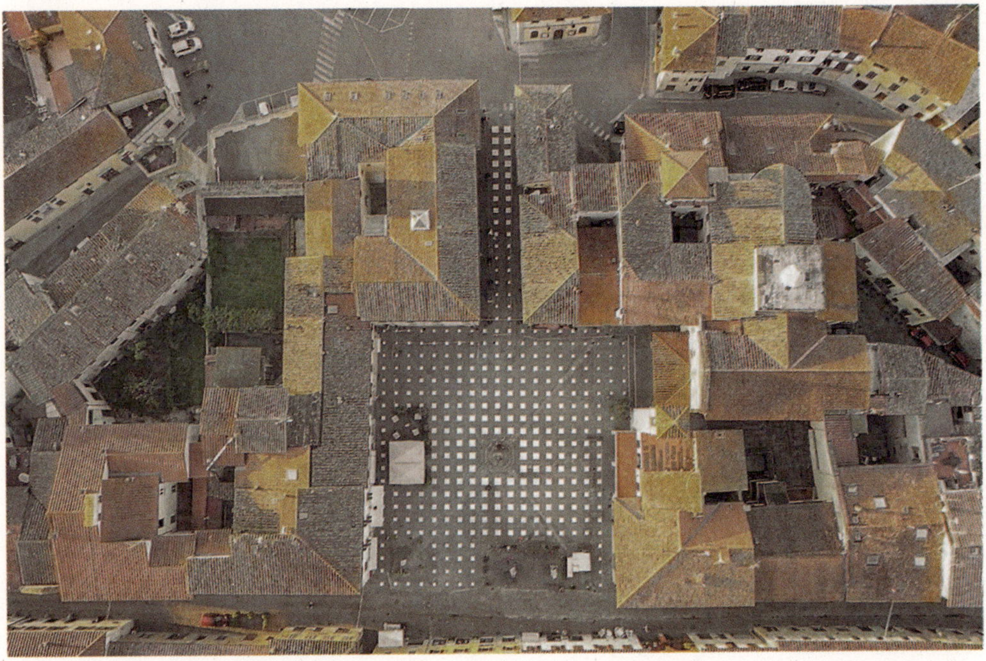

White squares painted on the paving of Piazza Giotto in Vicchio by Caret Studio for their project StoDistante.

KEFFIYEH MASKS

How a face mask made from a popular textile signifying resistance and solidarity reflects the intersectional crises many marginalised groups face

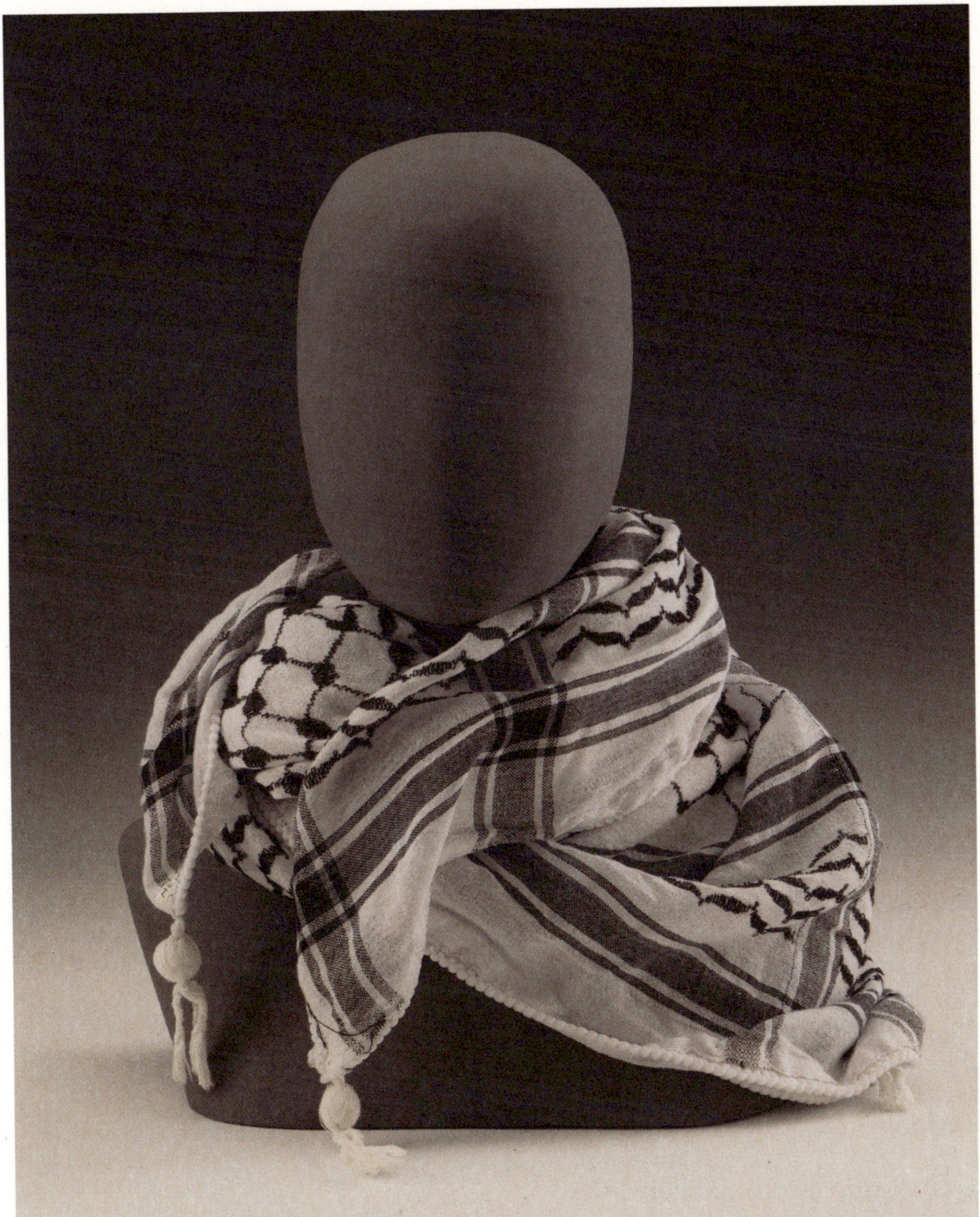

A keffiyeh manufactured at the Hirbawi textile factory in Hebron, Palestine.

April and May 2021 saw an escalation of violence in Israel and Palestine. Unrest was sparked by the forced displacement of Palestinian families from their homes in the Sheikh Jarrah neighbourhood of East Jerusalem, and the storming of Al-Aqsa Mosque by Israeli forces while Muslims were gathered to pray on the last Friday of Ramadan. On 10 May, Israel launched airstrikes on the Gaza Strip for 11 days, killing 253 Palestinians (including 66 children) injuring more than 1,900 and displacing 107,000 Gazans from their homes. Retaliatory rocket strikes by Hamas killed 12. By the time the ceasefire was negotiated on 21 May, there had been widespread destruction of infrastructure in Gaza, including damage to the already fragile healthcare system.

When demonstrations took place around the globe to express solidarity with Palestinians following this latest assault on their lives, the keffiyeh – an iconic symbol of support for Palestine – was ubiquitous. However, in the era of Covid-19, a new twist on this icon could also be seen: the keffiyeh face mask is an example that shows how long-established symbolic objects can find new forms of expression to meet the demands of a pandemic compounded by a wider political and humanitarian crisis.

The keffiyeh (or *kufiya*, as it is properly transcribed from classical Arabic) is a metre-square piece of cloth, usually woven from cotton, with a distinctive black-and-white checked or houndstooth pattern. It is typically worn on the head, folded in half diagonally and held in place by a head-rope (*agal*), which would originally have been made from goat or camel hair or wool. The keffiyeh can also be wrapped around the eyes and nose to keep dust out of the face. Until the 1930s, this cloth was the characteristic head covering of the Bedouin, or Arab nomads. Worn by men, it provided protection from the elements and visually distinguished them from those who lived in more settled environments like villages or towns.

The keffiyeh was politicised due to the important role of peasant farmers (*fellahin*) in the Great Arab Revolt of 1936–39, an uprising demanding Arab independence from the British Mandate government of Palestine. It came to be widely adopted by urban dwellers as a symbol of Arab and Palestinian identities and an expression of nationalism.

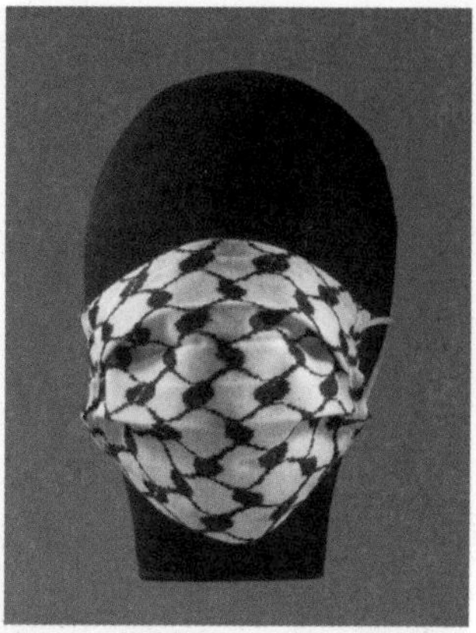

This symbolism only grew more powerful as these struggles intensified. The state of Israel was established following the war in 1947–48 and 770,000 Palestinians were expelled from their homes, events known as the Nakba to Palestinians. Further dispossessions took place following the Israeli occupation of the West Bank and Gaza in 1967. In Palestinian nationalist poetry and rhetoric, this sparked the use of symbols connected with a rural way of life; the peasant farmer, the keffiyeh, the olive tree, the cactus and traditional crafts such as embroidery all became, as Ted Swedenburg has put it, 'allegories for Palestine, the land, and the people's intention of remaining permanently on the land'.

A keffiyeh mask designed by Mohammed Musallam.

Yasser Arafat – chairman of the Palestinian Liberation Organisation from 1969, as well as the president of the Palestinian National Authority from 1994 until his death in 2004 – adopted the black-and-white checked keffiyeh to signify that he was a man of the people. He wore the keffiyeh in every public engagement, such as the signing ceremony of the Oslo Accords in September 1993 and the ceremony in which he accepted the Nobel Peace Prize in 1994 alongside Israeli Foreign Minister Shimon Peres and Israeli Prime Minister Yitzhak Rabin.

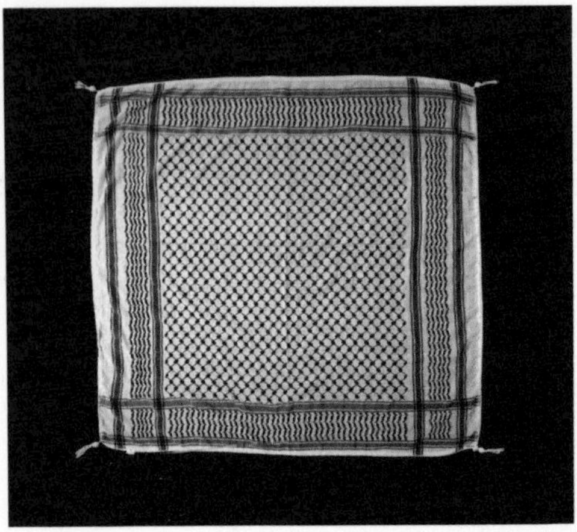

A keffiyeh made at the Hirbawi textile factory in Hebron, Palestine.

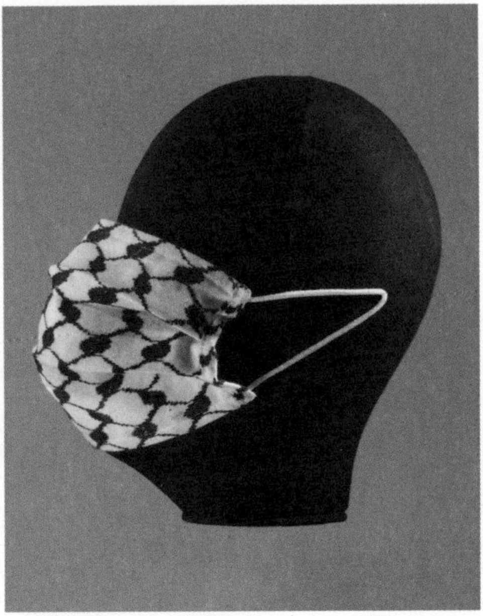

A keffiyeh mask designed by Mohammed Musallam.

Arafat's use of the keffiyeh as his permanent head covering cemented its status as a global icon of Palestinian nationalism and resistance. Guerilla fighters could conceal their identity by wrapping the cloth completely around their face. Having been an exclusively male garment, it was adopted by women, such as the resistance fighter Leila Khaled, who wore it in an iconic head-scarf fashion. During the First Intifada (1987–1993) and Second Intifada (2000–2005), it came to be worn worldwide as a symbol of protest, resistance and solidarity with the Palestinian people.

More than 30 factories once operated across Palestine producing keffiyehs. Today, only one survives: the Hirbawi factory in Hebron, the largest city in the West Bank. Founded by Yassar Hirbawi in 1961, the factory houses 15 antique machine looms, though by 2010 only four remained in operation as sales have been in steady decline since the 1990s. This is a result of foreign-made imports, primarily from China, which are cheaper though also inferior in quality to the Palestinian-made originals.

Although the keffiyeh face mask rose in popularity during the Covid-19 pandemic, it was originally developed in 2015 at a workshop organised by the Belgium-based not-for-profit association Disarming Design from Palestine (DDFP). DDFP develops

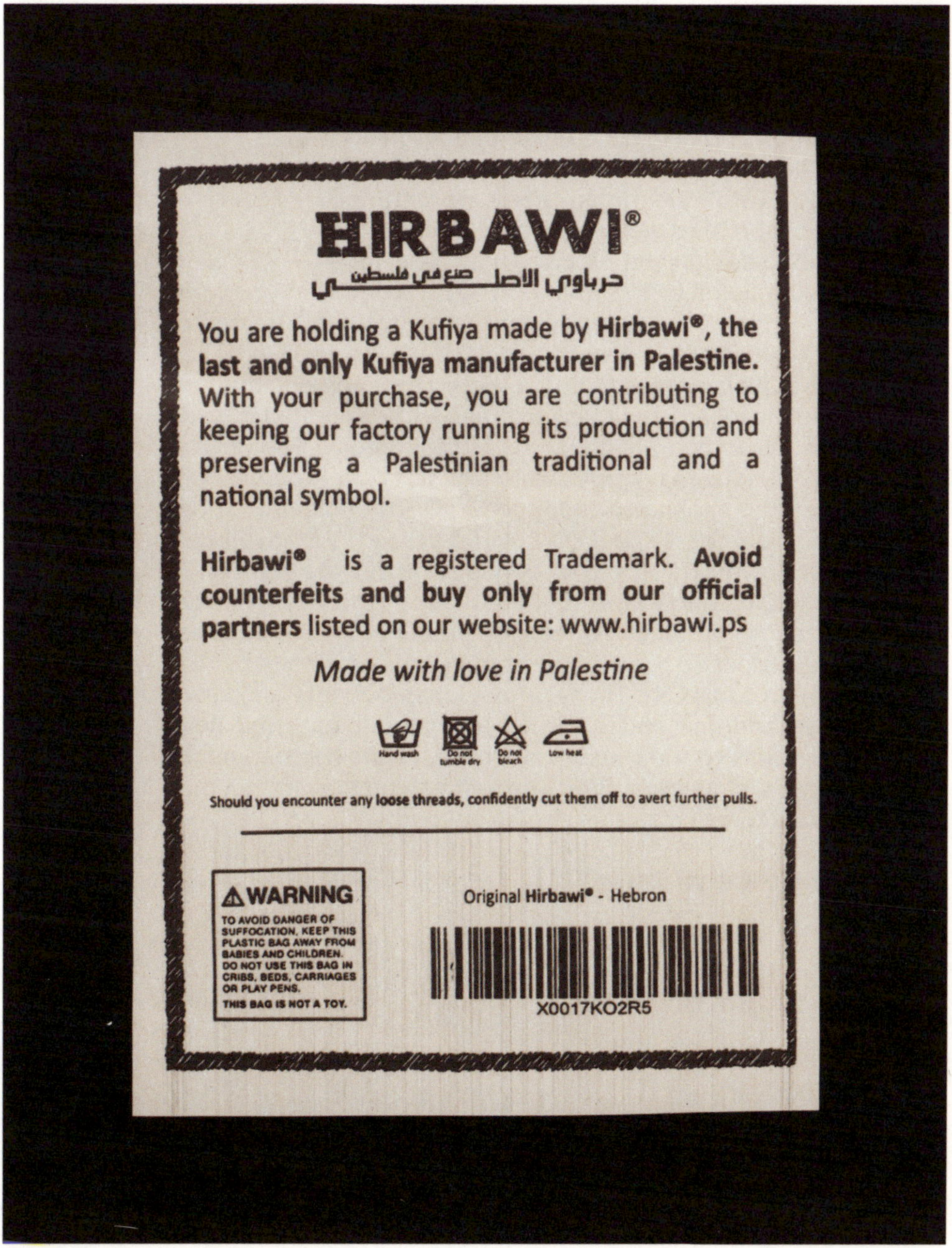

Label from a keffiyeh (also transcribed as *kufiya*) manufactured by Hirbawi.

contemporary designs based on manufacturing processes from Palestine, employing local Palestininan resources and techniques. The group aims to use these designs to connect consumers with craftspeople, providing work and fair pay, as well as preserving the heritage of making. During a DDFP workshop in 2015, Palestinian artist Mohammed Musallam collaborated with Gaza-based tailor Abu Alaa Ghaben to design and produce a surgical face mask from keffiyeh fabric. This proposed a unique Palestinian version of an object worn by medical staff to protect them from disease; in the words of DDFP, it 'symbolise[d] the need of Palestinian identity to be protected from the occupation'. According to Musallam, the mask expresses the idea that identity is the defender of the Palestinians and their cause. The project appears on his website under the title 'Our ID is our Protection'.

Mural depicting Leila Khaled on the separation wall in Bethlehem, 2018.

The keffiyeh mask was first used in Gazan hospitals under siege. Of course, the impact of Covid-19 could not have been foreseen when the project was conceived, but the pandemic prompted Musallam to return to the concept. Now living in exile in Canada, where he received refugee status in 2018, Musallam oversaw from afar the production of hundreds of masks by Abu Alaa Ghaben in Gaza City. The face mask has become an icon of the Covid-19 pandemic and textile artisans around the world have turned their skills to the mass production of masks, especially amid shortages of medical PPE. The keffiyeh masks are not only worn for safety but also as a symbol of solidarity.

Text by Mariam Rosser-Owen

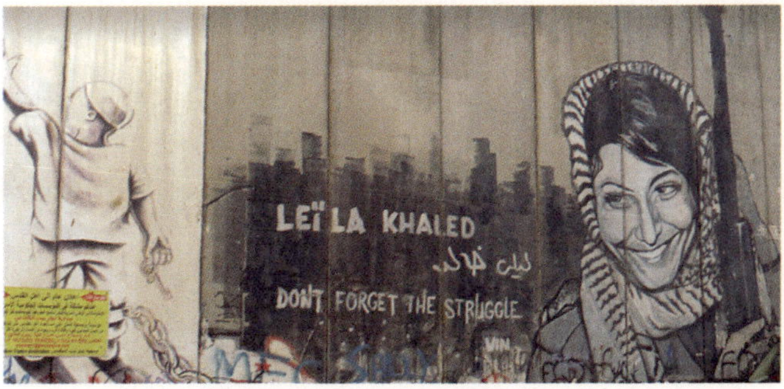

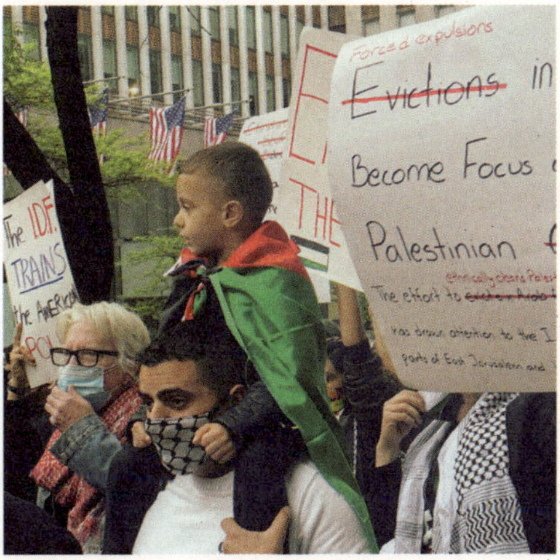

Pro-Palestinian protest in New York City, May 2021.

JAPANESE MEASLES PRINTS

Utagawa Yoshifuji,
Defeating the Measles Demon,
Edo (Tokyo), 1862.

What Japanese woodblock prints from a 19th-century measles outbreak can tell us about the public perception of an epidemic

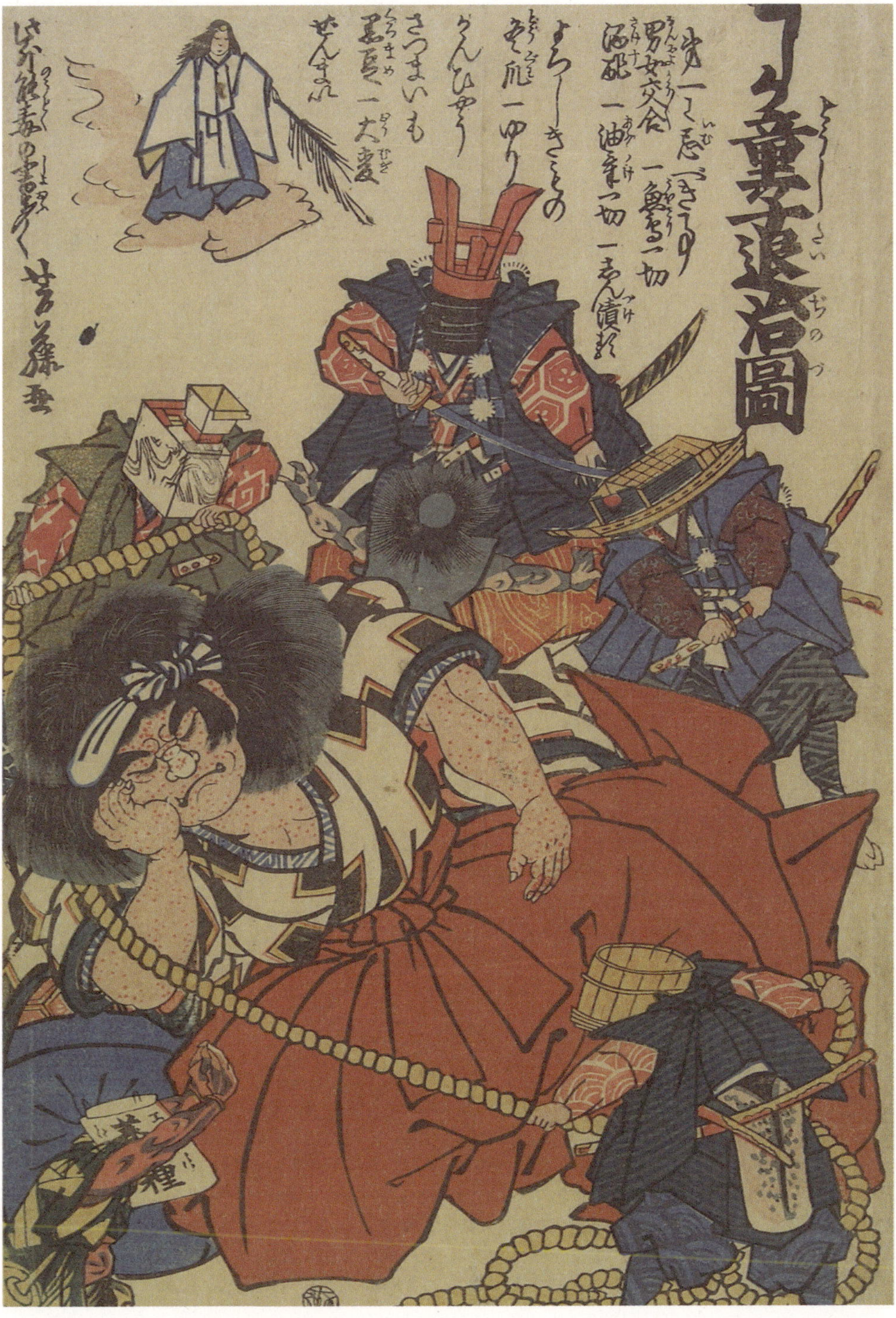
童子退治圖

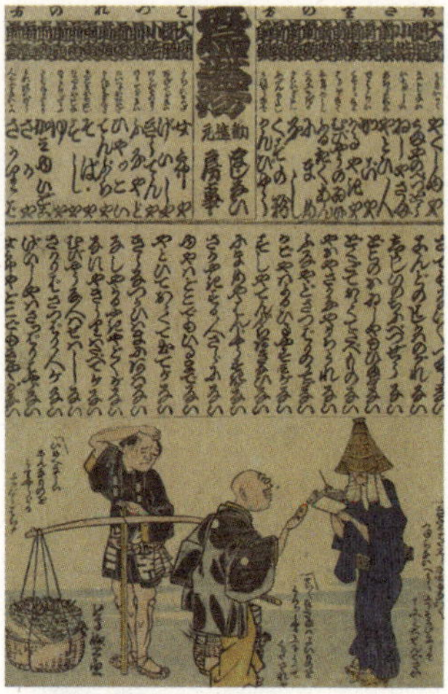

Japanese woodblock prints produced during the Edo period (1615–1868) are known as *ukiyo-e* (pictures of the floating world). Distributed in the thousands, these affordable pictures played a significant role in distributing information in bustling cities, with subject matter ranging from the latest fashion trends to new forms of entertainment.

As the Covid-19 pandemic swept the world, a lesser-known genre gained renewed relevance. *Hashika-e*, or 'measles prints', were mass produced at the height of an exceptionally severe outbreak of measles in 1862. Measles was a common infectious disease in Japan, and an epidemic struck every 20 to 30 years during the Edo period. The devastating crisis of 1862 is thought to have claimed tens of thousands of lives in the city of Edo (present-day Tokyo) alone. Outside the field of medical history, these relatively rare prints received little attention until 2020.

Measles prints first reached Europe during the age of Japonisme, a period in the 19th century when many artists and connoisseurs in western Europe took great interest in art and design from Japan. The most curious examples found in the V&A collections are social satires of the epidemic, which portray the perceived winners and losers of the crisis. The virus was often depicted in a human-like form: in one print by Utagawa Yoshifuji, entitled *Defeating the Measles Demon*, four figures representing businesses severely affected by the disease are tying up a sleeping demon covered in a measles rash, in an attempt to bring the outbreak to an end. The 'losers' here include a sake seller with a two-handled sake barrel head and a party boat owner with a boat-shaped head. They were both victims of a public warning against drinking during the epidemic. In contrast to the four 'losers', the pharmacist, who had notoriously prospered from the epidemic, is shown in the lower left-hand corner on his knees, imploring the others to spare the demon.

Almost every measles print included textual information with dietary advice or instructions about what not to do while recovering from the disease – sometimes of a dubious nature. Sexual intercourse and greasy food were often cited as things to avoid. The print *Harmful Things in Treatment* by Utagawa Yoshimori criticises the greedy beneficiaries of the epidemic economy by depicting the virus – this time as a deity dressed in a yellow kimono – protected by a medical doctor in a black jacket and a

Utagawa Yoshimori,
As Regards Measles,
Edo (Tokyo), 1862.

pharmacist in a blue-striped kimono. Meanwhile, the courageous men of Edo are seen attempting to kick the deity out of the city. The picture intimates people's dissatisfaction with medical doctors and the inaccessibility of overpriced remedies as, due to the long intervals between measles epidemics, most doctors were inexperienced in treatments for the disease.

Another print by Yoshimori, *As Regards Measles*, provides further details of the epidemic economy. Modelled on the way ranking lists of sumo wrestlers were traditionally presented, it shows a ranking of two groups – 'those for whom the epidemic is a blessing' and 'those for whom it is financial hardship'. The biggest winner is the pharmacist, followed by the stable keeper (due to the popularity of horse-related magical rites believed to alleviate symptoms, such as placing an empty horse-feeding bucket over the head of a sufferer) and the medical doctor. In the other column are the brothel owner, the geisha performer and the moxibustionist (a traditional healer who uses incense on the patient's body), all professions whose work relied on physical contact. The illustration shows a news-sheet seller, notorious for peddling inaccurate information about the disease, offering overpriced news-sheets. A street grocer makes a pained expression as he witnesses the unsavoury transaction.

Published a century and a half ago, these measles prints reveal surprisingly similar social changes to those that emerged during the Covid-19 pandemic. While the pandemic has been an existential threat to modern-day small private businesses, both e-commerce companies and healthcare companies providing Covid-19 testing clearly experienced huge growth in revenue. Similarly, the 1862 measles epidemic drastically transformed the economy, leaving obvious beneficiaries, who could be satirised, and victims, with whom audiences could commiserate.

The Japanese publishing industry was a remarkable winner in the crisis. It kept producing full-colour woodblock prints filled with healthcare information throughout the epidemic. The medium may have evolved, but the thirst for information at a time of health crisis is unchanged; the proliferation of these prints mirrors the relentless daily news updates seen during Covid-19.

Text by Masami Yamada

Toyohara Kunichika,
Full Recovery from Measles,
Edo (Tokyo), 1862.

Utagawa Yoshifuji,
Defeating the Measles Demon,
Edo (Tokyo), 1862.

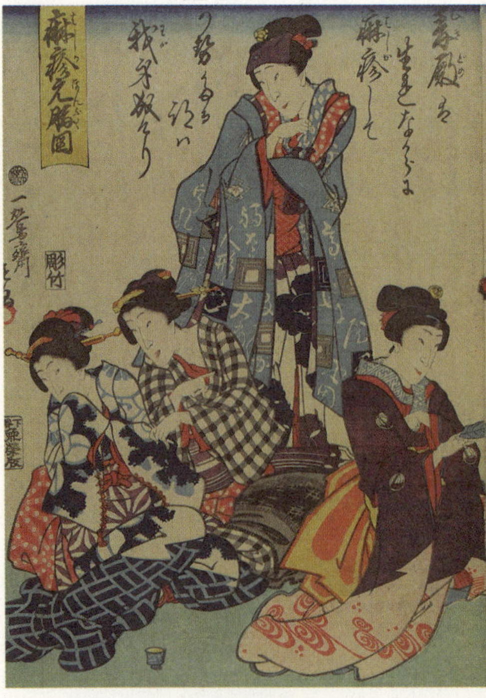

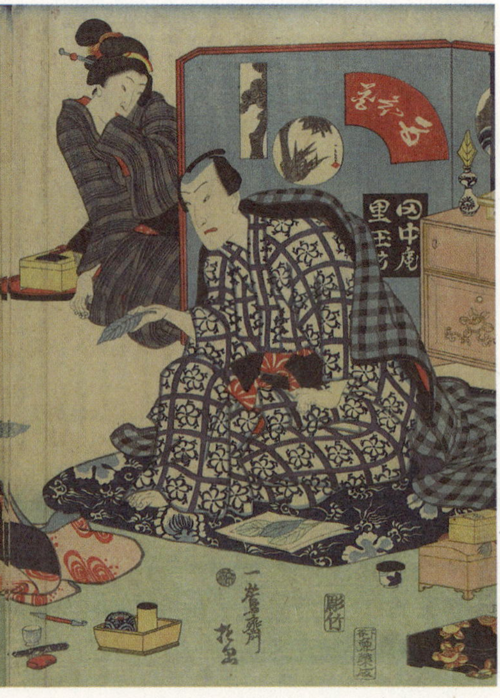

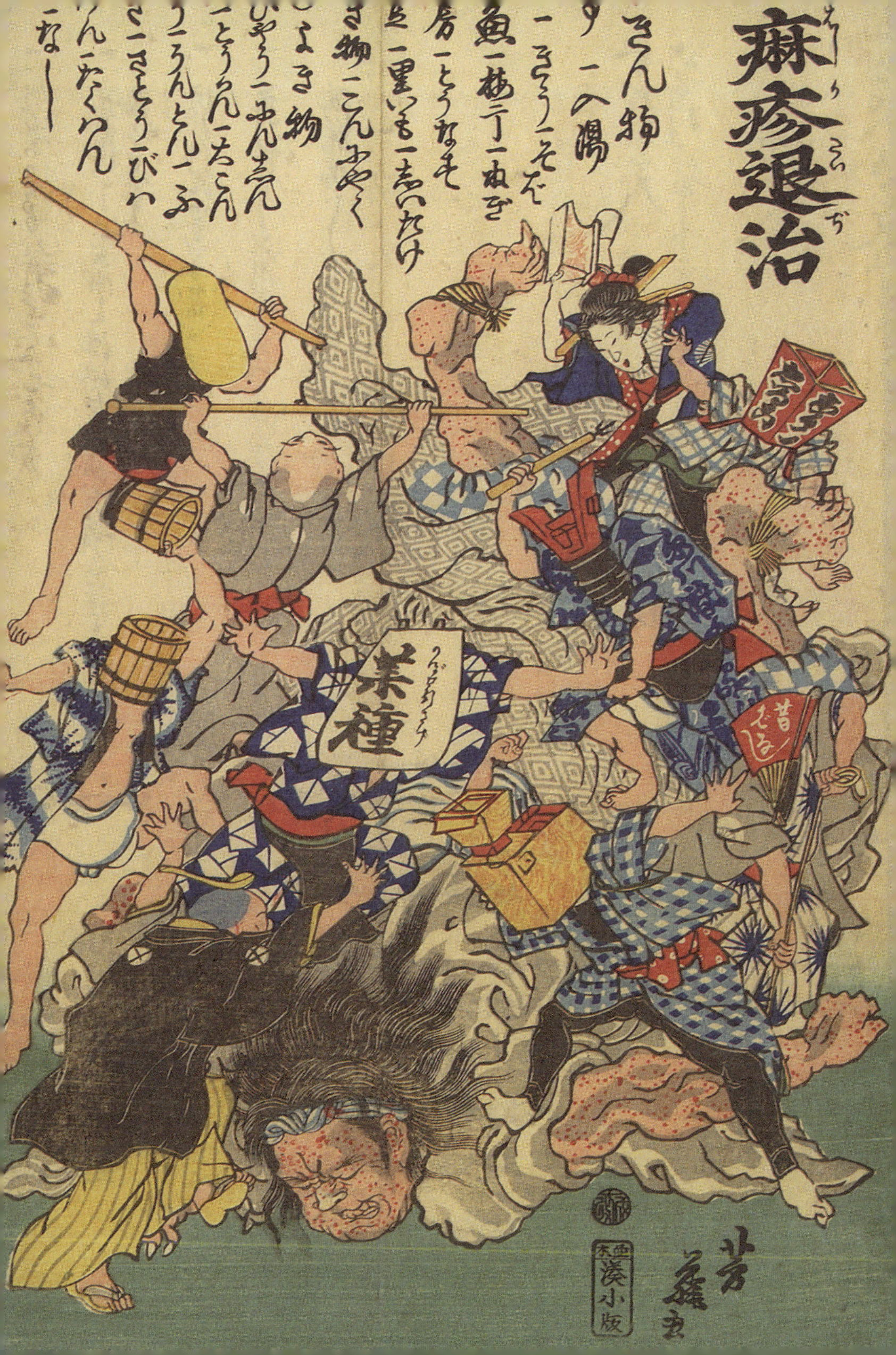
麻疹退治
よき物
芳藤画
湊小版

HIV / AIDS POSTERS

Be a Good Sport, designed by Gary Martin, UK, 1992–93.

How a global collection of posters from the HIV/AIDS pandemic reflects the challenges for the creation of effective communication campaigns against a virus

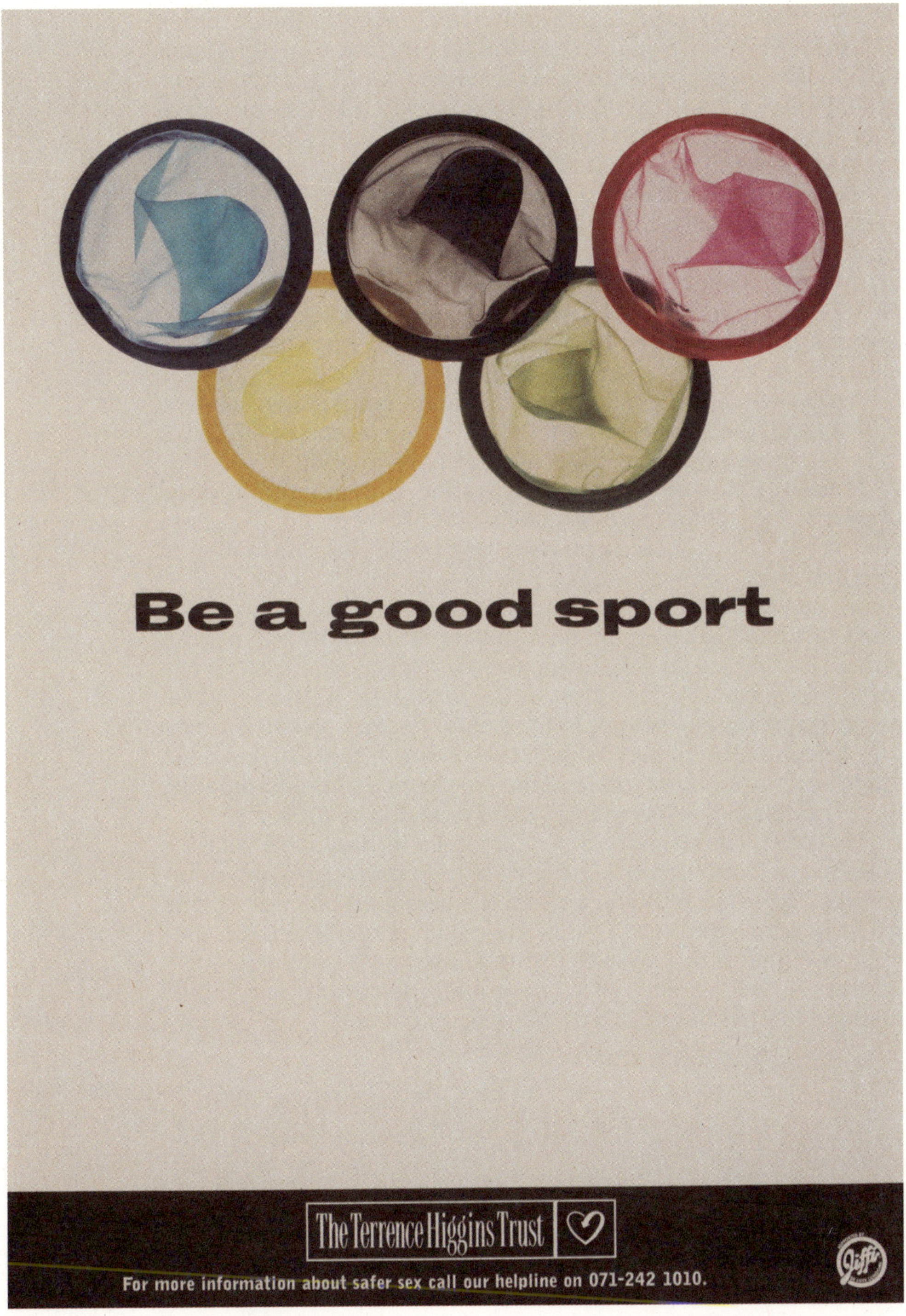
Be a good sport
The Terrence Higgins Trust
For more information about safer sex call our helpline on 071-242 1010.

When the World Health Organization first declared the outbreak of Covid-19 to be a global pandemic, there was a significant uptick of interest in pandemics and plagues of the past. Works of fiction such as Albert Camus' *The Plague* (1947) and Gabriel García Márquez's *Love in the Time of Cholera* (1985) experienced massive resurgences in sales, while John Barry's 2004 historical account *The Great Influenza: The Story of the Deadliest Pandemic in History* shot to the top of the *New York Times* Best Seller list in April 2020, remaining there for several weeks. There was hope that we could learn from these past events. Yet while the Spanish Flu received repeated attention in the search to find clues for how to manage the crisis, another global pandemic that still currently exists received scant reference: HIV/AIDS.

While Covid-19 and HIV/AIDS have differed in their patterns and spread, the contemporaneity and global reach of HIV/AIDS provides many useful perspectives for thinking about the Covid-19 pandemic. It is all the more frustrating that, despite obvious overlaps, the continued marginalisation of HIV as an important case study still echoes the historic and tragic marginalisation of the virus itself.

The V&A has a substantial collection of print material on HIV/AIDS, the result of an urgent show put together at the museum by curator Shaun Cole in 1996 called *Graphic Responses to AIDS*. The exhibition was particularly progressive for its time, as the depiction of gay men and gay culture in the poster designs risked breaching Section 28 of the UK's Local Government Act, which had been introduced in 1988 and banned local authorities from 'promoting homosexuality'. The law was only fully repealed in 2003.

Cole collected more than 100 works for the show with the intention of exhibiting how graphic design could play an important role in the larger battle against the disease. Looking at these works now, one can sense many connections relating to the situation presented by Covid-19 in the challenges and issues they address, as well as clues as to how graphic design can and should respond to a pandemic in a contemporary context.

Perhaps the most important role of graphic design during the rise of HIV/AIDS was to communicate how to prevent the spread of the disease. Pamphlets and posters urged people to practice safe sex and to use clean needles, often using humour and visual puns borrowed from the advertising world to catch the viewer's attention, such as condoms forming Olympic rings or in the shape of a lifebuoy. Similarly, with Covid-19, we saw national campaigns urging prevention techniques such as handwashing, mask wearing and social distancing, as well as a host of more humorous graphic responses taking on and challenging the sceptics.

With any novel virus, one of the biggest dangers is the amount of misinformation that can circulate. With HIV/AIDS, one of the most problematic misunderstandings was how the disease was transmitted, with misinformation being disseminated that implied a passing touch or a kiss on the cheek could result in a lifelong infection. Many poster campaigns aimed to counteract this by providing reminders of not only what was safe, but more importantly what the real risks were. Similar issues emerged during the Covid-19 pandemic, where competing sets of 'facts' shaped people's attitudes and behaviours and caused confusion about face masks, social distancing, vaccines and fringe treatments.

Blaming and shaming also prevailed during the Covid-19 pandemic. A nasty tendency was to place the blame on China, with derogatory and racist terms such as the 'China virus' or 'Wuhan flu' being used by unscrupulous people. With HIV/AIDS, the blame was violently targeted at the gay community, giving most people false moral license to turn a blind eye to the disease. With HIV/AIDS, several posters tried to correct this inaccuracy by highlighting what is true of most diseases – that a virus does not discriminate, even if people do. Another poster reminds people of the statistics: that 75% of all HIV infections were from heterosexual sex, while yet another depicts a pointed finger, saying 'anyone can get AIDS'.

Many of the HIV/AIDS posters in the V&A exhibition attempted to overcome the incredible stigma cast on people living with the virus by creating a sense of empathy, deploying powerful tools of allegory and portraiture to create human connections. A photograph of two men embracing with the phrase 'My boyfriend is HIV positive, I love him' provides the content for one poster, while another bears the figure of a boy, the accompanying text foretelling the suffering he will endure growing up simply because of his sexuality.

What does empathy look like today? During the pandemic there were exceptional moments of unity and an outpouring – even if purely symbolic – of support for the NHS and key workers through rainbow signs (see Rainbows p18) and clapping on Thursday evenings (see Hands p338). However, as the number of people succumbing to the virus increased, a creeping sense of apathy about rates of infection also began to emerge, detached as these figures were from the lives of the people affected (see Lists p60).

Graphic Responses to AIDS was especially impressive in its geographical breadth. Cole was able to bring together work not just from Britain but also from the US, Sweden, Germany, Uganda, Canada, Kenya, Italy, South Africa, Nicaragua and more. One thing we have learned from the Covid-19 pandemic is that local circumstances and responses have varied significantly from one place to another. Looking at these HIV/AIDS posters, a similar sense of the specificity of local context is apparent, depicted through many different settings and challenges, from a crowded Danish bar to a Ugandan rest stop to a lido in Toronto.

Above all, *Graphic Responses to AIDS* reminds us of the vital importance of collecting designed objects and materials that have borne witness to historical moments, challenges and crises, so that we can better understand the role objects play in mediating our everyday lives.

Poster designed by artist collective Gran Fury and published by ACT UP, 1989.

Text by Brendan Cormier

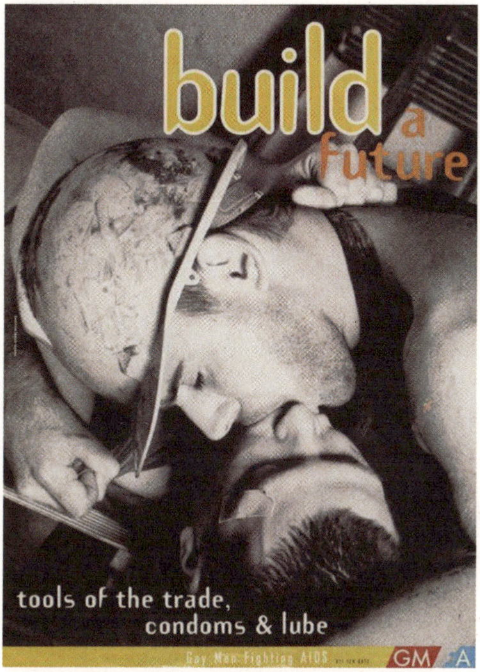

Poster designed by Declan Buckley featuring photography by Hywel Williams, UK, c1992.

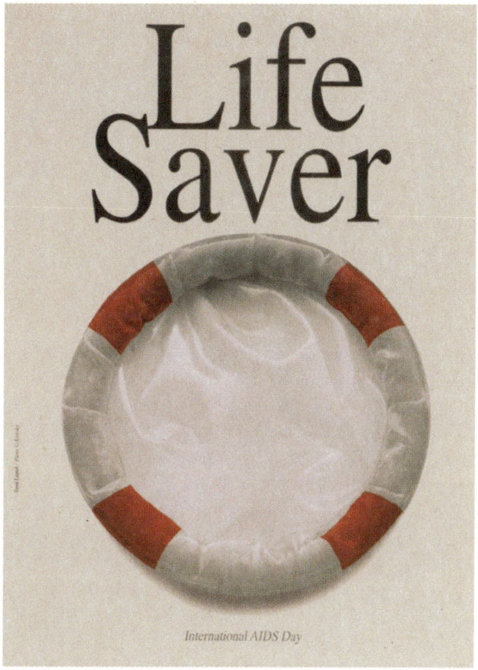
Life
Saver
International AIDS Day

Poster designed by Yossi Lemel with photography by G Korisky, 1993.

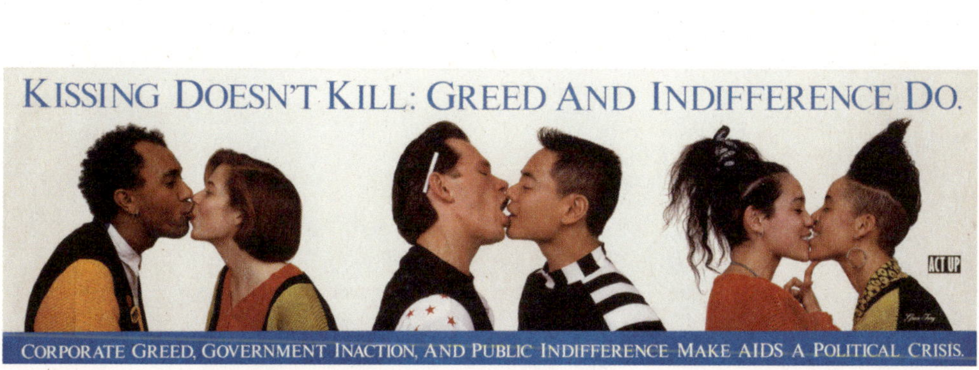
KISSING DOESN'T KILL: GREED AND INDIFFERENCE DO.
ACT UP
CORPORATE GREED, GOVERNMENT INACTION, AND PUBLIC INDIFFERENCE MAKE AIDS A POLITICAL CRISIS.

02

DOCUMENT

Covid-19 has been the most widely documented pandemic in human history. Prior to the outbreak, the proliferation of smartphone ownership already enabled five billion photos to be taken every day. Widespread social media use further encouraged many to document their everyday experiences of lockdown, a way of sharing with others while in isolation.

While certain images quickly became tropes (selfies with masks on, screengrabs of Zoom calls), many photographers, both amateur and professional, set upon more discrete documentation techniques, focusing their lens on the people cohabitating on their street, on the cast-away detritus of personal protective equipment (PPE) or a simple gaze out towards the sea while on a daily walk. These pictures gave us a rich sense of some of the commonalities of the pandemic experience, as well as the particularities – to each person their own pandemic.

The paradox of documenting a virus resides not only in the invisibility of the disease itself, but also in the fact that many aspects of the pandemic's impact remain difficult to visualise. Information designers grappled with finding effective means to convey the cold hard statistics of daily deaths and infections, while activists railed against the disproportionate and often unrecognised toll that the virus took on vulnerable communities. This came at a time when people had more technology than ever to sense, see and track human activity, whether through drones, Bluetooth tracking apps, surveillance cameras or myriad other tools. The pandemic fanned the flames of the privacy debate – about what should be seen and what should not – and confronted people with the uncomfortable dilemma of what we can divulge of ourselves to the public realm.

LISTS

The front cover of *The New York Times* on 24 May 2020.

How a simple list of names captured the scale of a tragedy

PANDEMIC OBJECTS

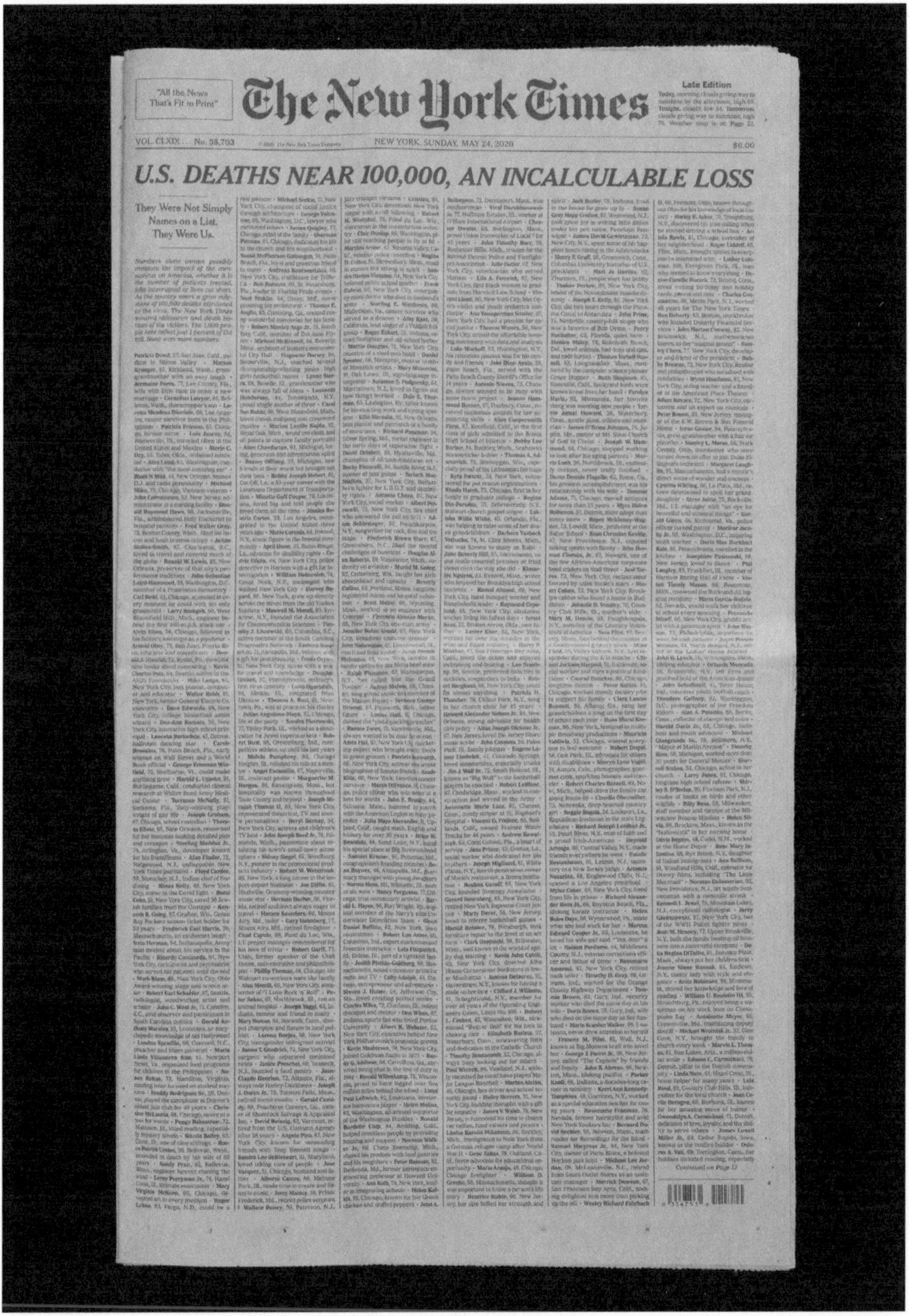
"All the News That's Fit to Print"
The New York Times
Late Edition
VOL. CLXIX . . . No. 58,703
NEW YORK, SUNDAY, MAY 24, 2020
$6.00
U.S. DEATHS NEAR 100,000, AN INCALCULABLE LOSS
They Were Not Simply Names on a List. They Were Us.
Continued on Page 12

DOCUMENT

How can one really understand the scale of a pandemic and grasp the meaning of its numbers? During the course of the Covid-19 pandemic, the barrage of daily figures dissolved into a haze of cold abstraction that left many with a sense of helpless indifference. Information design was put to the test during this crisis, charged with untangling and communicating in real time the daily evolution of an extremely complex condition. Some notable efforts quickly became go-to resources for millions looking for clarity in numbers. The Johns Hopkins dashboard, for example, was a useful early resource that conveyed the globality of the crisis in macabre hues of red and black. Originally run by a three-person team, the site saw a billion visits a day by April 2020. The *Financial Times*, like many major newspapers, also released a steady stream of graphics of all kinds. However, it was the logarithmic chart comparing daily deaths per country that most resonated with the public, and was widely shared and regularly updated.

As the shape of the pandemic changed, information design also had to keep changing tack in order to better map its course. Over time, the Johns Hopkins dashboard's use of proportional circles to show the location and intensity of outbreaks became a relatively useless world map filled with red blotches. *Süddeutsche Zeitung* once published each country's 'doubling rate' – the number of days it would take for the total deaths to double – but eventually retired this as infection rates slowed.

The Johns Hopkins Coronavirus Resource Center dashboard, captured on 1 June 2020.

Several months into the pandemic, a palpable sense of data fatigue set in. Just how often could one check a dashboard or look at a logarithmic chart without it becoming a kind of dull routine? *The New York Times* saw this problem coming. As the US approached the grim milestone of 100,000 Covid-19 deaths, the paper wrestled with the question of how to claw back a sense of meaning from these figures. How can one fully comprehend and convey what 100,000 deaths looks like and means? To do so, it resorted to one of the most basic forms of information design one can find: a list.

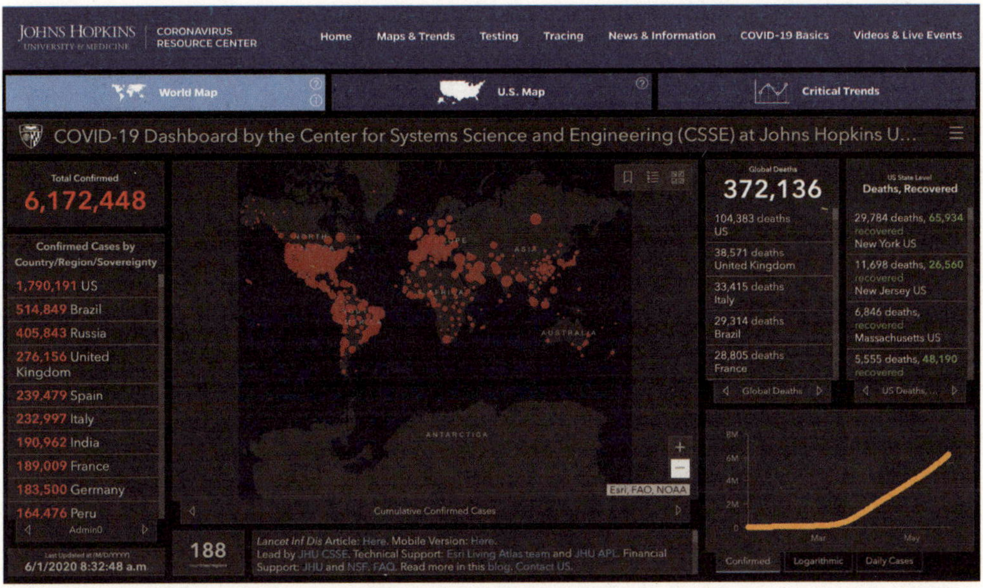

On 24 May 2020, in its Sunday edition, *The New York Times* covered its front page with a list of 1,000 names of people who had died from the virus in the US. The list marked the name of the deceased, their age, place and, when available, a short statement taken from their obituary. The stunning simplicity of the list yielded one of the most powerful expressions of the extent of loss and tragedy that the US – and the rest of the world – had just witnessed. *The New York Times*' version may have been the most publicised, but other publications published their own versions. A few weeks prior to *The New York Times*' piece, *O Globo* in Brazil ran a similar list to memorialise the first 10,000 deaths in Brazil. In Bergamo, the epicentre of the outbreak in Italy, the local newspaper expanded its one or two-page obituary section to ten pages.

The list is an underrated form of information design. Graphic designers today have increasingly advanced tools at their disposal and are capable of processing and rendering complex datasets that often veer towards the virtuosic, rather than something as simple and pedestrian as a list. But lists also have impressive precedents. Consider Maya Lin's Vietnam Veterans Memorial, as perhaps the most famous example, where the names of 58,320 US soldiers who fought and died in the Vietnam War are etched into polished granite. Or think of the writing of Walt Whitman, which consists in large part of lengthy and poetic enumerations of things.

The New York Times only printed 1,000 names. What would it have looked like if 100,000 names were printed – or, for that matter, every name of every victim from around the world? Such a book of names would be a monument in its own right.

In the mobile version of their editorial, *The New York Times* did something equally remarkable: they visualised each person with a tiny silhouetted figure. Readers were compelled to endlessly scroll as more and more figures appeared and an essay slowly unfurled on their phones, contemplating the tragedy of the event and the challenge of fully understanding the scale of 100,000 lives lost. Towards the end, the essay asked readers to contemplate an entire city – roughly of equal population – simply disappearing.

The New York Times editorial was powerful and moving, yet even that could not hold our attention for too long. As the pandemic continued, the US steadily trudged forward with new death milestones. When it recorded 1,000,000 deaths on 19 May 2022, *The New York Times* did not opt for a list on its front pages but instead ran more standard analytical pieces. Slowly, newspapers stopped the regular publishing of statistics altogether; the public appetite had changed. Despite continued infections and deaths, the statistics became a matter for policy wonks and the medical profession, rather than a monument for public grieving and concern.

Text by Brendan Cormier

The Vietnam Memorial
in Washington DC designed
by Maya Lin Studio.

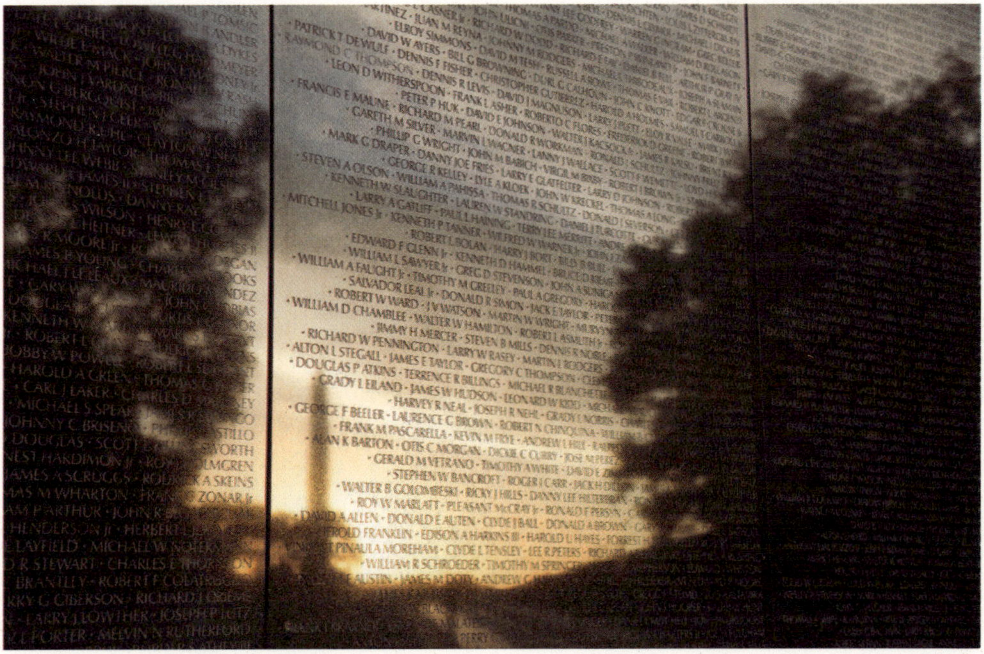

DRONES

How drones gave us a new way to see the pandemic and sparked essential debates about privacy

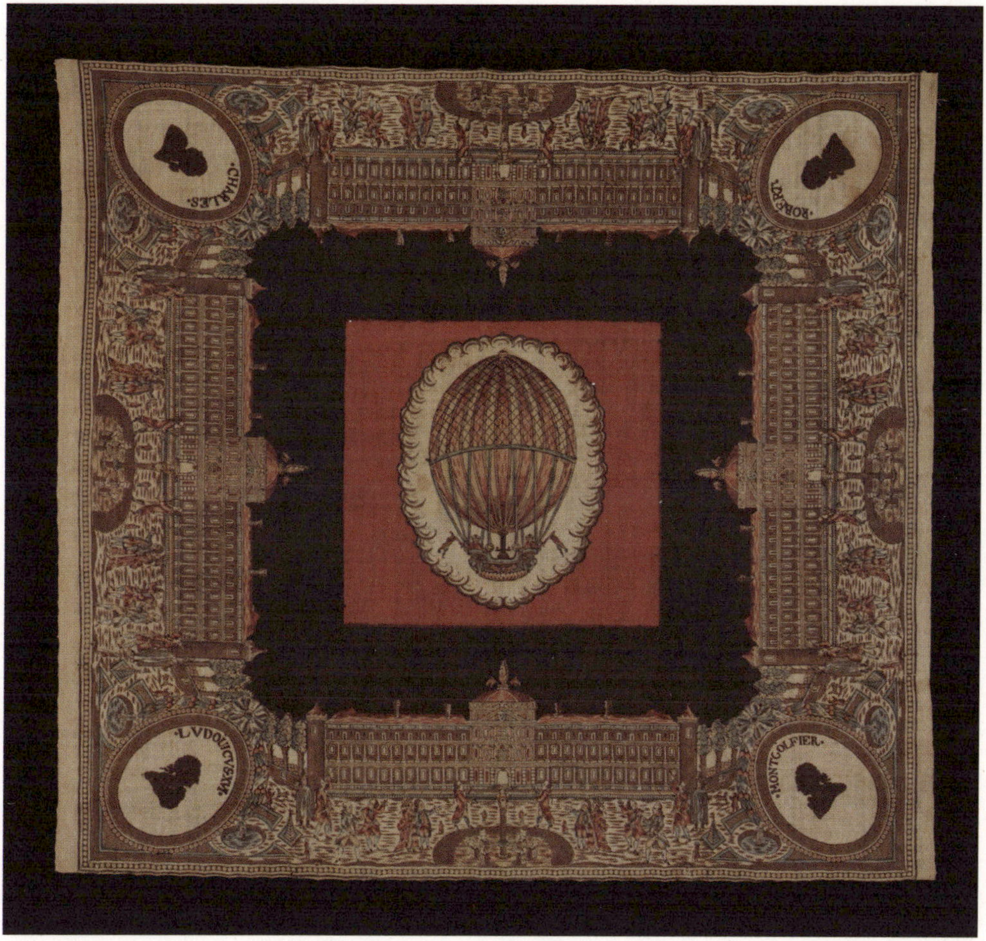

Handkerchief featuring a hot air balloon,
Alsace, c1783.

A drone is used to remotely distribute disinfectant in Seongnam, South Korea in March 2020.

In Ladj Ly's short film for the 2020 Netflix series *Homemade*, a young boy named Buzz finds some solace during lockdown by flying his drone. His lofty perambulations take place in the neighbourhood of Montfermeil, an eastern suburb of Paris densely populated with several high-rise apartment blocks and badly affected by Covid-19. The drone's gaze captures glimpses of the lives of residents stacked on top of each other as they while away the hours: a father trying to teach his young boys, a child staring out a window, a group of young men on a roof, a quarrelling couple on a balcony. Later, the drone moves through the streets observing residents who are waiting anxiously in long queues to access the open-air food market.

Drone imagery was plentiful during lockdown. For some, it provided a valuable form of escapism. In the BBC documentary *Three Years in Wuhan*, which was fortuitously still filming when the outbreak began, we meet an entrepreneur named Huang Tiesen who talks about the stress he endured cooped up in his small apartment. In one scene, he takes to the roof of his apartment to fly his drone and marvels at the emptiness of the city while enjoying a few precious minutes of fresh air, away from the interminable screen time of his computer and phone.

In March 2020, the internet was quickly inundated with viral videos of drone footage recording empty cities, streets, squares and piazzas around the world. A surge in illegal drone usage was documented in the UK, with users breaching the rule of being at least 150m away from built-up areas (yes, even drones have their own social distancing rules). More comical and light-hearted uses included a drone walking a dog in Cyprus and students using a flying device to deliver flowers on Mother's Day in Lebanon.

Tech entrepreneurs also accelerated their drive during this period to popularise and implement more drone-based services. Up until the pandemic, these ambitions had been beset by regulatory issues and community concern. A debatable selling point was the drone's ability as a contactless delivery system – producing newsreel fodder like Zipline drones delivering personal protective equipment (PPE) to hospitals or those deploying disinfectant in markets in Delhi – countered by its capacity as a tool for mass observation. In March, public outrage erupted when it emerged that UK police were using drones to shame people who were flouting the rules by going for walks in the Peak District. Meanwhile drones were also tested to combat the virus through remote fever detection, although the efficacy of this technology has been seriously questioned.

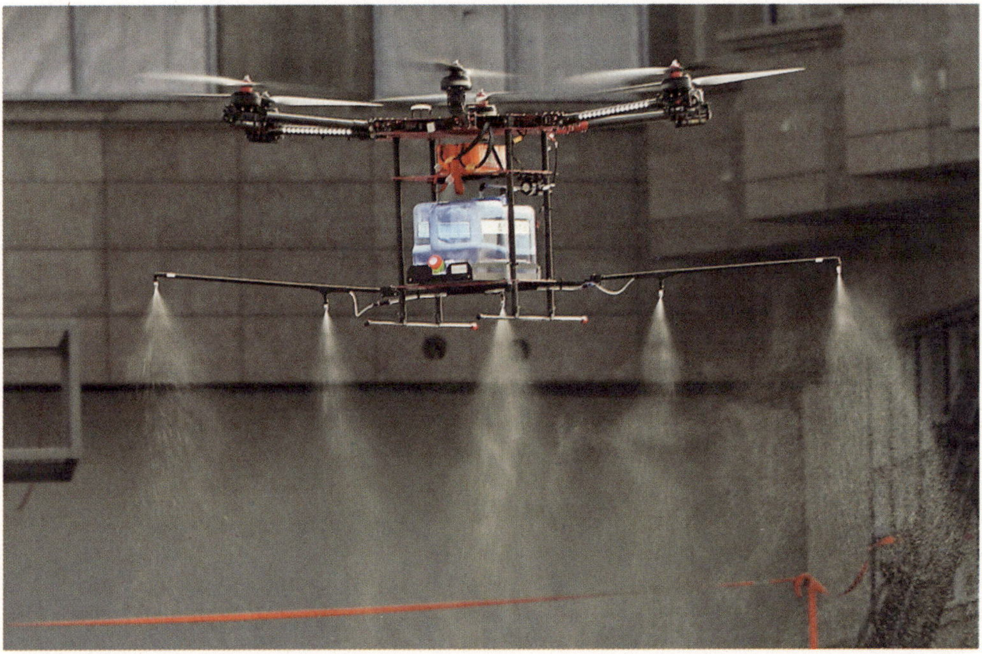

The drone's rapid rise from a tech hobby to a commonplace object is remarkable. Its relative success can be attributed primarily to the pioneering work of Shenzhen-based startup DJI in the early 2010s, whose Phantom drones were the first to hit the market with an accessible design and affordable price point. The DJI drone was not so much a new technology as it was a clever assemblage of pre-existing off-the-rack technologies (a Go Pro camera, a gimble, GPS software, remote-controlled flight) that together produced something altogether new. It gave the user a superhuman power, offering a seductive new way of seeing. Drone sales correspondingly soared, turning DJI into one of China's most successful tech companies.

Drones are incredibly ambidextrous; they can be deployed both as a tool of subversion and of control. In 2014, in one of the first recorded 'drone protests', a drone descended on a football match between Serbia and Albania carrying a 'Greater Albanian' flag to assert ethnic Albanian presence and rights across the Balkans. In 2018, hundreds of flights were disrupted at Gatwick Airport, when reports of drone sightings close to the runways caused the airport to shut down for days. On the other hand, police forces and militaries around the world have snapped up drones in large quantities, creating small fleets for monitoring crowds and other surveillance activities – a looming menace in the skies. At the core, drones raise the fundamental conundrum of who has the right to see and who has the right not to be seen. It is a tension between data collection and privacy, which has been brewing in the tech world for the last decade, and which plagued the development of contact tracing apps in the UK during the pandemic.

Returning to Ladj Ly's short film, a suggestion for another use of drones emerges. At the end, an intertitle reads: 'If the current times are tough, for who is it so?' By focusing his gaze on a suburb mainly inhabited by working-class immigrants and people of colour hit hard by the virus, Ly is addressing a central problem of the pandemic: the invisibility of marginalised communities and the structural inequities leading to their plight. The drone is thus politicised as a tool to render visible; to make people see uncomfortable truths about the kinds of cities we have built and the spatial organisation of our societies, and to question how we might want to live together in the future.

Text by Brendan Cormier

Phantom drone, made by Shenzhen-based manufacturer DJI, 2013.

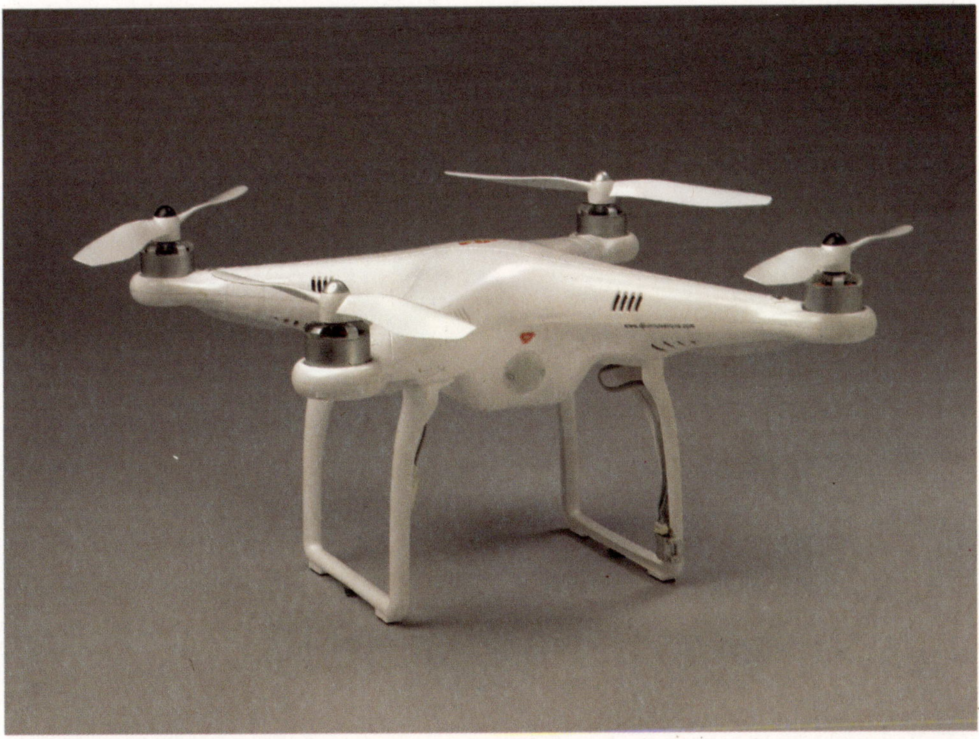

FAMILY PORTRAITS

How a series of portraits depicting cohabitants in lockdown together provide images for the diverse forms a family can take

PANDEMIC OBJECTS

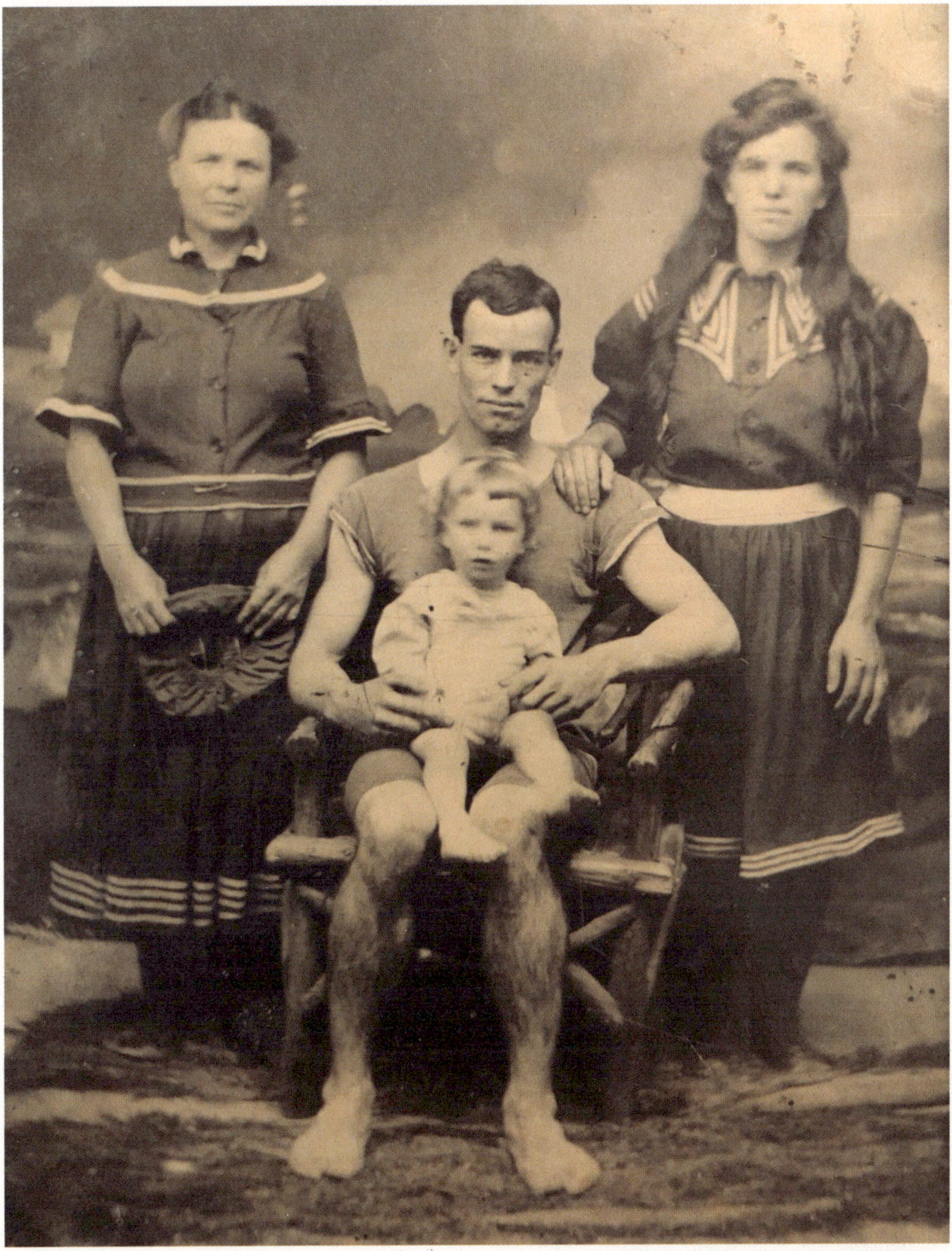

Tintype family portrait, c1900.

During the UK's first lockdown, writer and photographer Eithne Nightingale produced a series called *Life Under Lockdown*, photographing people in two neighbouring streets and on her local estate in Hackney from May to June 2020. She asked the people living in each residence to stand in their doorways and hold an object that helped sustain them during lockdown. The result is a series of 'family portraits' that expands the notion of what a family looks like, brought together in the book *Life Under Lockdown: on Mehetabel Road and Isabella Road in Hackney, 2020*. We see a group of flatmates who met at a Bulgarian music festival; a group of Australian paramedics living together; older couples whose children have left the house; and people living alone and shielding, relying on neighbours to do their shopping. The objects, such as a sewing machine, a camera and a microphone, enrich the story as well, giving a sense of how each family member spent their time under lockdown and the powerful role objects played in sustaining people's moods and perseverance.

Text by Brendan Cormier

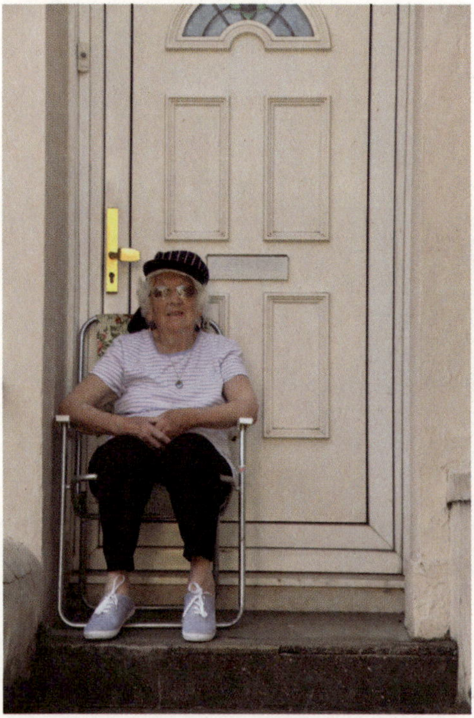

[1]

Photographs by Eithne Nightingale.

[1]
Elsie: Sun hat. As the weather has been good, I've been sitting in the garden wearing my sun hat.

[2}
Ila: Bottle of chimichurri. I was using this Argentinian condiment when I was locked down for two months with my boyfriend in Buenos Aires. We spent our days cooking and eating.
Maya: SLR film camera. I've been learning how to use this manual camera through online videos. It's much more fun than press and shoot but, because of lockdown, I can't get the films developed.

[3]
Lawrence: Loaf. I run Hackney Bread Kitchen from home.
Helen: Sewing machine. This is my first sewing machine, bought during lockdown.
Iris: Our cat. The household is not complete without Mouse.
Stella: Patchwork. I've made this quilt with my mum, using her new sewing machine.

[4]
All: Uniforms. Four of us work as paramedics and one as an occupational therapist.
All: Flag. We are Australians who've been living in London for the past few years.
Christina: Pasta machine. We have a meal of homemade pasta when we're all at home.
All: Our dog. Baloo, a rescue dog, has seen us through our worst days.

[5]
Shahbana: Qu'ran. Although not in the picture, the Qu'ran has been important to me.
Laibah: The computer. I have used this for school and for staying in contact with my friends.
Maariya: 'Lockdown' poster. When I'm bored, I do calligraphy.
Adil: Bike. When I'm bored, I ride my bike.
Sulayman: Bike. When I'm bored, I, too, ride my bike.

[6]
Harriet: Plant and tools. Tending to my new vegetable patch is my early morning task.
Iona: Bear. Cuddles, a present from Karim, has been helping me sleep.
Elektra: Wooden spoon. Iona and I are writing a cookbook, *Soup for Soul*, which is being sold in aid of the Trussell Trust, who support food banks in the UK.
Jacqui: Speaker. We're a house full of life and music.
Karim: Coconut sugar. An excellent alternative to sugar for my cinnamon buns and cookies.

[7]
Becca: Masks, plants, scones, wine and Rex-u-Bastard. I've been making masks, gardening, making distance cream teas and drinking wine. Rex-u-Bastard was bought by my mum, Sue Chester, who used to live here.
Steve: Rex, my dog and brandy. Rex was part of my cabaret act moons ago, reminding me of freer times. Brandy is my self-medication for lockdown melancholia.

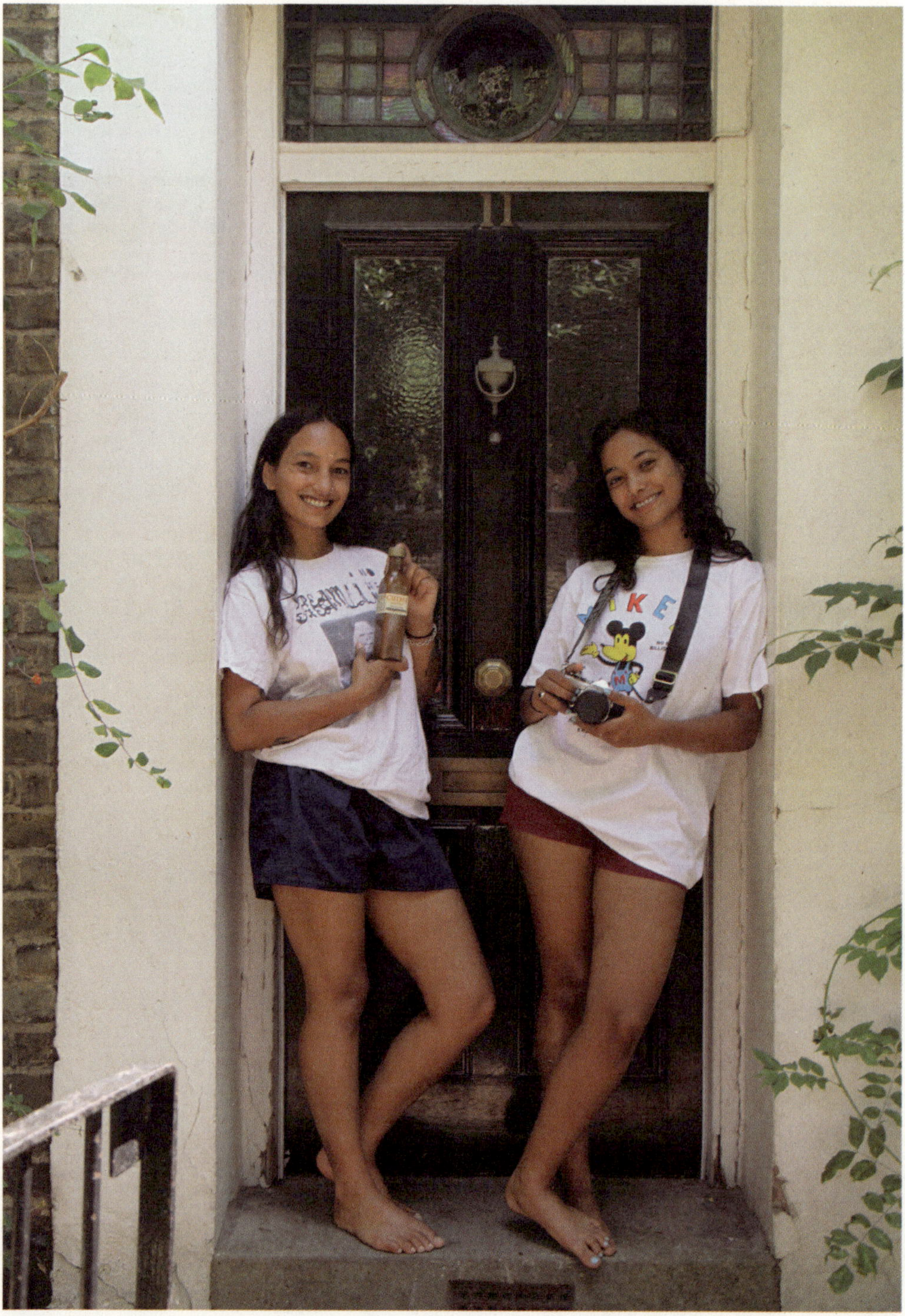

[2]

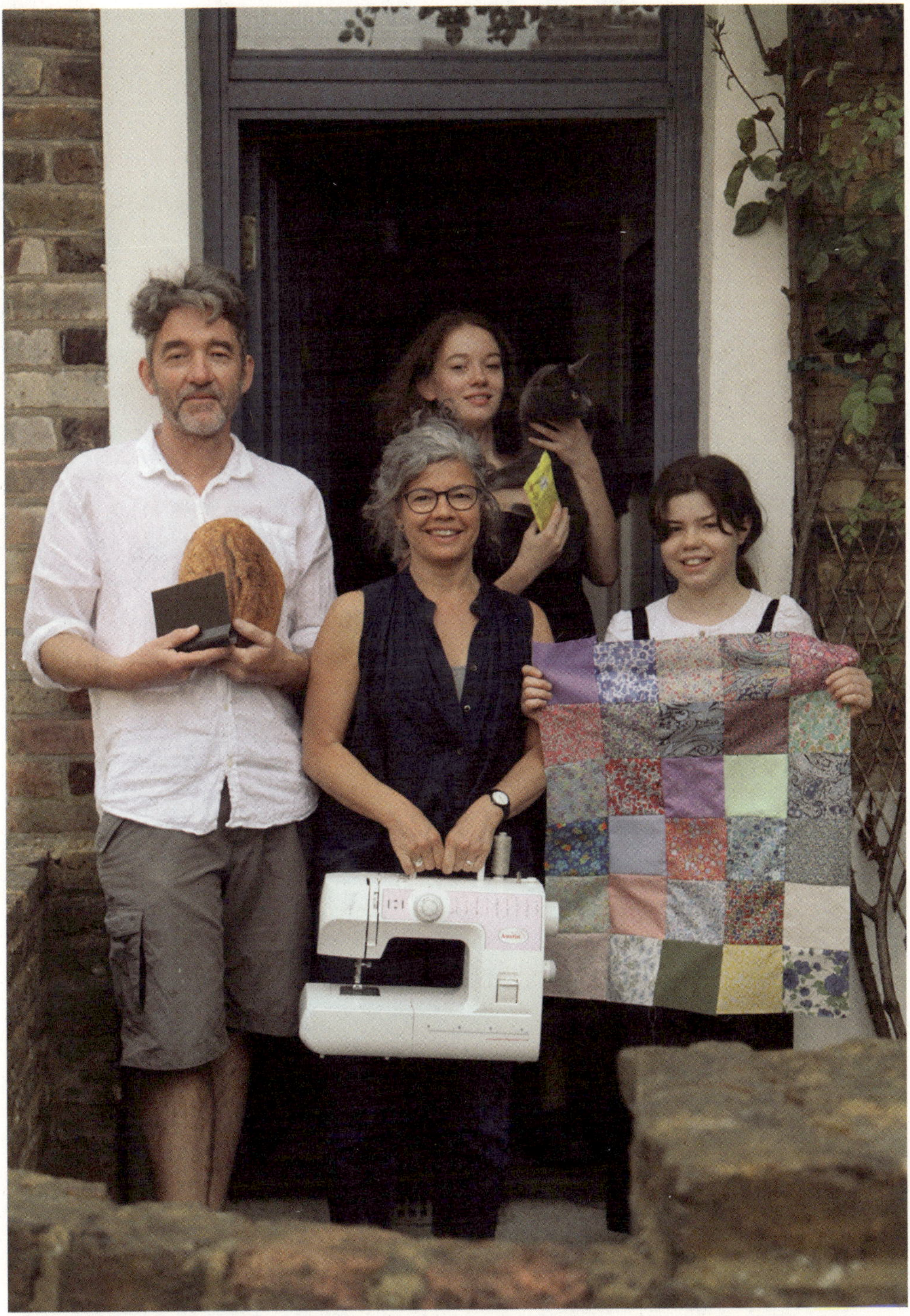

[3]

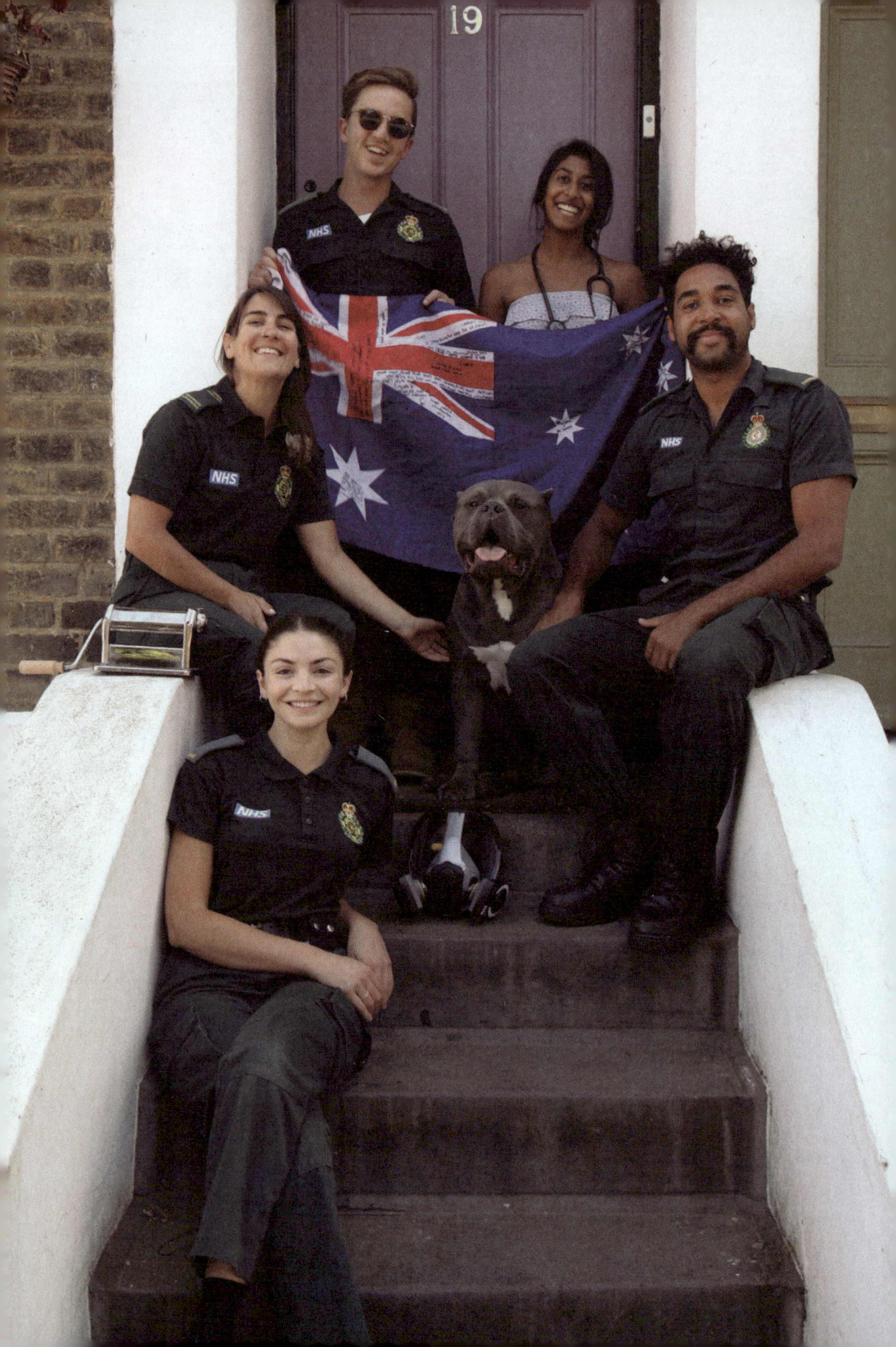
19
NHS
NHS
NHS
NHS

[4]

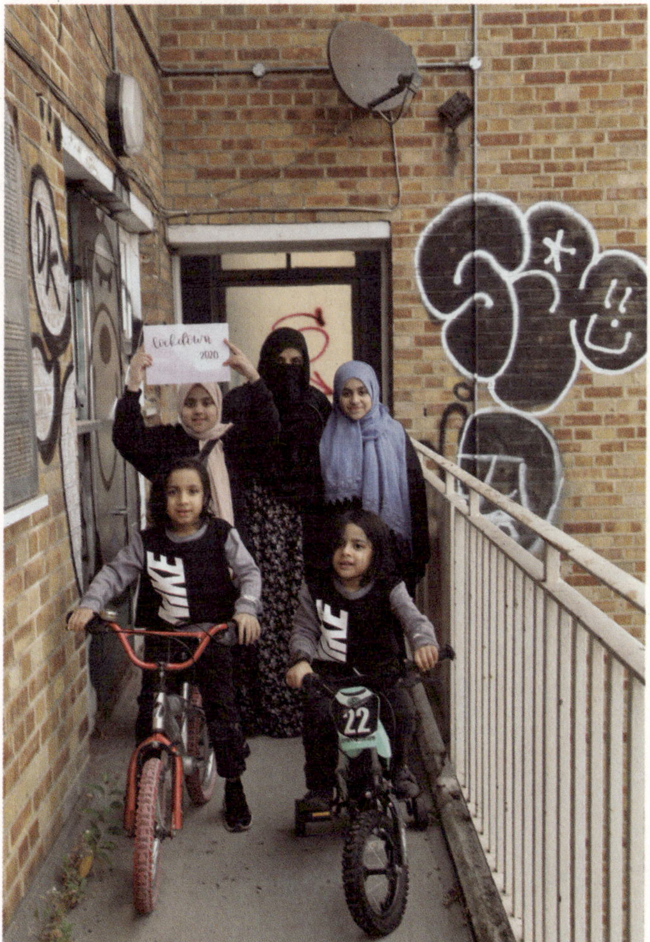

[5]

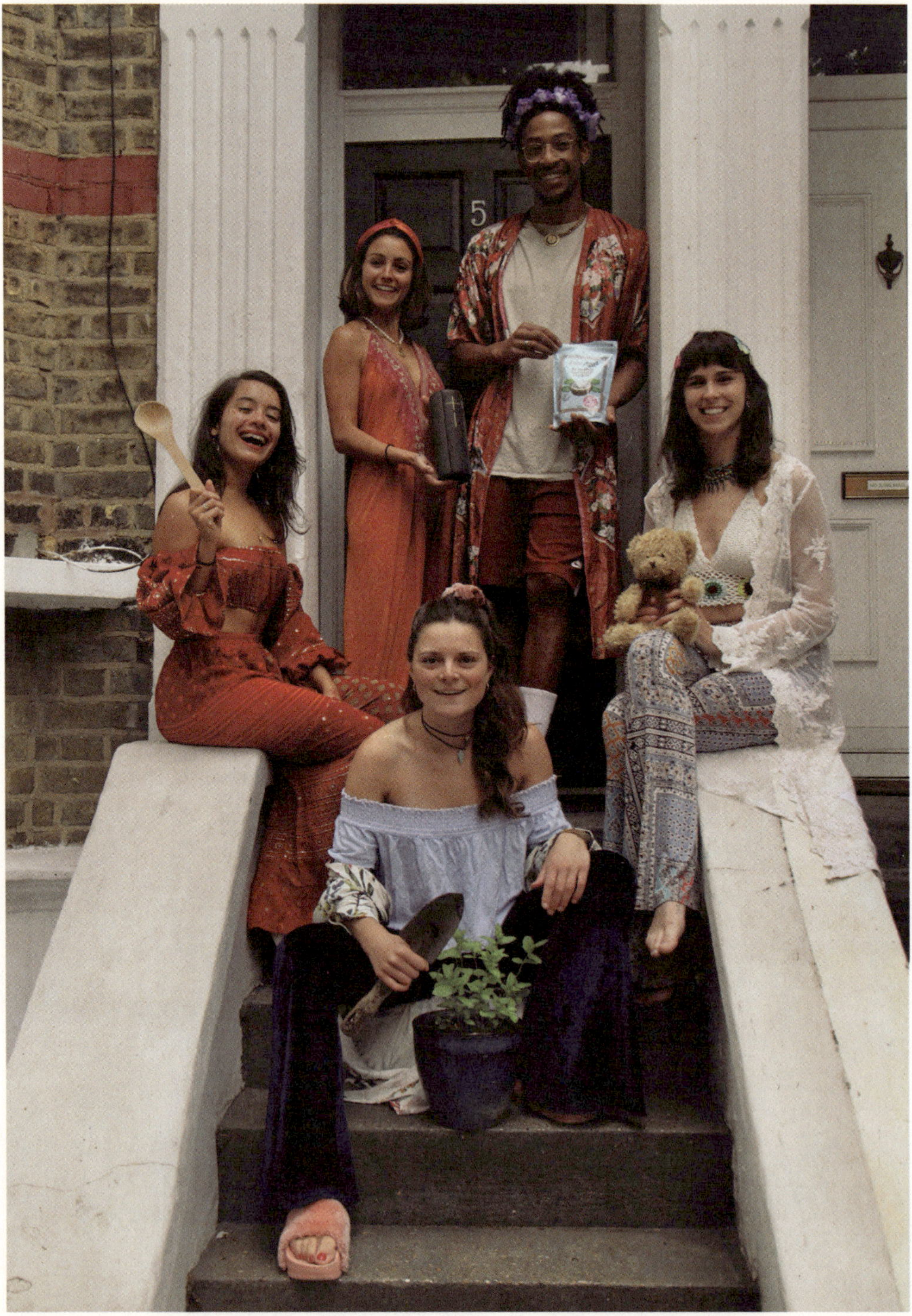

[6]

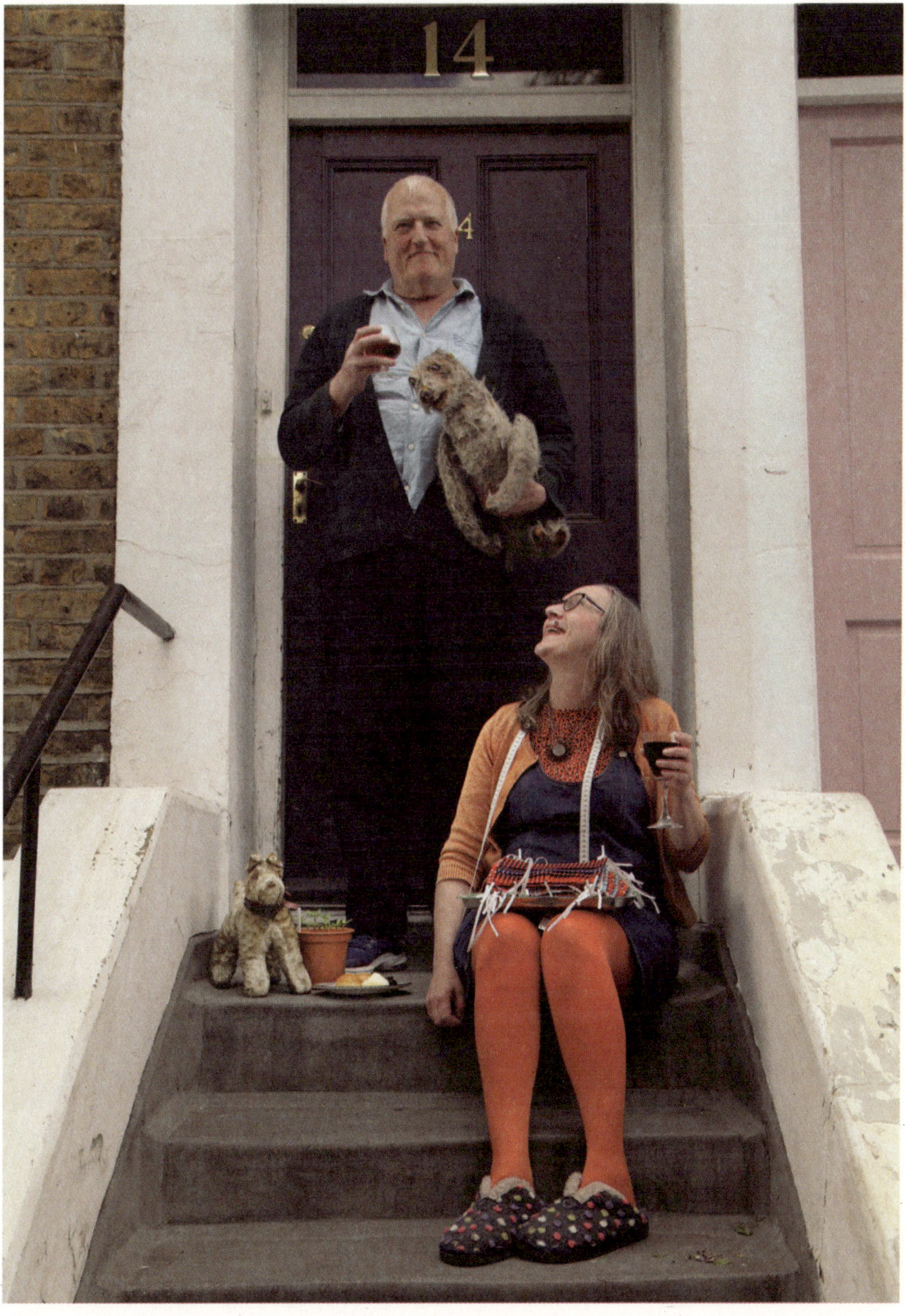

[7]

BARRICADES

How barricades recall the ways in which space can be reorganised through everyday objects

PANDEMIC OBJECTS

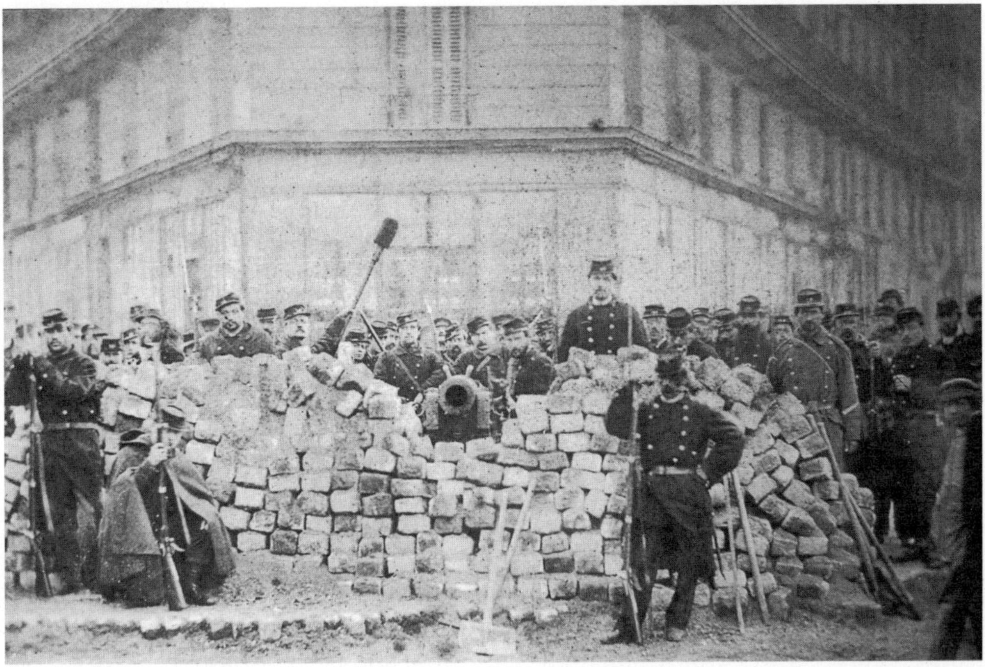

Road barricade in Paris during the Paris Commune, 1871, captured by Bruno Braquehais.

The barricade is an object steeped in urban history. In contrast to its use for top-down control, managing parades, protests and, more recently, as a preventative measure against terrorist acts, it has also been deployed paradoxically as an act of bottom-up resistance. Uniting these differing motives is an association with past and potential violence. During the pandemic, ad-hoc and temporary barriers were deployed in cities around the world, either to ward off the use of public spaces or to dissuade vehicle entrance onto newly pedestrianised streets.

The photographer Shashank Peshawaria documented the streets of Amritsar, India after curfew had been imposed in the state of Punjab. Made from an array of at-hand materials – road signs, discarded carts, even a piece of rope strung across a side street – the barriers were built to limit the movement of vehicles during certain times, allowing people to access essential goods and services, as well as to keep people within their neighbourhood.

The photographs reflect a recurring thread which played out in different ways throughout the world: lacking resources, make-shift solutions are sought. There is a latent potential of any object on the street to be turned into an organising force. Trash cans, parked cars, paving stones: all form a material library of potential use, whether for control or critique.

Text by Brendan Cormier

Photographs by Shashank Peshawaria.

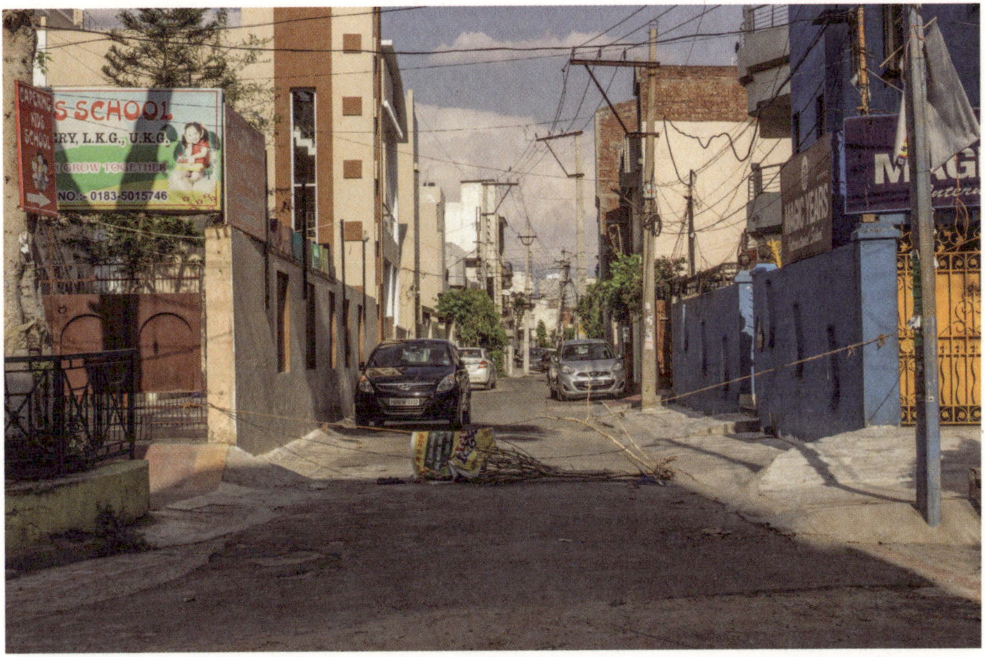
S SCHOOL
ERY, L.K.G., U.K.G.
NO.:- 0183-5015746

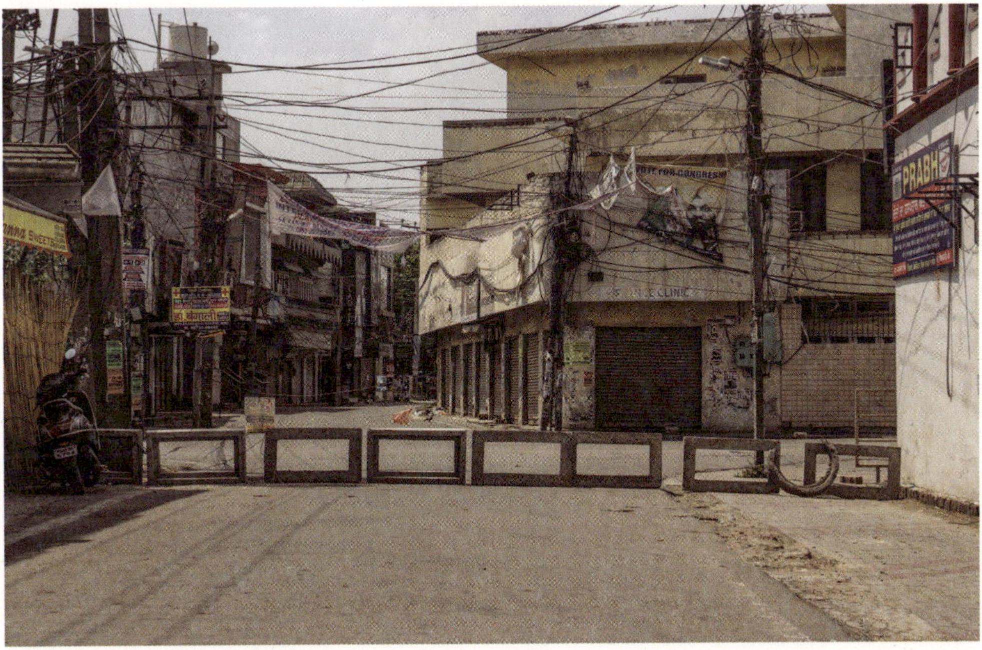
PRABH

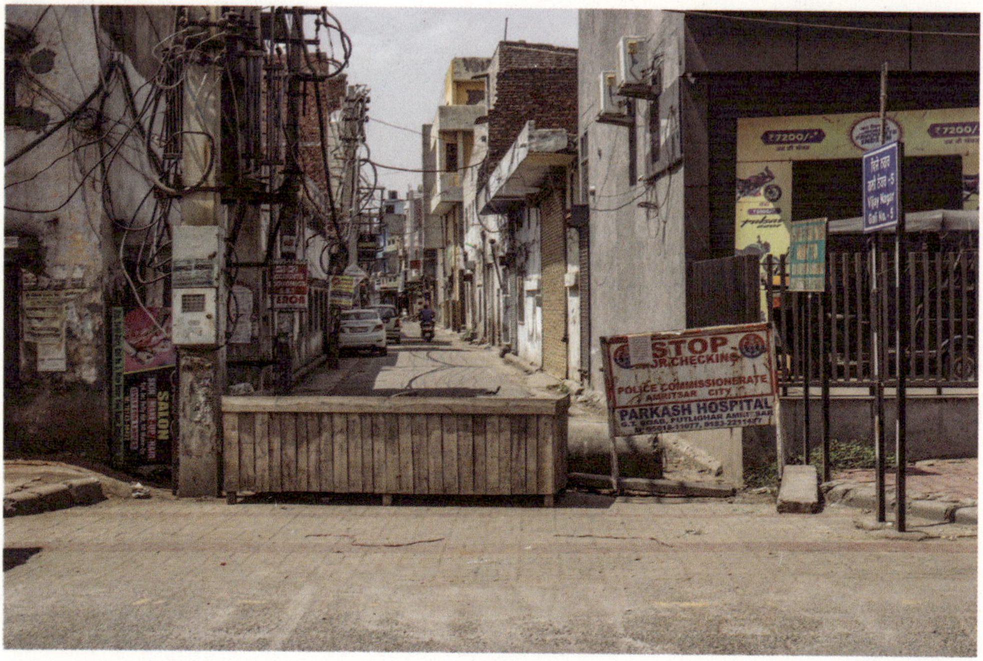
STOP
R CHECKING
POLICE COMMISSIONERATE
AMRITSAR CITY
PARKASH HOSPITAL
Vijay Nagar
Gali No. - 5

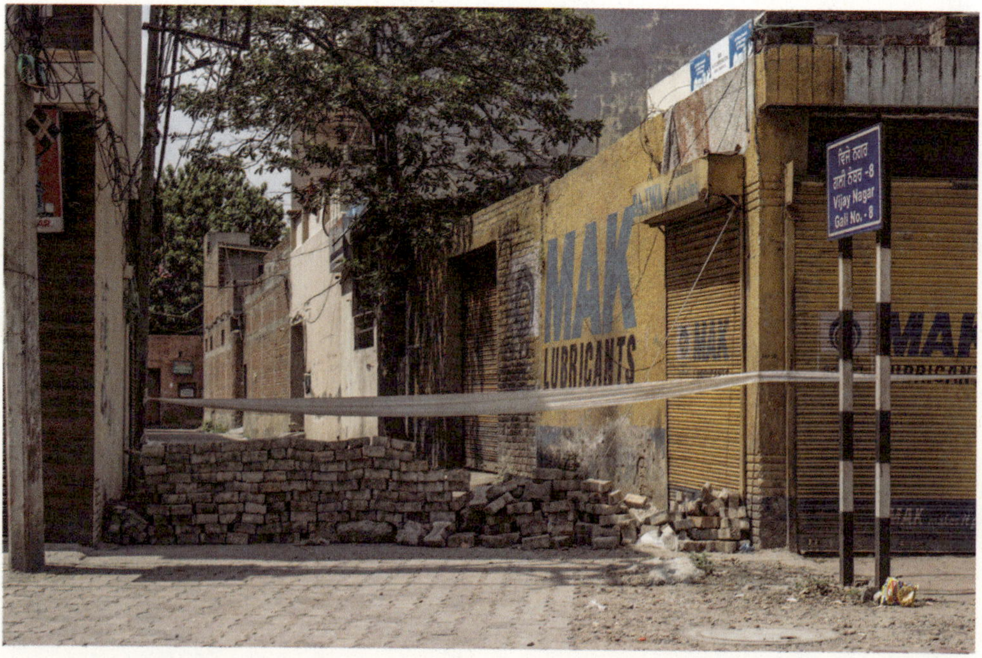
Vijay Nagar
Gali No. - 8
MAK
LUBRICANTS

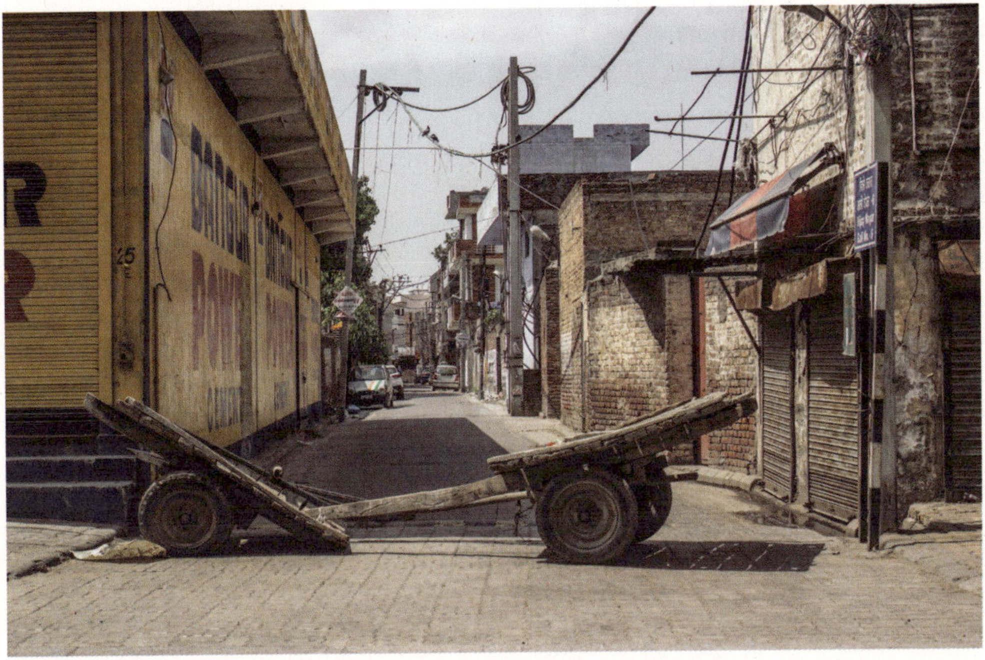

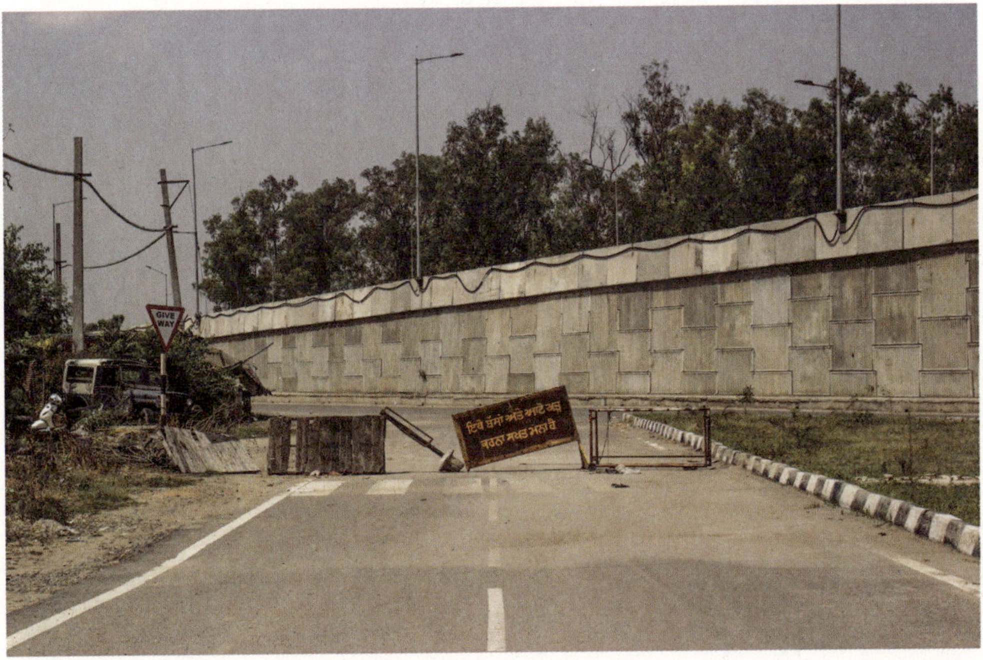
GIVE
WAY

POSTCARDS

How a series of photographs documented the new environmental detritus of the pandemic, appearing as postcards from a particular time

PANDEMIC OBJECTS

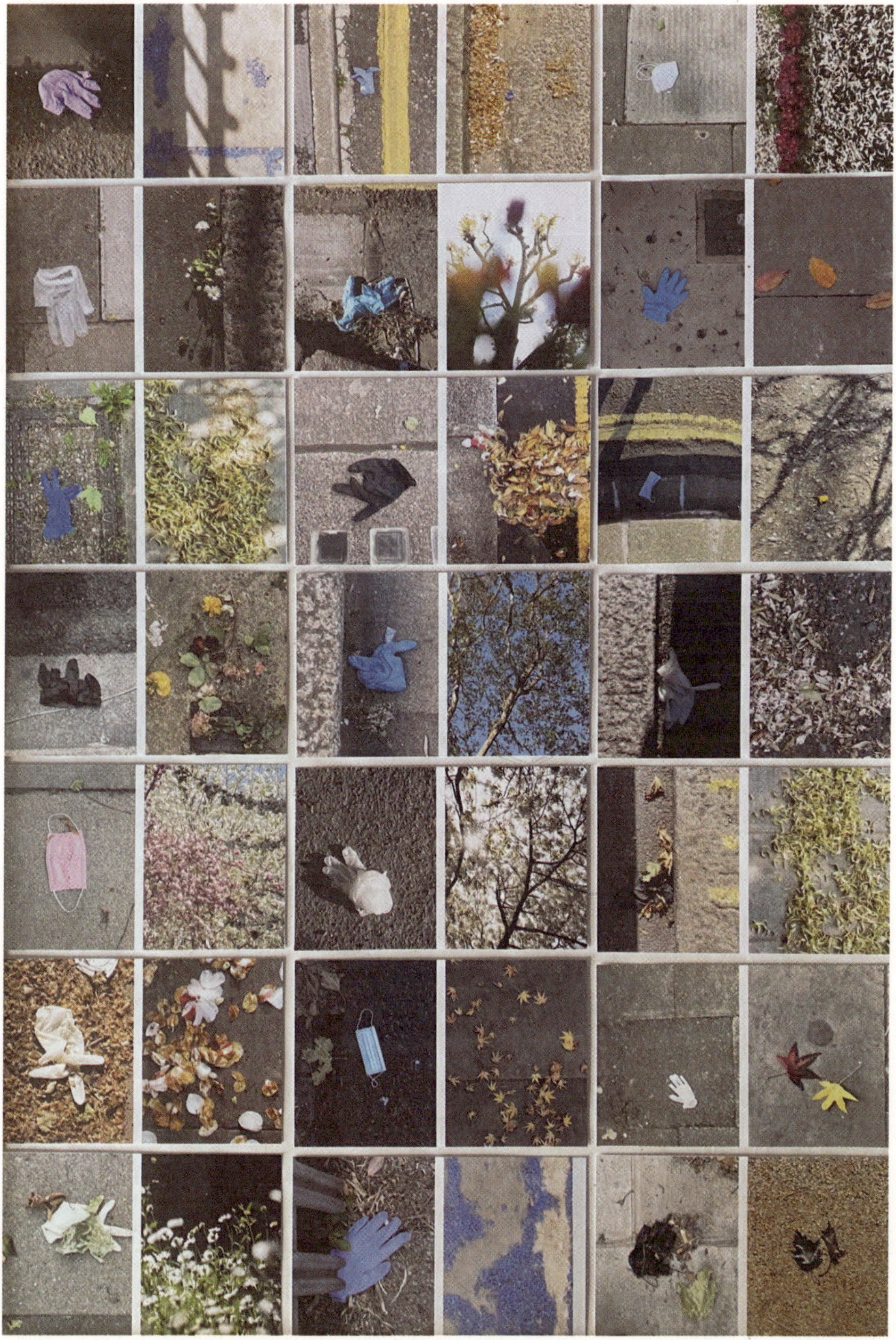

The first picture postcard was sent and received by the same person: Theodore Hook, in 1840. The card featured a caricature of a postal worker, most likely meant as a practical joke by Hook about the postal service itself. The legacy of his trick turned out to be longlasting, as he unwittingly sparked a booming industry that would continue to flourish until the turn of this millennium, only to fade out with advancements in technology and the rise of social media.

A postcard is an image from another place, a trigger to think about where someone has been, evoking an alternate universe of sights, sounds and encounters. The first few months of the Covid-19 pandemic now feel distant as well – not just historically distant, but like another space altogether. This distance gives Natasha Durlacher's photographic series *Postcards from the Pandemic* (2020) extra heft. Shot in postcard format during the unusually warm and sunny days of the first months of lockdown, Durlacher paired images of the detritus of nitrile gloves and face masks found strewn on pavements everywhere with flower petals and blossoms in complementary colours. The contrast between the idyllic weather and the alien intrusion of the glove seems especially jarring now, recalling the anxiety and uncanniness of the period. The postcard may be a dying medium, but it finds a renewed expression here – recalling a collective memory, not from a far-off place but from our recent past.

Text by Brendan Cormier

Photographs by Natasha Durlacher.

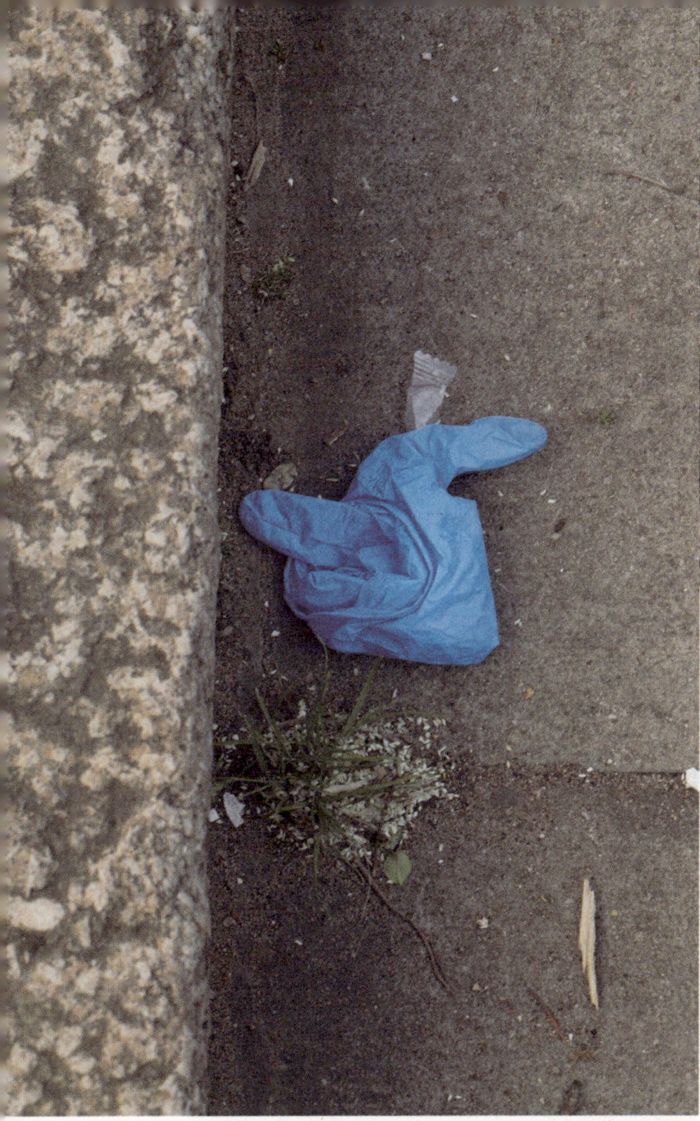

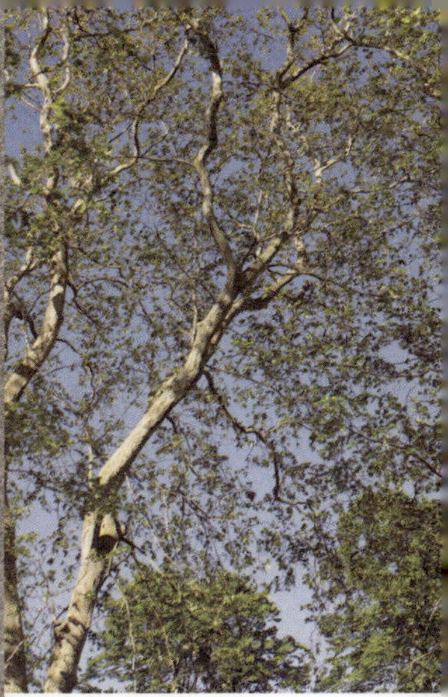

DOCUMENT

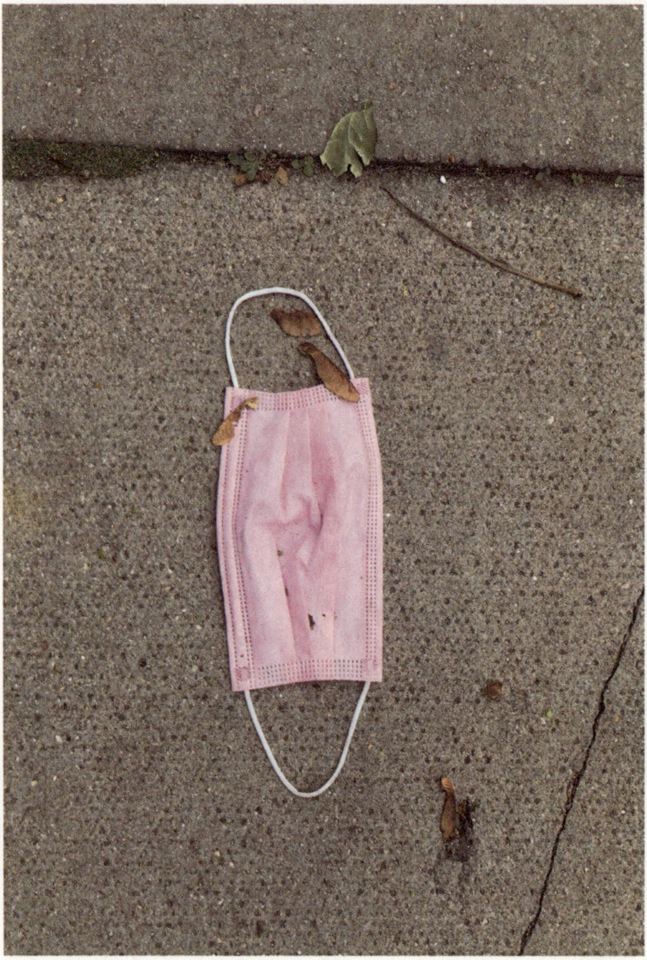

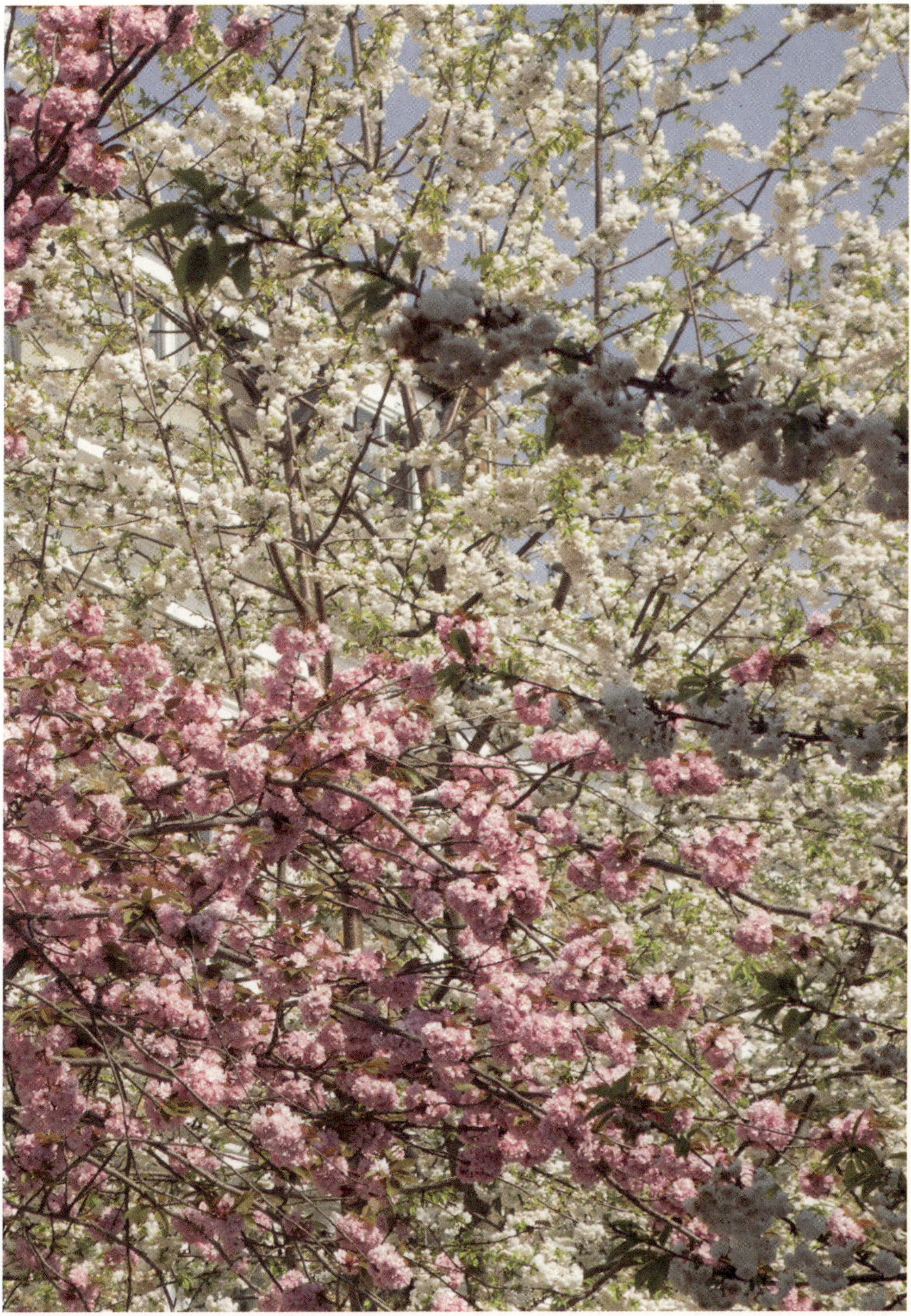

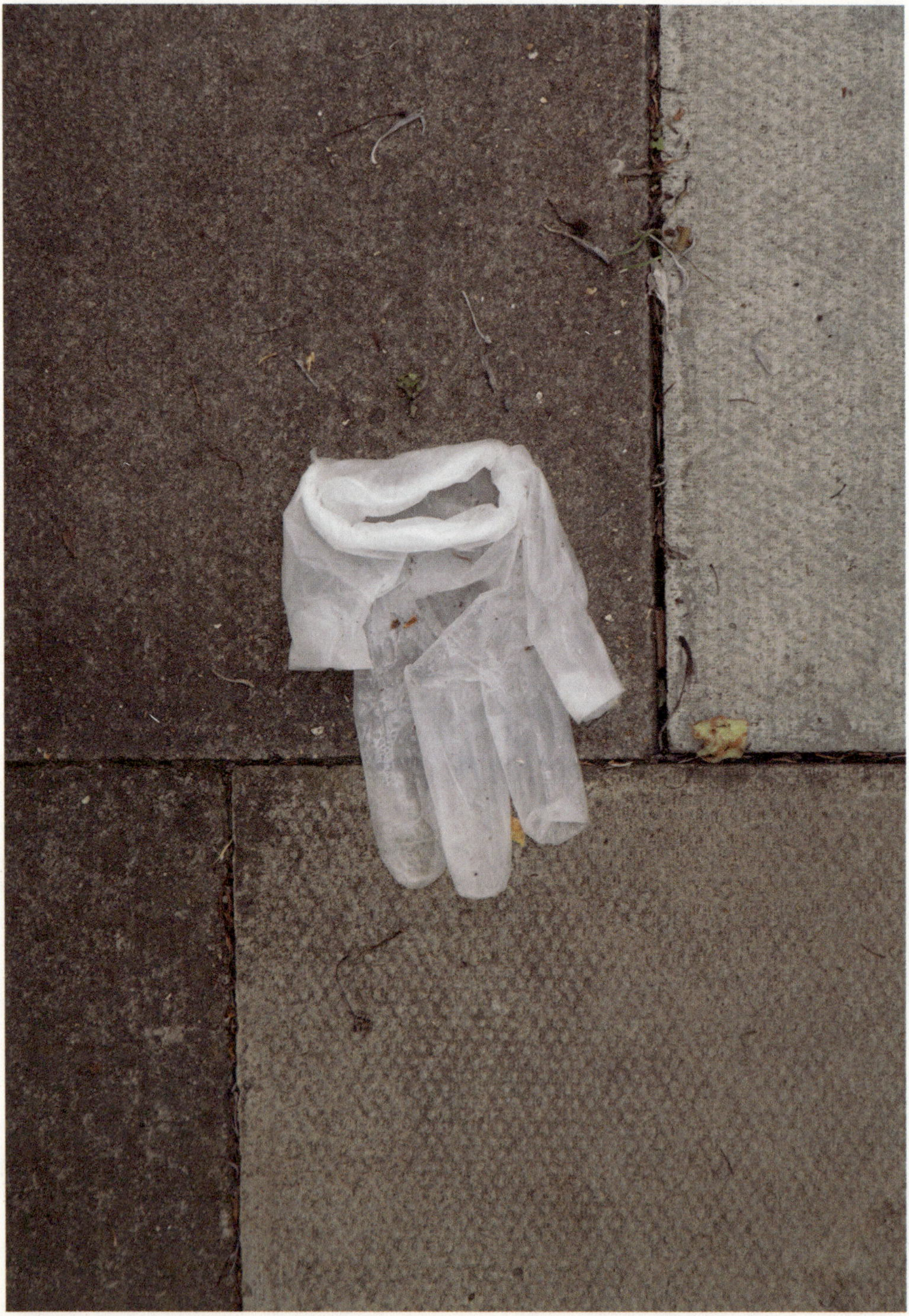

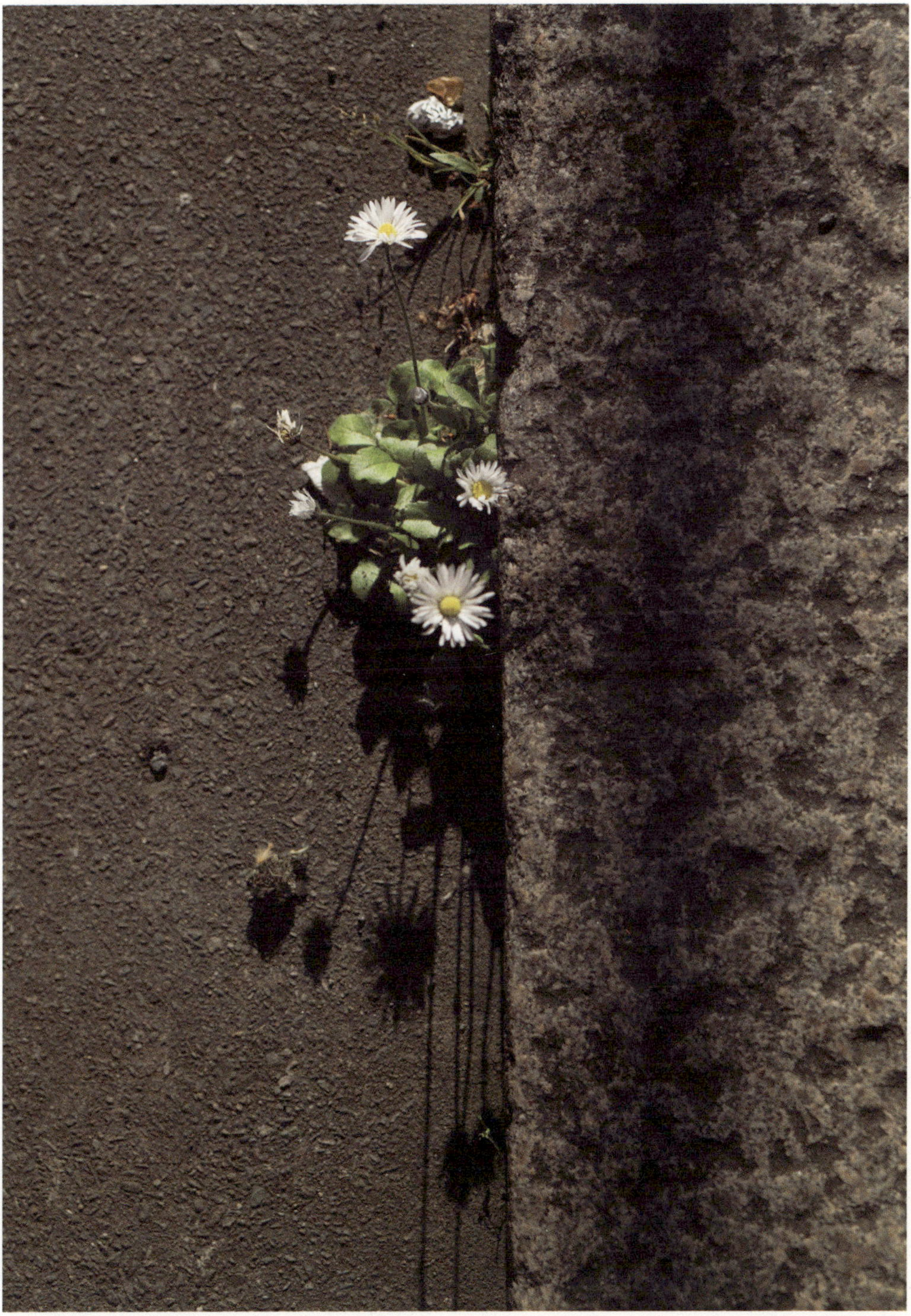

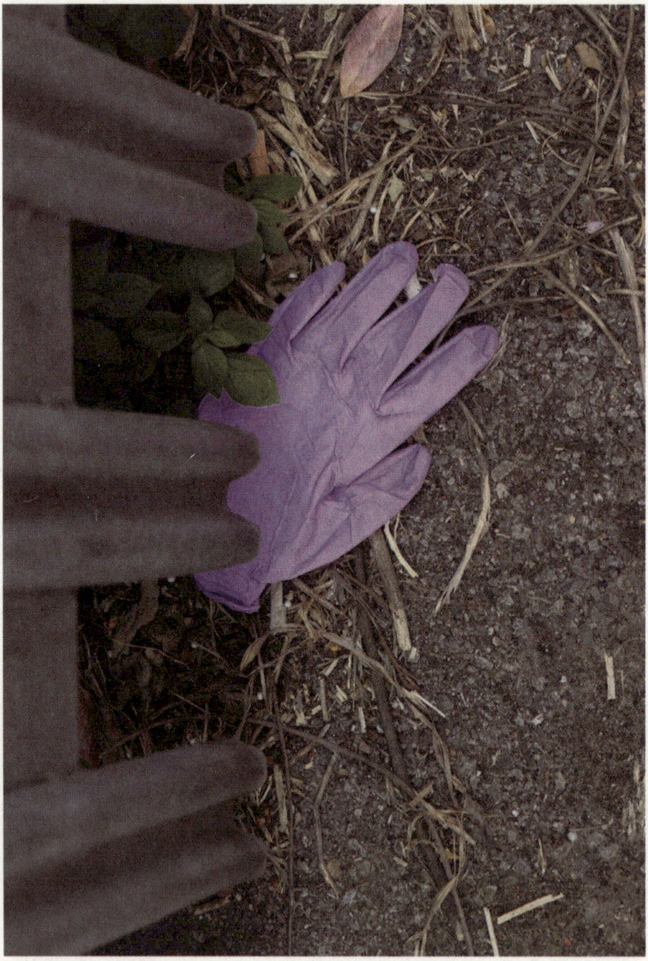

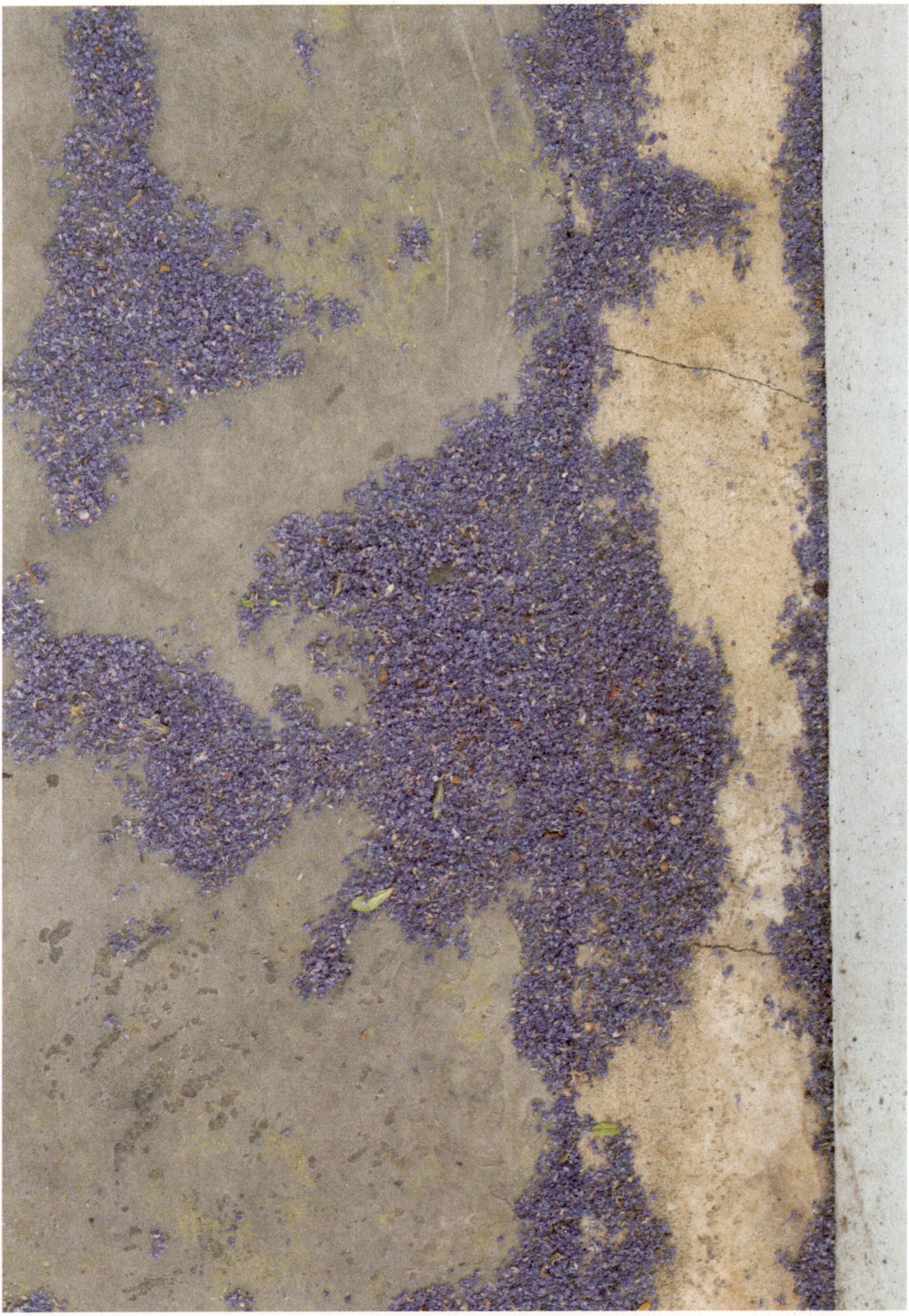

THE SEA

How a daily photography project offered a collective meditation on the expansiveness of the world, while raising funds for the NHS

[01]

Simon Roberts, *Day 52, 9 May 2020, 346 deaths (31,586 cumulative)*

Invisible, your clocking tides
Break on the lovebeds of the weeds;
The weed of love's left dry;
There round about your stones the shades
Of children go who, from their voids,
Cry to the dolphined sea.

Dylan Thomas
extract from *Where Once the Waters on Your Face*

From the series *A Daily Sea*, 2020, by Simon Roberts.

DOCUMENT

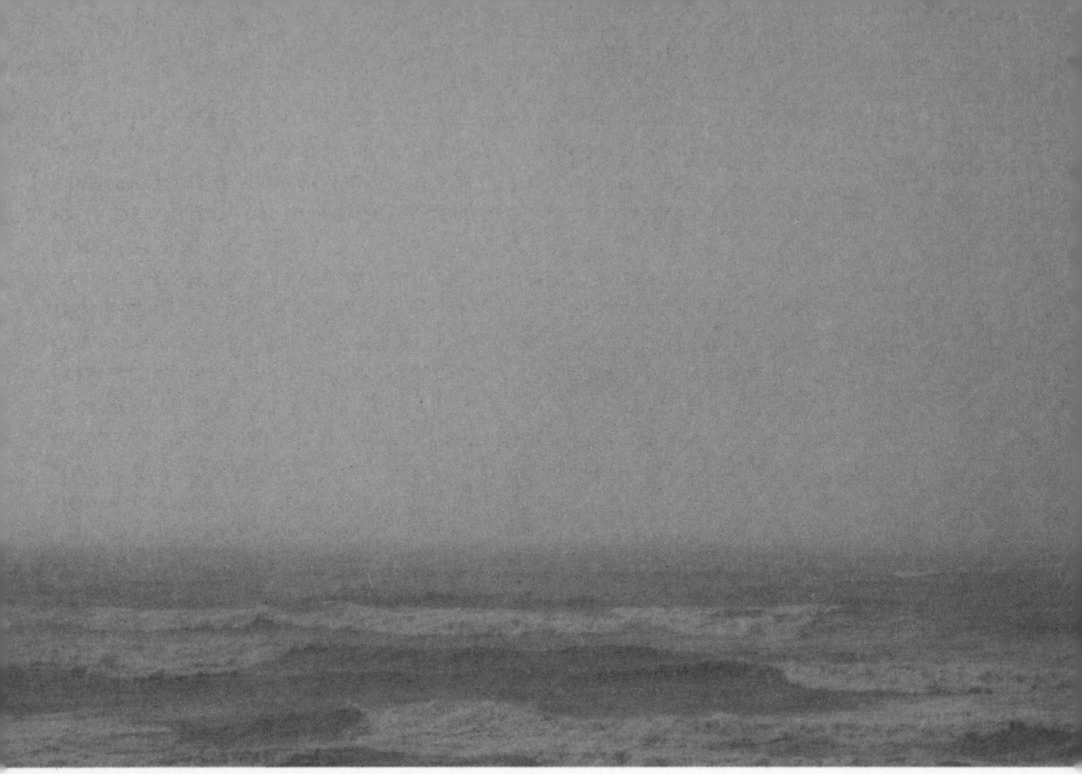

[02]

Simon Roberts, *Day 1, 19 March 2020, 43 deaths (158 cumulative)*

For whatever we lose (like a you or a me),
it's always ourselves we find in the sea.

ee cummings
extract from *maggie and milly and molly and may*

[03]

Simon Roberts, *Day 13, 31 March 2020, 382 deaths (2,425 cumulative)*

There is a pleasure in the pathless woods,
There is a rapture on the lonely shore,
There is a society, where none intrudes,
By the deep Sea, and music in its roar:
I love not Man the less, but Nature more,

Lord Byron
extract from *Childe Harold's Pilgrimage*

[04]

Simon Roberts, *Day 36, 23 April 2020, 727 deaths (21,787 cumulative)*

Look at that sea, girls – all silver and shadow and vision of things not seen. We couldn't enjoy its loveliness any more if we had millions of dollars and ropes of diamonds.

Lucy Maud Montgomery
extract from *Anne of Green Gables*

[05]

Simon Roberts, *Day 22, 9 April 2020,*
1,103 deaths (9,608 cumulative)

You are the moon, dear love, and I the sea:
The tide of hope swells high within my breast,
And hides the rough dark rocks of life's unrest
When your fond eyes smile near in perigee.
But when that loving face is turned from me,
Low falls the tide, and the grim rocks appear,
And earth's dim coast-line seems a thing to fear.
You are the moon, dear one, and I the sea.

Ella Wheeler Wilcox
Moon and Sea

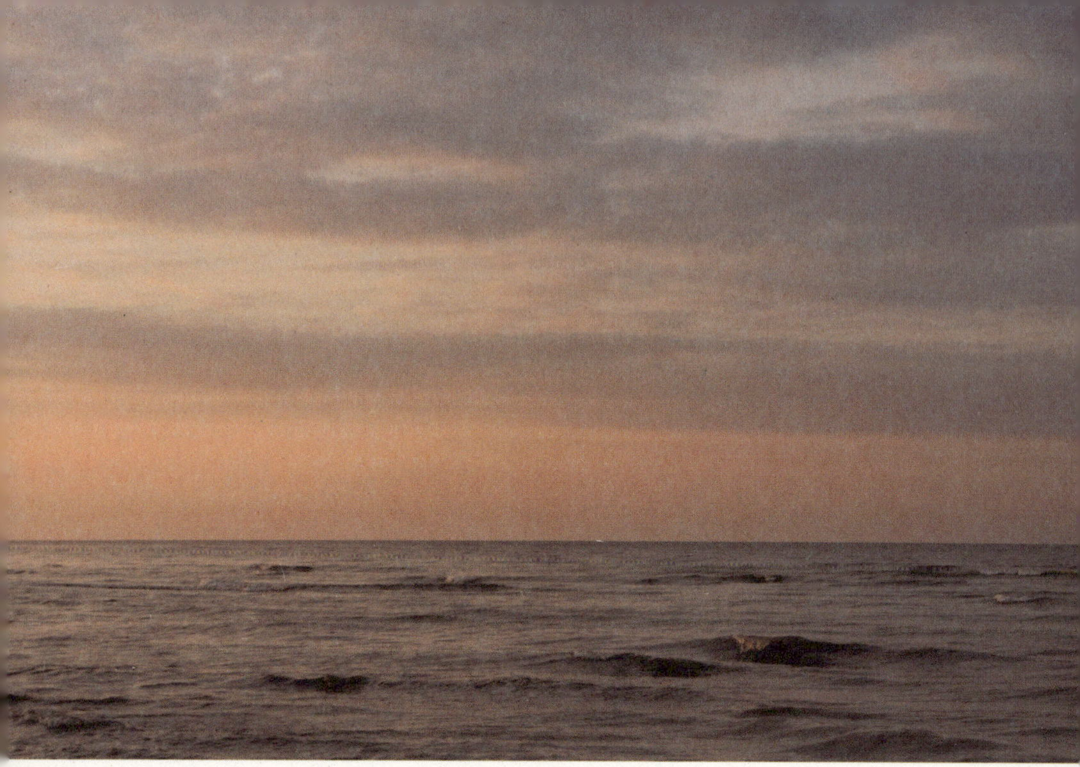

[06]

Simon Roberts, *Day 56, 13 May 2020, 494 deaths (33,186 cumulative)*

Now, voyager – once resigned
Go forth to seek and find
The hazy days you left behind
Right there in the back of your mind
Where lucid dreams begin
With rolling dunes and rattling shale
The shoreline then a swollen sail
Picked out by a shimmering halo
That's where the sea comes in...

Dr John Cooper Clarke
extract from *Nation's Ode to the Coast*

A Daily Sea is a meditative series of 56 photographs of seascapes by Simon Roberts, taken every day over the course of the first Covid-19 lockdown in the UK. Instinct brought Roberts to the sea at the start of the outbreak, when much of the world was overwhelmed by the uncertainty that lay ahead. Driven by the need for personal respite, and for a practical use of his daily permitted exercise, he began photographing the sea once a day from Brighton beach, a mere 200m from his home, and sharing the images on his Instagram page.

Humans have always sought solace from the sea. The mysteries that exist beyond the horizon and below its surface seem to provoke an endless capacity for personal reflection and metaphor. Roberts is no different, stating in an interview with photographer Jim Grover that, 'for me, water provides a great sense of release...emotionally and physically'.

Comments on his Instagram posts reveal that Roberts' seascapes resonated with audiences. For many, they offered a delightful break in their feeds from the monotony of upsetting news and forays into home baking (Flour and Yeast, p108). Instead, these posts offered a moment to consider life outside the confines of one's living room and to ruminate on the vastness of Covid-19's impact. It was this response from his audiences, paired with a desire to do something meaningful, that led Roberts to take the project further, making the series available as limited-edition prints, with funds earned from the sale going to support the NHS's Covid-19 Urgent Appeal.

Each photograph is accompanied by a sea-related text and daily figures of Covid-19 mortalities from the Office for National Statistics. 'I consider the portfolio box of all 56 prints as a kind of memorial piece,' Roberts notes. 'I wanted people to consider the emotional significance of this time for those families who'd lost loved ones. The work isn't just about these bucolic scenes, it's also rooted in a significant national moment.'

The images are spectacular when seen together. Through the variations in hues and weather patterns, both stark and subtle, Roberts' series enables us to relive the changing seasons, the shifts from morning to afternoon to nightfall. The images are measures of time that, during the tedium of lockdown, started to blend together as the days began to feel increasingly similar. The photographs function as a visual record, providing us with a means to reflect on and distil this strange period in a series of frozen moments.

Text by Hana Kaluznick

03

SELF-CARE

The pandemic focused attention on the body in unprecedented ways. While notions of wellness and self-care have been rapidly gaining traction over the course of the past decade, Covid-19 accelerated the urgency of taking care of oneself. It was not just the virus that we needed to shield from; the pandemic was a cluster bomb of psychological pressures that came from the grieving of lost loved ones, isolation and anxieties about the future. This was exacerbated by lockdowns that cut people off from so many services that could help fulfil their wellness needs.

Domestic spaces had to work overtime. Not only were they now offices, schools and homes all at once, they needed to provide room for physical and mental recuperation. New household objects came into popular use: hand sanitiser became a modern-day talisman to ward off disease and many people adopted potted plants, bringing a sense of the outdoors in. Where the space of the home found internal limits, digital space became a vital form of escape, from passive activities like watching Netflix to more engaged forms of worldbuilding, as evidenced in the huge success of Animal Crossing.

The drive for self-care revealed an ongoing social divide where those with access to bigger spaces, more amenities and certain devices had more opportunity to find peace, solace and wellbeing during the darker days of the pandemic in contrast to others with limited area and resources. Despite this, and with a little ingenuity, many were able to reassess the objects they had at hand to harness their therapeutic effects.

FLOUR AND YEAST

How a lockdown hobby revealed the grounding effect of baking while shining a light on the importance of understanding food supply chains

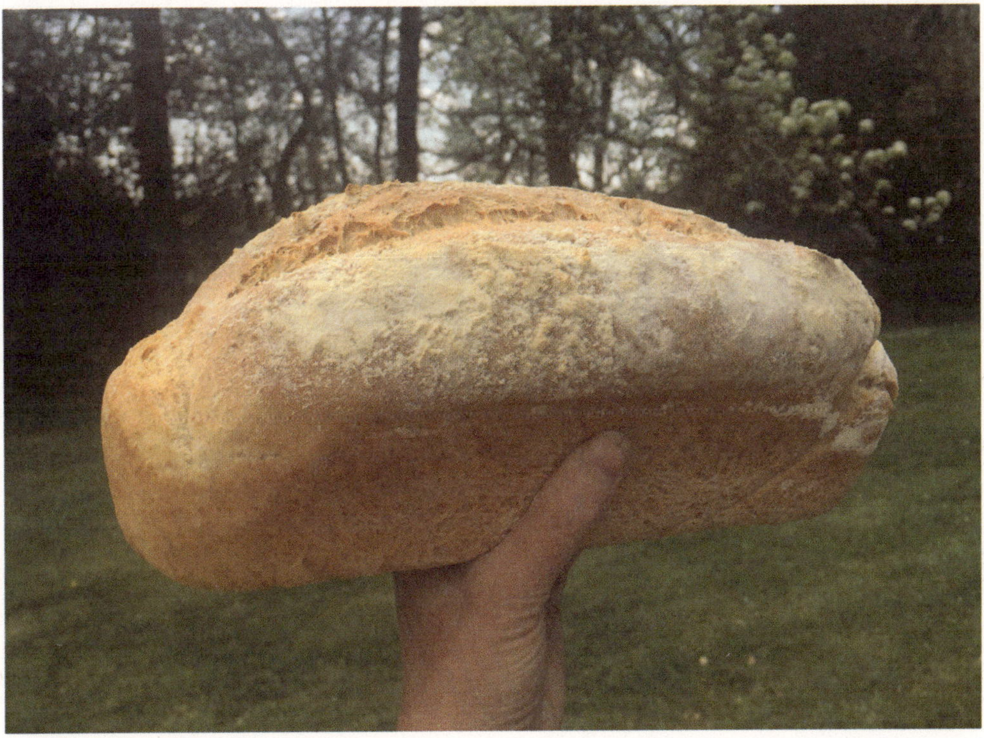

One of the author's attempts at making bread during lockdown.

In many parts of the world, Covid-19 lockdowns brought about a mass resurgence in home cooking as the hospitality sector pulled down its shutters and left people largely to their own culinary resources. Initially, it was dried pasta – a go-to ingredient for quick meals – which disappeared from supermarket shelves, causing minor hysteria alongside a toilet paper shortage (see Toilet Roll p306). In the following weeks, however, flour and yeast became newly discussed scarcities as many suddenly turned their hand to baking their own bread. In the UK, grocery sales of flour increased by 92% in March 2020 in comparison to the same period the previous year. In the midst of a public health catastrophe, a craze for baking felt like an incidental phenomenon. It did, however, reveal something about both our behaviour during the pandemic and the ever-evolving significance of bread as a cultural object.

Bread is a classic comfort food, not only full of serotonin-boosting carbs but also rich in symbolism. One of the most common and ritualised foods throughout history, it is synonymous with physical and spiritual sustenance. In the broadest sense, bread can embody a reassuring notion of continuity and human resilience in the context of crisis and uncertainty, 'a kind of promise that we'll get through it', as Steven Kaplan, a historian who specialises in bread, declares. Beyond that, there are a number of reasons why the making of bread at home flourished during lockdown.

First, there is something to be said for the tactile pleasures of making bread during a time of social distancing, when physical contact became the object of regulation and fear. Bread has long been associated with bodies, from Jewish texts that liken humans to Challah dough as a combination of body and soul, flour and water, to bread transforming into the body of Christ in the Holy Communion of the Catholic Church. On an earthier level, there are instances of priests in the Middle Ages complaining about women kneading dough on their naked bodies before baking and serving it as an aphrodisiac, while today bread can be used as slang for desirable, nicely rounded parts of the body: 'buns' in English, or 'miche' in French. Folding your hands into pliant, pillowy dough clearly has both spiritual and sensual potential. Kneading feels good and releases tension. The alchemy of transforming flour, yeast and water into a gloriously risen loaf is also creatively satisfying; a tangible result you pull from the oven, taste and ingest. The lockdowns meant that our lives were more digitally mediated than ever, social interactions reduced in large part to heads on screens; perhaps, on the most visceral level, making bread was a way to reaffirm our bodily existence.

Then there is the smell: warm, slightly heady and redolent of all things homely. The aroma of baking bread is powerfully associated with a wholesome ideal of home, even if it has never featured in a person's home life. It is cliché that having bread baking in the oven helps to sell a house by subliminally presenting it as a home. Baking, indeed, slipped easily into comforting fantasies of domesticity and self-sufficiency – embodied in trends like 'cottagecore' – that developed through the 2010s but grew wings during the pandemic as people were forced to make home the centre of their world.

The practical process of making bread also fits well with the directive to stay at home. Baking a basic loaf isn't labour intensive: overall the prep takes less time than watching an episode of *The Great British Bake Off*. But it does require you to be in one place for several hours, ready to intervene at the right moment in the various stages of kneading, proofing and baking. The rhythm of bread making can feel impossible to square with the frenetic pace of modern life. But when schedules vanish overnight, the opposite is true: making bread can create a structure and routine – one of the reasons it is often taken up by people when they retire. Arguably, making bread during the pandemic was less about filling time, and more a response to an altered sense of time.

In another sense, however, making bread feeds into the familiar pressure to always be producing, consuming and communicating. People did not just bake loaves; they photographed and posted them on Instagram. Baking bread, especially complex sourdoughs, became a favoured method of showing the world that you were having a 'productive lockdown'. With so many activities commonly used for communicating status and identity via social media suspended, others took their place. According to Andrew Potter, author of *The Authenticity Hoax*, when you share images of your sourdough efforts, you are also signalling that you have the privilege and resources to develop new skills during lockdown as opposed to simply surviving. The issue of inequality becomes even clearer when we consider that the sudden boom in recreational baking meant that workers packaging flour for retail were having to work overtime on factory lines operating around the clock to meet demand.

The most radical result of the pandemic's disruption to our food consumption should be that people take more notice of where their food comes from, how it reaches them and who produces it.

Text by Catherine Flood

A WhatsApp conversation on home baking between curator May Rosenthal Sloan and her father.

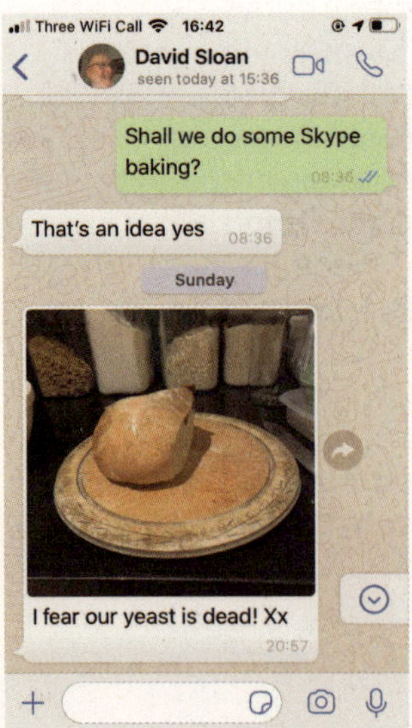
Three WiFi Call 16:42
David Sloan
seen today at 15:36
Shall we do some Skype baking? 08:36
That's an idea yes 08:36
Sunday
I fear our yeast is dead! Xx
20:57

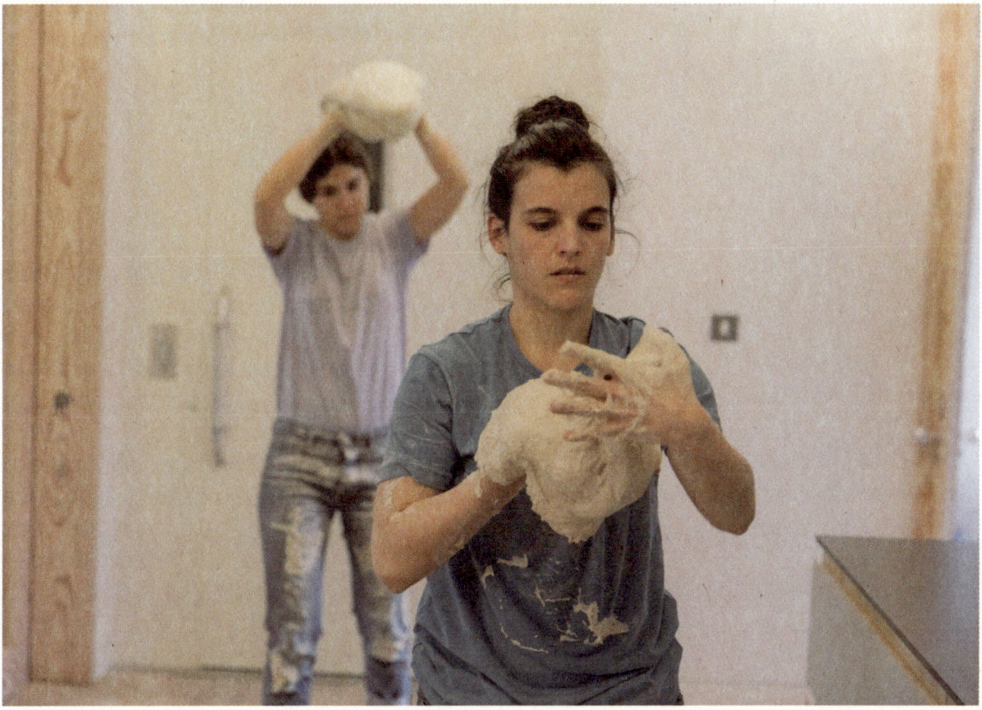

A performance of *Rolling* (2017) by Laura Wilson, performed by Elina Akhmetova, Iris Chan, Nick Keegan, Eliza Soroga and Piedad Seiquer. Commissioned by Delfina Foundation and the Curating Contemporary Art MA Programme at the Royal College of Art, and photographed by Jan Naraine.

GARDENS

Illustration from *A Floral Fantasy in an Old English Garden*, Walter Crane, Great Britain, 1899.

How the garden became a focal point in discussions of social disparity, and what its long history in visual and literary culture can ask of the future of wellbeing

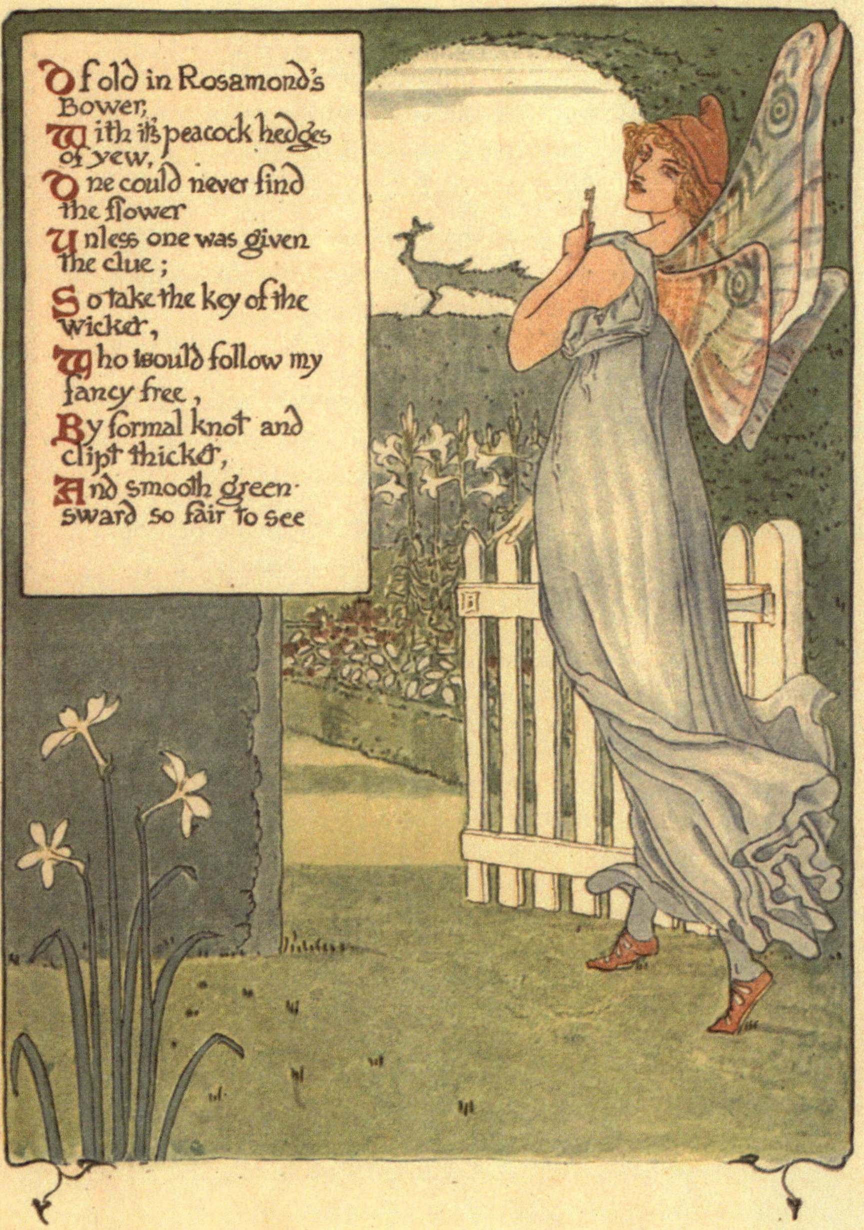
Of old in Rosamond's
Bower,
With its peacock hedges
of yew,
One could never find
the flower
Unless one was given
the clue;
So take the key of the
wicket,
Who would follow my
fancy free,
By formal knot and
clipt thicket,
And smooth green-
sward so fair to see

In the face of confinement and uncertainty during the pandemic, many people across the world dialled up their horticultural aspirations. Google searches for 'gardening' doubled compared to prior years, and there was record demand for seeds and compost in the UK in the months following the country's first lockdown. Green-fingered journalists leapt from their trowels to their keyboards to convey the considerable benefits of gardening, including physical and mental wellbeing, encouraging others to have a go at growing their own life-affirming 'victory garden'.

This was a new leisure pursuit for many, as they made the move from just about keeping houseplants alive to making their first purchase of seeds online. Some were lucky enough to have a patch of soil to call their own; some utilised less favourable spaces: a modest patio, a balcony or a small rooftop spot. For others, cultivating a piece of nature for themselves remained an unattainable luxury.

In May 2020, the Office for National Statistics released data revealing that 21% of households in London, compared with 12% across the country, were living without access to private outdoor space. In some areas of the capital where high-density living is typical, this figure was more than 70%. The data also revealed a huge racial disparity, with white people four times more likely than Black people to have private access to outdoor space.

The results of this survey came at a time when access to green outdoor space was more crucial than ever. With no choice but to stay at home, many people's daily lives and mental health were largely shaped by their personal domestic environments and immediate surroundings. These, in turn, were shaped by where they sat on the country's widening social spectrum, with the urban working classes disproportionately punished by the measures taken to prevent the further spread of Covid-19. Adding insult to injury, those without gardens had to face the moral panic and stigma over how – as well as for how long – they used public parks (p214). While the UK government wanted us to believe that we were 'all in this together', the inequalities that many people experienced in their access to space – and outdoor space in particular – were not easy to ignore.

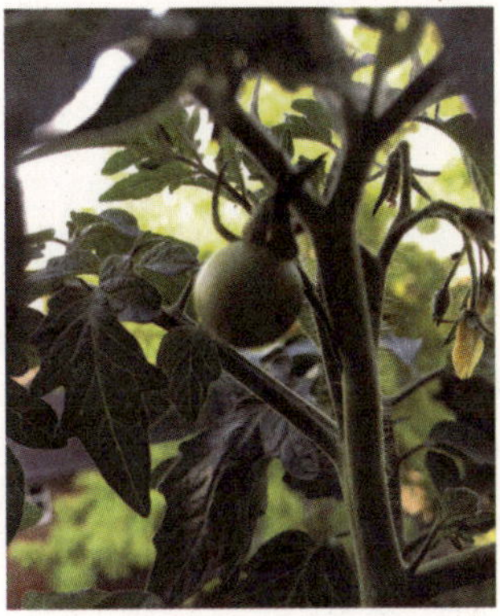

From mid-May 2020, after more than six weeks of the initial lockdown, the government's list of 'reasonable excuses' to leave the house was expanded to make spending time in public parks acceptable again. Though undoubtedly a huge relief for those cooped up in flats without green spaces at home, these places were no substitute for the private garden as a site of personal agency. As the horticultural boom suggested, there is more to garden access than simply having space to get fresh air, relax and sunbathe.

Since antiquity, the garden has offered refuge from the trials and tribulations of everyday life. Our relationship to these spaces is often seen as apolitical and escapist, but as places of both physical labour and aesthetic choice, they have the power to fulfil aspirations as much as recreational needs. This power has long been expressed in visual and literary culture, with the garden having held symbolic weight throughout history as a vehicle for utopian thought. When writer, philosopher and social critic Voltaire wrote his signature work *Candide, ou l'Optimisme* (*Candide, or The Optimist*) in 1759, the garden was a recurring motif used to reflect his aversion to the social inequalities inflicted by the church and aristocracy, and to further his call for radical social reformation during the Enlightenment. The narrative's final assertion is that in order for people to seek a peaceful existence they must cultivate their own gardens – a private and productive act that promises to nurture the soul.

A century later, as the significance of access to green spaces for public health gained traction in 19th-century Britain, the garden was used heavily in the rhetoric of socialism. In response to the 'brutalisation' of the working classes wrought by the Industrial Revolution, artist William Morris founded the Socialist League in 1884 and began to envision a pre-industrial Edenic idyll in which communities united by a shared purpose would be prioritised over class systems and corporate hierarchies. The workings of nature – as articulated in Morris's graphics, wallpaper and furnishing designs, as well as his novel *News From Nowhere* (1890) – became

The author's rooftop tomatoes.

emblematic of a utopian world in which 'useful toil' provided the antidote to the alienation of workers from the 'fruits of their labour' as induced by industrialisation. For Morris, the garden was a place in which all people could generate plenty and pleasure. Artist Walter Crane, an acquaintance and supporter of Morris, used his practice – which included designs for illustrated children's books – to espouse a specific politics based on nature. In *A Floral Fantasy in an Old English Garden* (1899), Crane depicts himself being led through an enclosed garden by a fairy wearing a 'cap of liberty'. The cap was a widely known symbol of the revolutionary ideals of liberty and equality, featuring prominently in Crane's work. Throughout the garden, Crane encounters a series of characters dressed in elaborate costumes of petals, tendrils and leaves, each personifying a different plant. The depiction of the enchanting garden setting, and its 'flowering' of humankind, condemned the greed and unjust social order of the world outside it. The inhabitants' jubilation over the arrival of spring expressed a vision of hope and renewal.

A week into the UK's first lockdown, it was announced that the pioneering garden of artist and filmmaker Derek Jarman had been saved from being privately sold, following a ten-week public fundraising campaign. Jarman's desire to cultivate a piece of overlooked and inhospitable land in Dungeness in the late 1980s and early 1990s grew out of a period of immense personal strife in which he battled with AIDS and campaigned for gay rights and social justice. In his book *Modern Nature* (1992), Jarman described the suspension of time he felt among his ravaged garden: 'The gardener digs in another time, without past or future, beginning or end'. For him, the garden – which provided the ideal set for his 1987 film *The Last of England* – was a liberating place; a sanctuary free of the capitalist constructs of time, where alternate realities could be imagined.

Research conducted by the University of Exeter and the Royal Horticultural Society, released in May 2020, found that people with access to a private garden have significantly higher psychological wellbeing than those without. Moreover, there is increasing evidence that gardening has an enormous impact on mental health, improving levels of confidence, concentration and self-belief, as well as helping people deal with loss, anxiety and depression.

Despite this, and as a result of population growth, housing demand and increasing land value, the number of households in the UK without gardens has increased from 1.6 million to 3.3 million in the last 25 years. The experience of lockdown during the pandemic, and the consequent mass movement towards horticultural pursuits, made urgent the need to rethink this trajectory. How might the redemptive power of the garden, as so often exhibited in the realms of art and literature, be appreciated and activated at the level of urban planning and policymaking for the sake of more equitable futures? Ensuring that the opportunities afforded by private outdoor space are enjoyed by all, as a right and not a privilege, remains a challenge for the future.

Text by Samantha Manton

POTTED PLANTS

How potted plants created a virtual outdoors in periods of confinement and a sense of agency in uncertain times

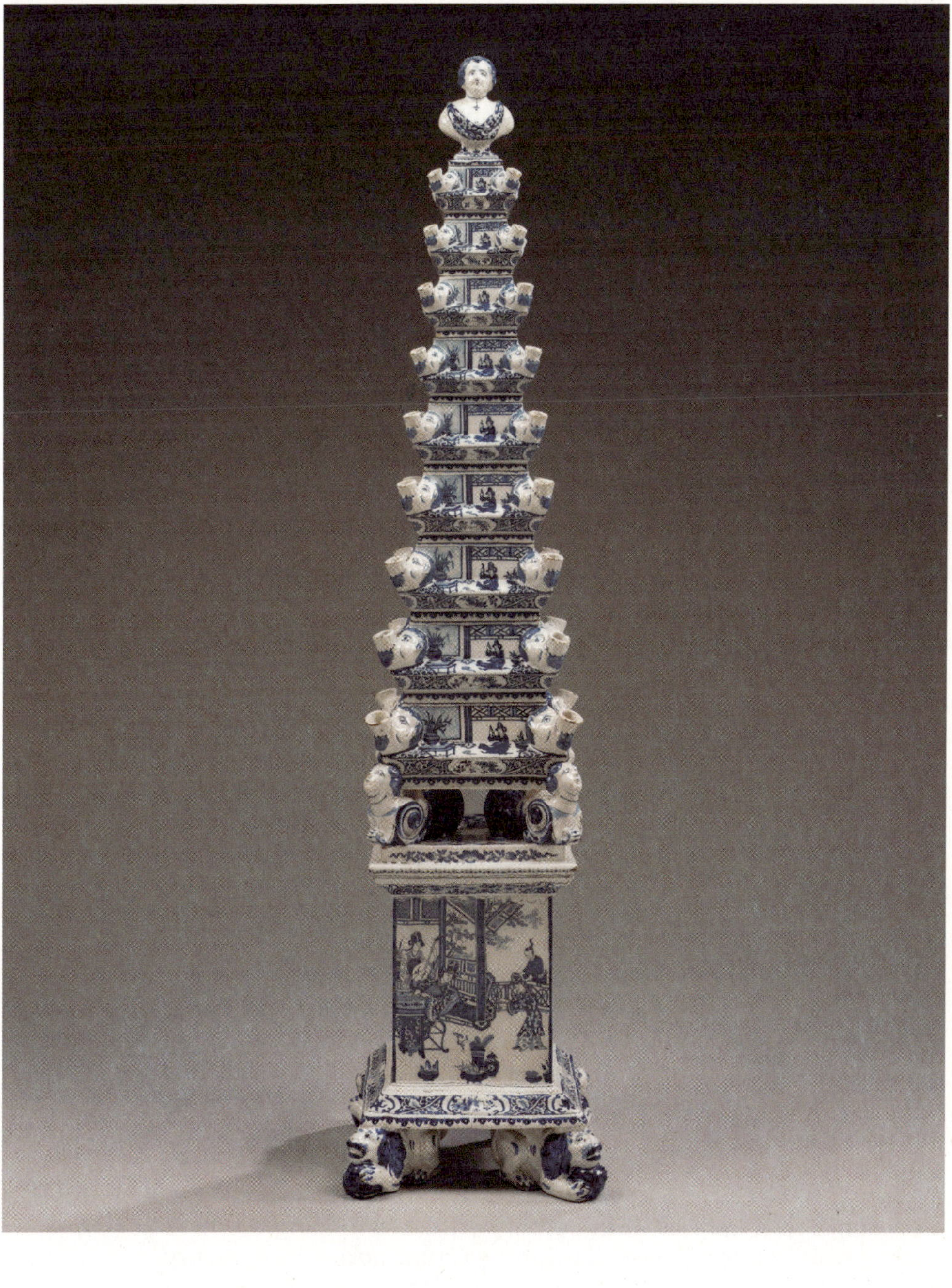

Flower pyramid, Delft, c1695.

Flower pot,
Derby Porcelain Factory,
Great Britain, c1765.

In recent years, houseplant hoarding has been the subject of ridicule as a millennial obsession. But has this perception shifted due to the pandemic? For those living in flats, without access to green outdoor space (see Gardens p114), being confined to our homes revealed a deep human attraction to nature. Houseplants became a saving grace for many people, allowing them to bring the outside in by injecting a tiny bit of greenery into their domestic spaces. Research by the Royal Horticultural Society confirms that certain houseplants can help improve air quality and even increase people's levels of concentration – especially useful for those working from home.

The potted plant industry flourished during the pandemic with evergreens, ferns, aloes and cacti ensnaring the attention of the masses. This saw the Horticultural Trades Association (HTA) launch a website called Plants Near Me, which helps users locate their nearest garden centre. In April and May 2020, the number of visitors to the HTA website more than doubled.

But what is the historical context of potted plants? Humans have been obsessed with bringing greenery into their homes for centuries, going at least as far back as the fabled Hanging Gardens of Babylon. These were thought by some to have been created around 600 BCE by King Nebuchadnezzar II of the Neo-Babylonian Empire as a botanical haven for his wife, Queen Amytis. Over the years, plants have continued to be seen as a symbol of wealth and power. In his 1652 treatise *The Garden of Eden*, the English agriculturist Hugh Platt encouraged the cultivation of indoor plants, especially during the winter months. This saw the wealthiest in English society start to build greenhouses and orangeries. Around the same time, 'tulip mania' – an intense period of speculative demand for bulbs – took over elite homes in the Netherlands and England.

In 18th-century France, the Age of Enlightenment ushered in new ideas about the natural world. Jean-Jacques Rousseau, a keen botanist and philosopher, believed that people are fundamentally better off when surrounded by nature. In his 1782 book *Confessions*, he fondly recalls witnessing the planting of a walnut tree as a child: 'every day, eager spectators of [its] watering, my cousin and I became more strongly convinced, as was natural, that it was a finer thing to plant a tree on a terrace than a flag upon a breach'. From the mid-18th century onwards, a rising demand for portable indoor flower gardens encouraged a new luxury goods market. Decorative pots of all shapes and sizes suddenly appeared, produced by ceramics factories such as Meissen in Germany, Sèvres in France and Wedgwood in England.

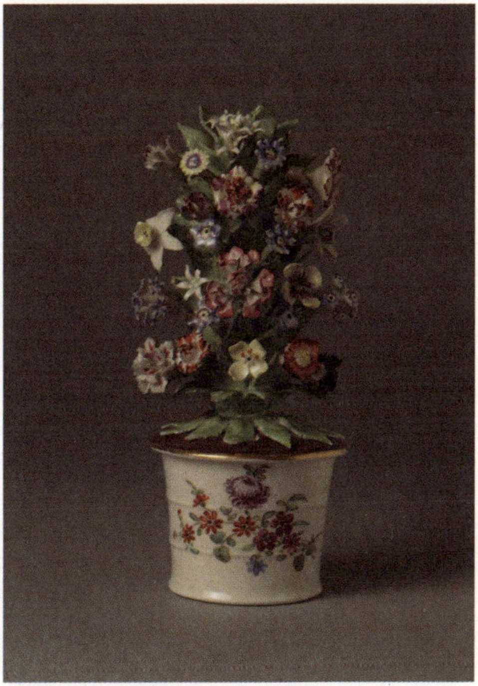

Despite this, plants were not always kept in specially designed pots. In fact, Madame de Pompadour, the famous mistress of King Louis XV of France, owned so many porcelain wine coolers that it is now thought she used them as flowerpots, filling them with bulbs and plants but also with artificial porcelain flowers. These porcelain flowers, to which perfume was added, were mounted on bronze stalks to create bouquets. The story goes, according to Cardinal Richelieu, that Madame de Pompadour once decorated her rooms with so many pots of realistically perfumed porcelain flowers that Louis XV tried to pick up a bunch.

Whether they are porcelain or real, houseplants have never truly lost that sense of artifice. Today, we add towering cactus plants and pots of perennials to our homes to help us construct an artificial green oasis, a calming illusion of access to the natural world outside. Taking care of potted plants can be therapeutic, helping one to feel a little bit more in control. Perhaps it is no surprise that their sales jumped during the pandemic, as people tried – as with baking (see Flour and Yeast p108) and gardening – to bring some sense of agency back into their daily lives, by recreating our own Hanging Gardens of Babylon.

Text by Caroline McCaffrey-Howarth

DOGS

Photograph of actor Ellen Terry from an album of ‘cartes de visite’ (small collectible prints) collected by Guy Tristram Little, Great Britain, 19th century.

How rising rates of dog ownership during the pandemic reflect a longstanding tradition of using pets to project a personal identity

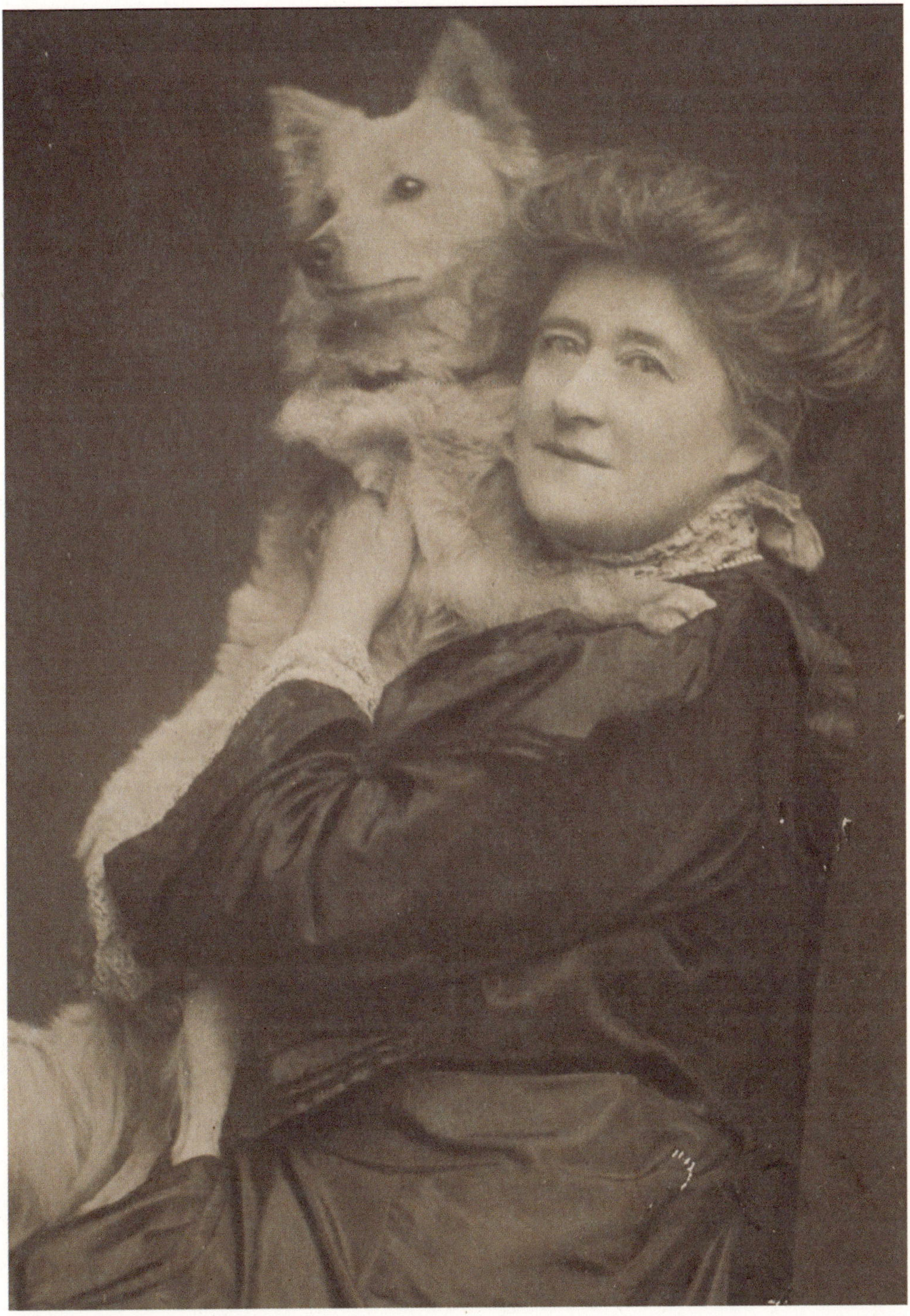

SELF-CARE

Dog ownership soared during the first eight months of the pandemic. Google searches for 'buy a puppy' increased by 166% as many rushed to pick up a canine companion to help them get through multiple lockdowns. The results were staggering: the number of pet dogs in the UK rose from 9 million in 2019 to 13 million by 2022.

The trend was perhaps unsurprising; the benefits of dog ownership have been well documented, with several studies indicating that it can lower anxiety, reduce feelings of isolation and help manage stress. With so many people working from home, thousands seized the opportunity to welcome a dog into their life.

The surge led to a shortage of puppies, particularly of the most Instagrammable and sought-after breeds such as dachshunds, golden retrievers, bulldogs and pugs – some of which saw price hikes of up to 89% in the UK from the beginning of the first lockdown. This rise in demand also resulted in an increase in criminality, with unscrupulous breeding, scams, puppy smuggling and dog thefts all on the up. Although many shelters also reported an increase in adoptions and fostering, the proliferation of pedigree and designer puppy sales suggested that many new owners wanted a dog which offered more than companionship or an excuse to get out on a daily walk.

Long before Paris Hilton brought fame to the handbag chihuahua with her many pocket-sized pals, patterns in dog ownership have been grounded in fashion trends, a propensity towards specific physical characteristics and the associations that certain breeds have with social status. Indeed, we have the Victorians to thank for pioneering and amplifying many of these tendencies, and for the array of dog breeds we have today.

The second half of the 19th century saw the development of what was then called 'dog fancying', taking ideas of ancestry and bloodline first used to grade horses and applying these to the breeding and showing of dogs. This focus on purity and pedigree appealed to middle-class town dwellers who were fixated with the kind of status and symbolism found in horse ownership but had no livestock through which they could demonstrate their social standing or wealth. Dog shows, the first of which was held in Newcastle in 1859, provided an opportunity for owners to gain prestige, where the quality of the dog was seen as reflective of the status and good taste of its owner.

These shows proliferated and came to popularise many of the dog breeds we know today, such as basset hounds and King Charles spaniels, providing categories and archetypes for dogs to be judged against. By the end of the 19th century, 'doggy people' (as they were known) had developed an intricate set of rules which were designed to enforce distinctions and standards between types of dogs – often entirely arbitrarily. This standardisation revolutionised the way people thought about the varieties of dogs and marked the first time that they were bred not for their function (working dogs, hunting dogs) but for their appearance (flat face, big eyes). Dogs were now bred either for uniformity, to change features according to popular taste or even to create new breeds entirely.

There was undoubtedly a market for these new fashionable dogs, with celebrity and royal influence making certain breeds popular middle-class pets. Much like Paris Hilton with her handbag chihuahuas, Queen Victoria is credited with popularising the collie, a former working dog which saw a surge in prominence as a pet thanks to her fondness for the breed.

While most people today are no longer attempting to manoeuvre their dogs around a show ring, the desire to showcase has not waned. Today, dogs fulfil the same image-making role but online, featured prominently on Instagram accounts and social media profiles as a well-filtered digital version of Victorian-era parading. This image-making function intensified during lockdown, as screens and social media accounts became the sole outlet to connect canines to a wider public. The medium may have changed, but the understanding that our dogs reflect our status and style has persisted through the 21st century.

Text by Jenna Mason

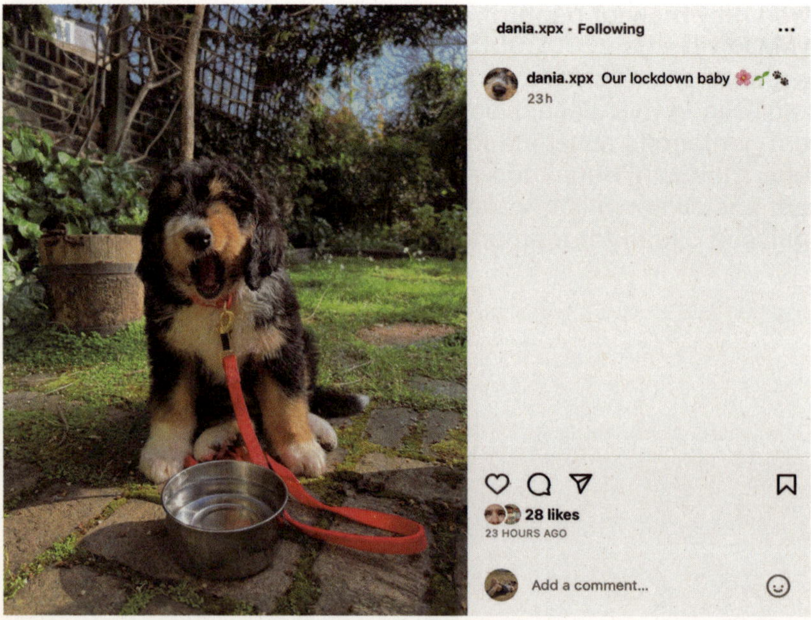
dania.xpx • Following
dania.xpx Our lockdown baby 🌸🌱🐾
23h
28 likes
23 HOURS AGO
Add a comment...

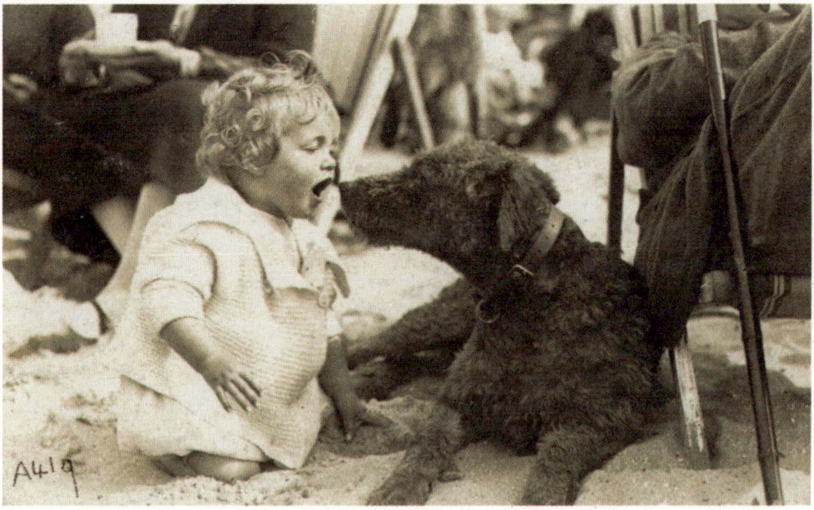

Photograph by Arthur Herbert Remington,
UK, 1920–39.

ANIMAL CROSSING

How a video game became an overnight hit during lockdown, and its connection to escapist imagery in art history

PANDEMIC OBJECTS

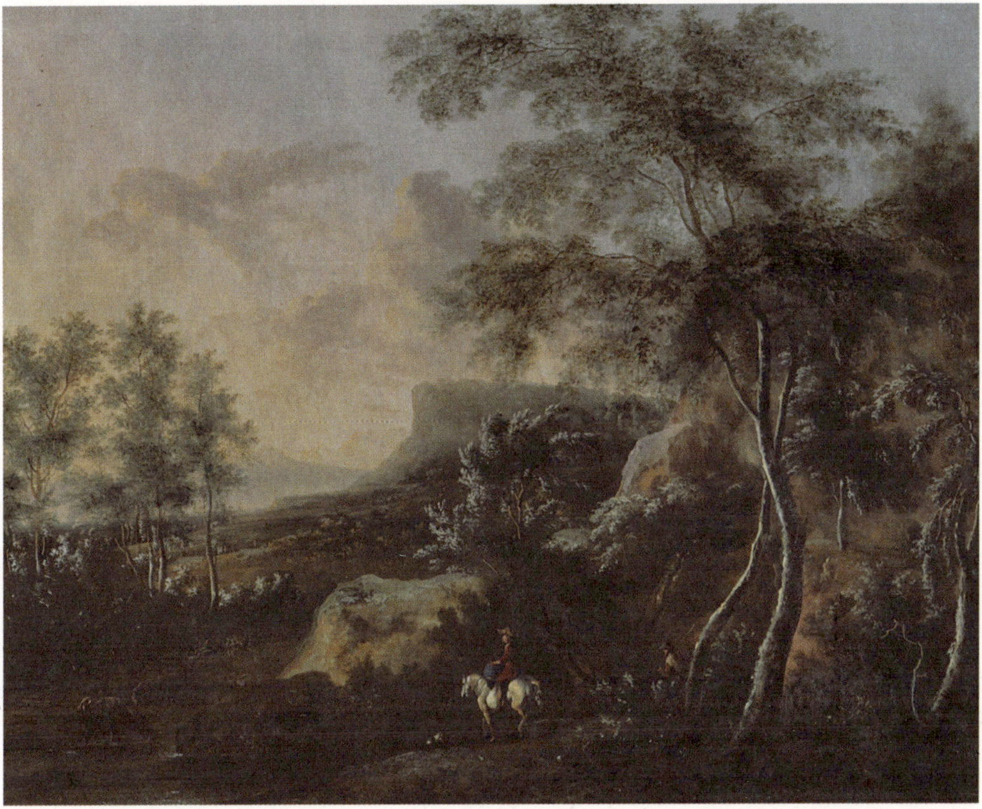

Frederik de Moucheron,
Rocky Landscape,
Amsterdam, 1660s.

New Horizons, from Nintendo's *Animal Crossing* series, was released on 20 March 2020, just three days before the UK's first lockdown began. Faced with the prospect of more time at home, consumers rushed online to purchase the game, which sold 11.77 million units worldwide in the first 12 days of release. It proved to be one of the most in-demand games of the pandemic, even luring in gamers more interested in high-intensity action, which *Animal Crossing* is definitely not. With many other games to choose from, what drew so many to *New Horizons*' basic premise of being cast away on a virtual island?

All *Animal Crossing* games start with the player being offered a special role in the development of a new settlement. In *New Horizons* you are solely responsible for the design, infrastructure and layout of a recently inhabited island. It is also your task to recruit new villagers, Sylvanian Families-like characters of which there are around 400 variations, each with their own personalities and catchphrases.

The premise sounds cute, but what made *New Horizons* so engaging? Part of the appeal lies in the open-ended quality of the game, and the fact that the construction of the island plays out in real time, the game encouraging recurrent gameplay through its slow pace. Perhaps the key to the game's success during the pandemic, however, was the way it offered players another world to which they could escape.

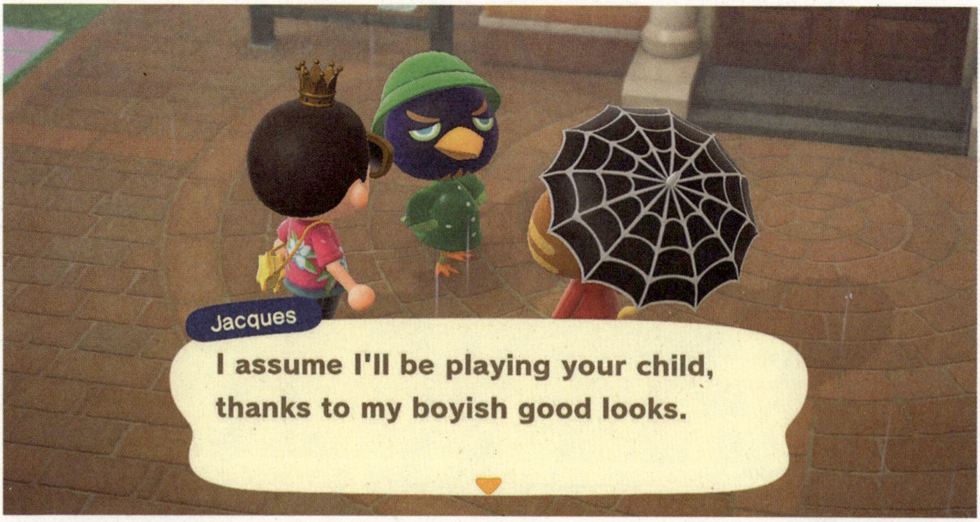
Jacques
I assume I'll be playing your child,
thanks to my boyish good looks.

For all the cartoonish appearance of *Animal Crossing*, there is something very thoughtful about the detail the game gives to the natural world. The weather changes, trees sway, your footsteps make a slight sinking sound when you run on the beach. The way the world of *Animal Crossing* both admires and idealises nature recalls something of Dutch landscape painting, particularly its emergence and popularity during the Dutch Golden Age in the 17th century. At that time, paintings that depicted idealised natural landscapes became popular among the Dutch bourgeoisie, creating an alternate narrative that obscured the crueller reality; a merchant who purchased a rocky pastoral scene of their famously flat country was investing in a vision of the world that glossed over the difficult realities of rural life and the harshness of agricultural work. Similarly, *Animal Crossing* players – particularly those in large cities – were more disconnected from nature than ever before. During the UK's first lockdown, many people were only permitted to leave their homes for essential shopping and daily exercise. Dwelling in nature, even in a city park, became in some cases a fineable offence. *Animal Crossing* reproduced an escapist version of nature at home, one where you could determine the shape of the land and where bodies of water formed.

New Horizons also provided a range of small daily tasks. You could find fossils, water your flowers and check the price of turnips, which in the *Animal Crossing* universe are traded like stocks, inevitably referred to as the 'stalk market'. While the pandemic affected almost every aspect of people's daily lives, *Animal Crossing* provided some routine and consistency.

One of the daily tasks was to develop relationships with your villagers, and many players even spoke of forming emotional connections with them. Villagers are all scripted non-player characters, but a wide range of dialogue options gives them some sense of depth. It is even possible to write them letters. Just as in childhood, when many of us develop inner stories and connections with toys in a world where we have little agency, social relationships with villagers in *Animal Crossing* offered a space away from endless discussions about the real-world health crisis. Many people also found communities of other players, visiting each other's islands and forming group chats exclusively for sharing turnip prices and discussing details found in the game: a moment to step away from the anxieties of the pandemic and keep in touch while isolated at home.

Screenshot from *Animal Crossing: New Horizons* taken by Alice Power.

Conversely, other people used *New Horizons* to promote urgent political issues that were taking place away from the screen, such as the pro-democracy movement in Hong Kong and the Black Lives Matter movement, congregating in digital protests. For some, the islands created in the game were escapist dream-scapes, but they were also operating as a para-reality, a form of connection in a largely atomised real-world space.

Text by Alice Power

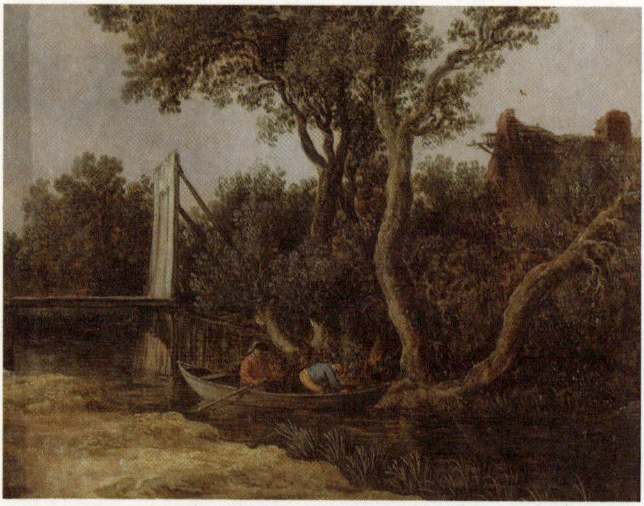

Jan van Goyen, *Landscape with Stream*, Leyden, 1628.

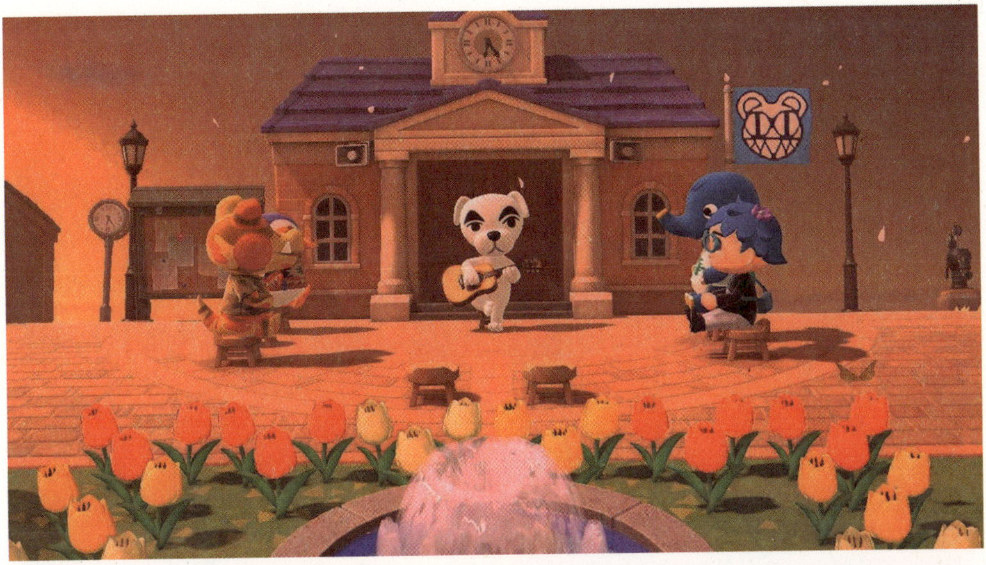

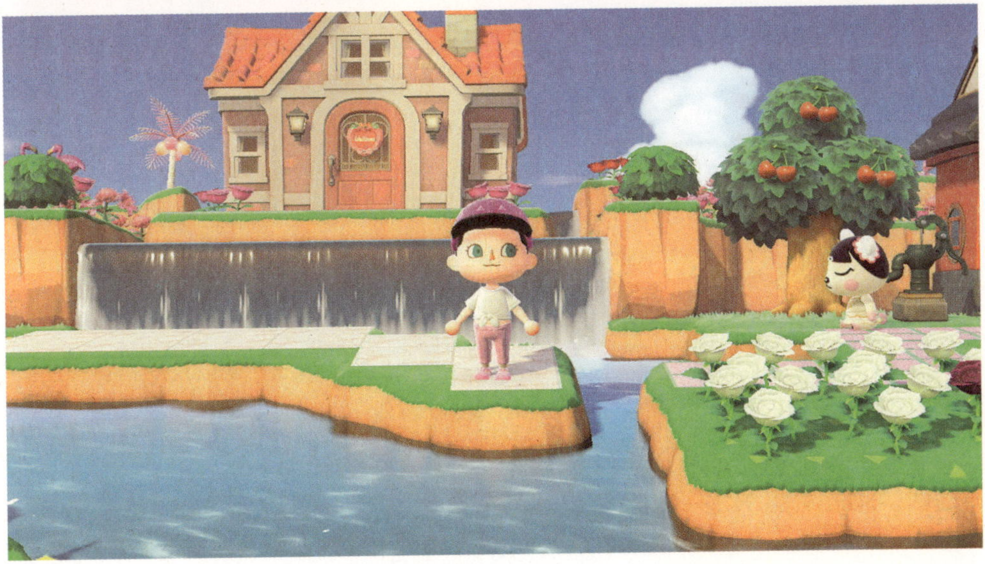

Screenshots from *Animal Crossing: New Horizons* taken by Alice Power.

TIKTOK

How viral dances link communities in times of crisis, and how TikTok capitalised on this phenomenon for the internet age

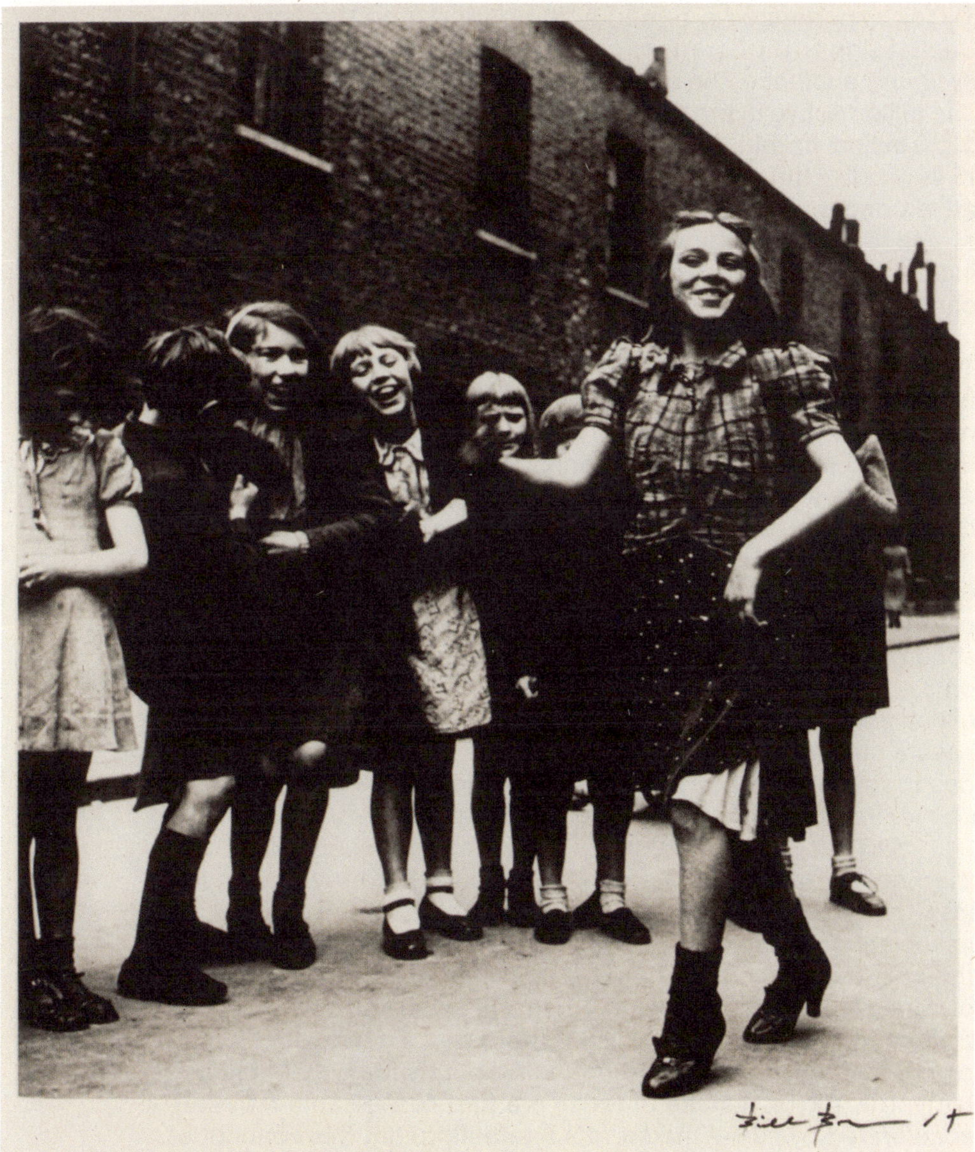

Bill Brandt, *East End Girl Dancing the 'Lambeth Walk'*, London, 1939.

TikTok experienced a remarkable boom during the pandemic. Capitalising on the boredom, creativity and savviness of its primarily young audience, the social media app now boasts more than one billion active users and its owner, ByteDance, is worth around $220 billion. Its initial premise – the sharing of short videos under 15 seconds – thrived during lockdown due to its playful, performative concept and its strict time limit. It is no coincidence that at a time when attention spans were shortened but leisure time increased, an app that packages succinct, constantly changing content thrived.

TikTok's 'staccato, no-explanations, absurdist flavour', as Tom Lamont described it in *The Guardian*, has been defined by its proliferation of viral dances, created by users using clipped or remixed songs and then copied worldwide. Popular TikTok dances from 2020 such as 'Say So', 'Cannibal', 'Renegade', 'Supalonely', 'Savage Love' and 'Attention' often catapulted both the TikTok choreographer and musical artist to new (or further) fame.

The commercial success of TikTok reached a new apex early in 2020 when rapper Drake joined the trend, asking TikTok celebrities Toosie, Hiii Key and Ayo & Teo to create a dance to accompany his new single. The song, 'Toosie Slide' was released on 3 April 2020 and sparked more than 4.5 million videos and 6.8 billion views on TikTok in just two months. The music video, which sees a masked Drake perform the dance throughout the numerous rooms of his empty Toronto mansion, was lauded by *Vanity Fair* for its zeitgeisty 'quarantine-core aesthetic'.

TikTok's viral dance sensations may seem superficial, but the novelty dance has a rich history, one that may have even inspired the concept of viral entertainment itself. Jason King, an associate professor at New York University (NYU), has compared the phenomenon of the 21st-century viral dance with the spread of dance crazes a century ago: 'To me, [it's] the same as the Black Bottom in the 1920s'. The Black Bottom was a dance step based on the same rhythm as the Charleston but overtaking it in popularity. The TikTok dances of today are part of the same tradition, accelerated by social media. 'It's interesting that this concept of virality is something that novelty dances actually prefigured,' King notes. 'The Charleston, in a way, was viral.'

It could also be argued that the dances of TikTok provided vital comfort and solidarity in a time of uncertainty – not unlike the dances popularised in the 1920s and 1930s. In 1937, for instance, the musical *Me and My Girl* premiered at the Victoria Palace Theatre in London, and included the song 'The Lambeth Walk', composed by Noel Gay. The number, featuring an exaggerated Cockney dance performed by Lupino Lane, spun off into its own dance craze. Its simplicity (in contrast to the conventions of formal British dances) and its Cockney roots appealed to all ages and classes across the country. As Lane described it: 'The "Lambeth Walk" has not only been the dance success of the year – it promises to continue indefinitely as one of our national dances. It is more than a craze, because it expresses the London spirit, and this Christmas it will be danced in homes all over Britain.'

While marketed as a British novelty dance to rival fads that had travelled over from the US, the 'Lambeth Walk' took on a new significance as Britain entered the Second World War. Much of the population continued to attend dance halls even under threat of bombing, including 'Gas Mask Balls' which encouraged attendees to bring face coverings in the event of attack. The performance of the 'Lambeth Walk' unified dancers across the country and demonstrated people's resilience and positivity in the face of uncertainty. With fascism creeping across Europe, one reporter from a 1939 edition of *The Dancing Times* saw the dance in political terms: 'No longer can we treat these dances as frivolities. They have become important, they are international, and truly democratic'.

Perhaps the dance's most enduring legacy is as a striking piece of wartime propaganda which capitalised on the nationalist themes of the song. In 1941, the UK government edited footage of the German 1935 film *Triumph of the Will* to the 'Lambeth Walk' song, making it appear that Adolf Hitler and Nazi soldiers were performing the dance. The film was packaged in news reels across the country. The sophistication and humour of the film eerily chimes with TikTok and the meme culture of the internet age.

While the period of social isolation during lockdown may have been the key to TikTok's ascent, the app has developed beyond the dance craze and now seems to be pivoting away from short-form, algorithmic entertainment. In February 2022, it announced that it would accept videos of up to ten minutes long, as well as exploring the realms of commerce, gaming and news. In July 2022, TikTok became the fastest-growing source for news in the UK that year, where 7% of adults used the app for news, up from 1% in 2020.

The expansion of the app is not surprising; it is comparable to YouTube's own development from a website composed primarily of cat videos to an information and entertainment media powerhouse. But what is notable is its evolution from being a tool used to distract from an unprecedented news cycle to another form of broadcast media.

Text by Harriet Reed

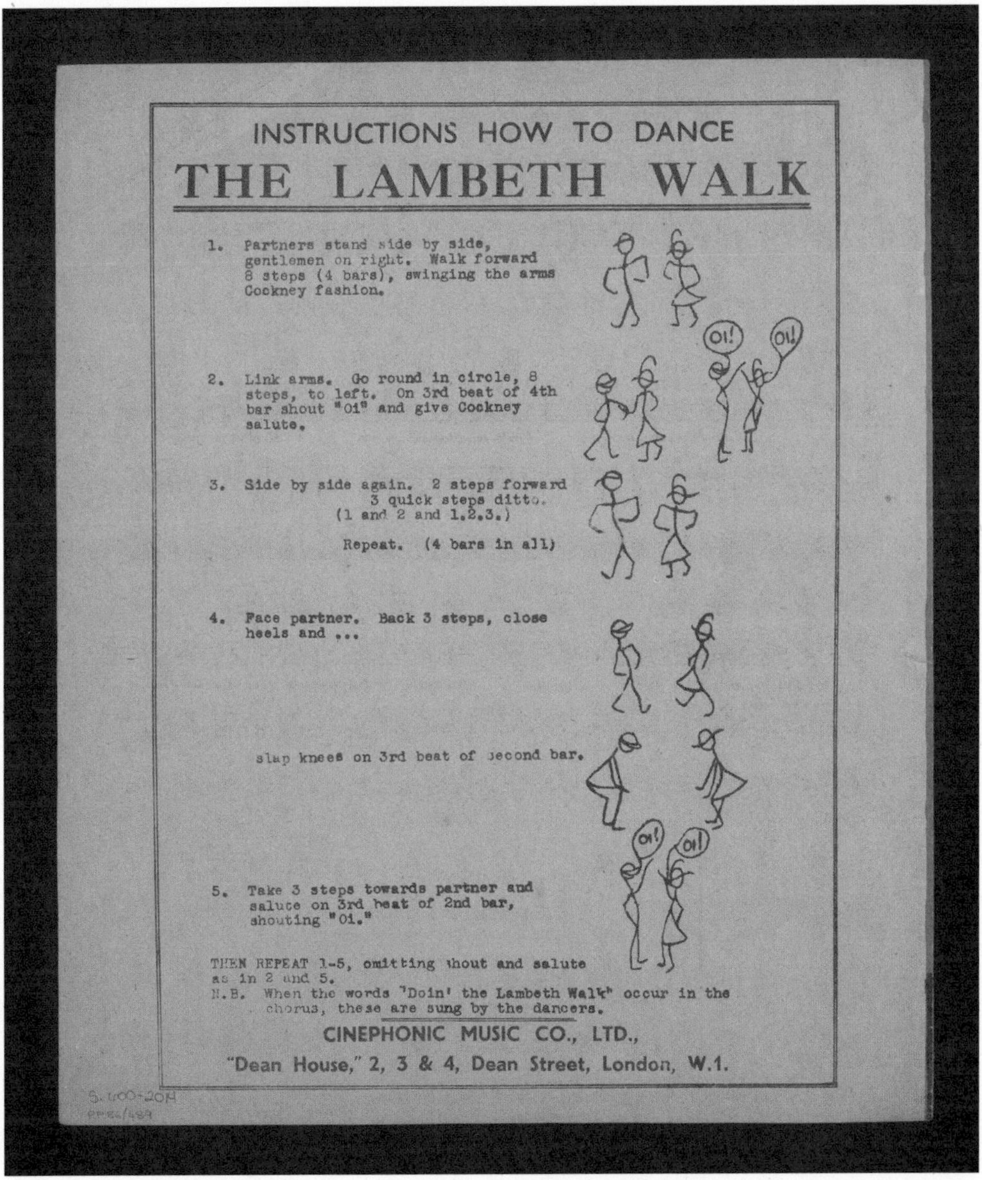

INSTRUCTIONS HOW TO DANCE

THE LAMBETH WALK

1. Partners stand side by side, gentlemen on right. Walk forward 8 steps (4 bars), swinging the arms Cockney fashion.

2. Link arms. Go round in circle, 8 steps, to left. On 3rd beat of 4th bar shout "Oi" and give Cockney salute.

3. Side by side again. 2 steps forward 3 quick steps ditto. (1 and 2 and 1.2.3.)

Repeat. (4 bars in all)

4. Face partner. Back 3 steps, close heels and ...

slap knees on 3rd beat of second bar.

5. Take 3 steps towards partner and salute on 3rd beat of 2nd bar, shouting "Oi."

THEN REPEAT 1-5, omitting shout and salute as in 2 and 5.

N.B. When the words 'Doin' the Lambeth Walk' occur in the chorus, these are sung by the dancers.

CINEPHONIC MUSIC CO., LTD.,

"Dean House," 2, 3 & 4, Dean Street, London, W.1.

Instructions on how to dance the 'Lambeth Walk', published in 1937 by the Cinephonic Music Company.

STREAMING SERVICES

'Videosphere' television set, made by JVC Ltd, Japan, 1970.

How the rise of streaming services during the pandemic shifted viewing habits from intentional to ambient and what we can learn from Muzak as the original streamed content

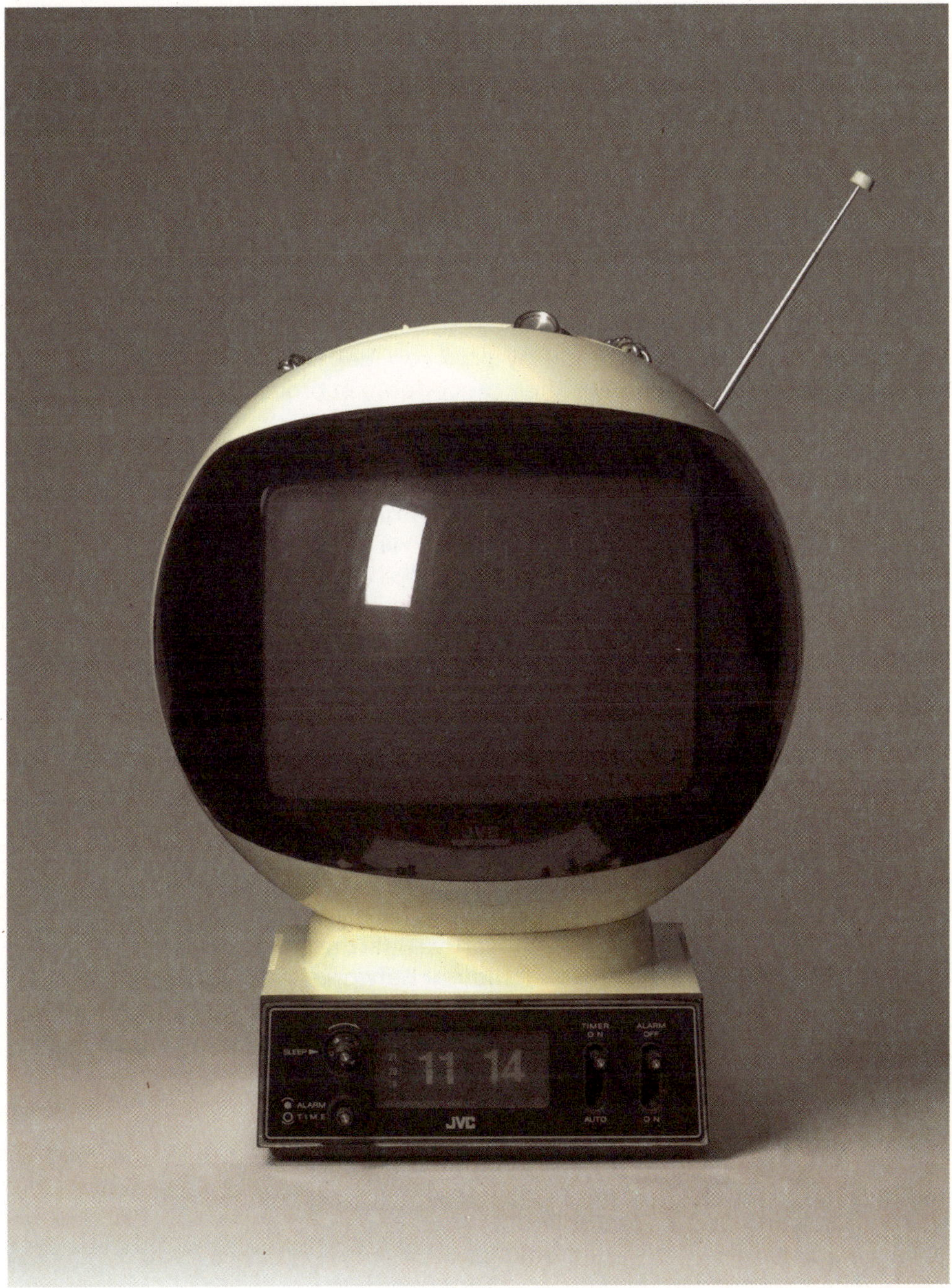
SLEEP
11 14
ALARM
TIME
JVC
TIMER
ON
AUTO
ALARM
OFF
ON

Lockdown shifted the media landscape, spurring an intensified use of streaming services and changing the ways people related to what they were consuming. The pandemic came at a time when almost any media was available on demand, an era of instant gratification through streamed media consumption that was already well established before lockdown brought about this particular intensification.

To trace a history of this period, one might start with YouTube, which launched in 2005 offering novel short-form homegrown video content. Spotify followed for music in 2006 and Netflix for professionally produced television and movies in 2007 (although it started in 1997 as a DVD rental-by-post service). However, the origins of these platforms have their precedents in broadcasting that go back nearly a century.

For a 20th-century proto-streaming service, consider George Owen Squier's 1922 patent for the transmission and distribution of signals over electrical lines. Squier's system was designed to pipe music through electrical wires directly into a home receiver, without the need for specialised radio equipment. Named Muzak, it could not compete with the eventual popularity of radio (p298), which took over the domestic market in the 1930s, and instead moved into public and commercial spaces. Muzak became synonymous with a particular type of music, due both to licensing rights and the development of a concept called 'stimulus progression'. This suggested that workers and shoppers would respond positively to music with a bright and breezy tone, and that a progressively faster and bouncier rhythm, without distracting lyrics, would encourage increased productivity.

The content Muzak supplied was, of course, curated and served whole to consumers without their agreement. Consumer choice in streaming technology did not arrive until the early 2000s. At this point, increased access to computer networks with higher bandwidth had changed the landscape of media. File-sharing sites such as Napster, a peer-to-peer service with which consumers could illegally share and download digital files of songs, came to the fore and changed the nature of the music business. No longer could songs be bought or sold as commodities; instead, they had become de facto public goods that anyone with access to the internet could have for free. Record labels grappled to save their business, and after a number of court cases, Napster ceased its peer-to-peer sharing in 2001. Instead, services such as Spotify emerged, building on licensing deals with major record labels

Poster advertising the Murphy television, designed by Abram Games, UK, c1951.

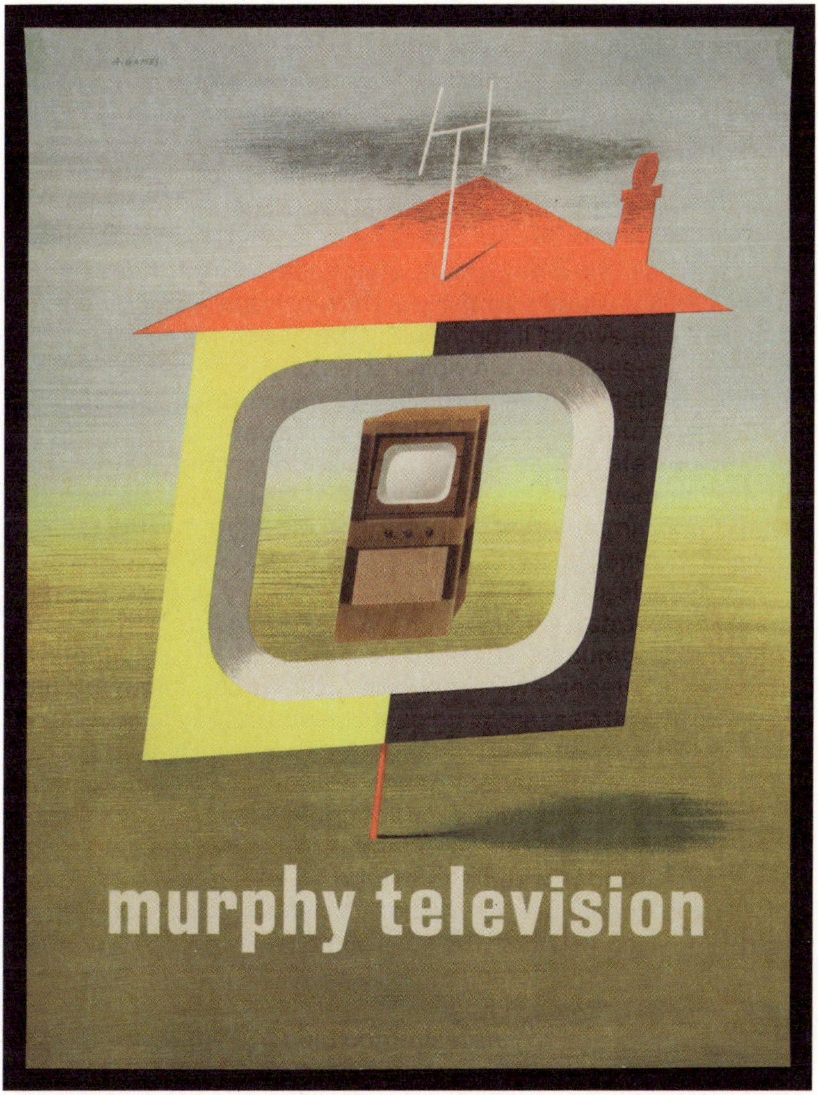
murphy television

and offering subscriptions to consumers for unlimited music, or limited free music with advertising. Spotify has since grown into the foremost music streaming service and, by 2018, music streaming was making more money than the combined sales of physical copies of music and digital downloads.

Like Muzak attempted many years earlier, streaming has changed our relationship to recorded music. Many musicians no longer focus on albums as their key artistic statement and now foreground singular streaming successes. In televisual terms Netflix – which, thanks to the pandemic, quickly became more valuable than oil giant ExxonMobil – has been noted for making high-production value television. Yet the kind of visionary filmmaking it has been lauded for producing became impossible during lockdown, and its successes during this period were defined through outrageous (and much cheaper) documentaries with viral contingencies such as *Tiger King*. These platforms have also defined and narrowed our tastes, encouraging myopic cultural cul-de-sacs through algorithms that point people towards similar attention-sucks or comfort food in the form of unchallenging retro programming. Is this all that different to churning out a kind of piped easy listening Muzak?

You might well be reading this while tuned into YouTube's live stream 'lofi hip hop radio – beats to relax/study to'. With more than 13 million subscribers it is among the service's most popular channels, dispensing live feeds of chill, downtempo hip hop 24/7, accompanied by a sleepy-looking anime girl studying at her desk. Many similar feeds have emerged in its wake, looking to help people focus on tasks at hand, with wordless regular beats that hope, just as Muzak did all those years ago, to increase productivity. This, though, came to the fore at a particularly distinct juncture in our lives when working from home became normalised and the need to focus was a difficult challenge.

For those furloughed during lockdown, temporarily freed from sitting at a computer screen, the pandemic gifted them with a plethora of televisual streaming services. Disney+ was a lucky early winner, launching in the UK on 24 March 2020, the day after the first lockdown was announced and just in time to mollify the children. However, as lockdowns eased in 2021, and with the market saturated with other streaming services, Netflix made their first announcement about losing subscribers, contrary to the continuous growth they had promised shareholders following rapid uptake during the pandemic. With traditional media companies making billion-pound investments into other streaming services, this decline was inevitable. Netflix has since responded with limits on password sharing and a commitment to bring back advertisements through a lower-priced service. It seems that streaming services, along with the age of bingeing on uninterrupted prestige television and of an endless loop of background chatter from reality TV show contestants, may be the next in a long list of technologies to become a thing of the past.

Text by Kristian Volsing

WINDOWS

How windows became a vital lifeline for people isolating indoors, and what they mean to the public health of a city

PANDEMIC OBJECTS

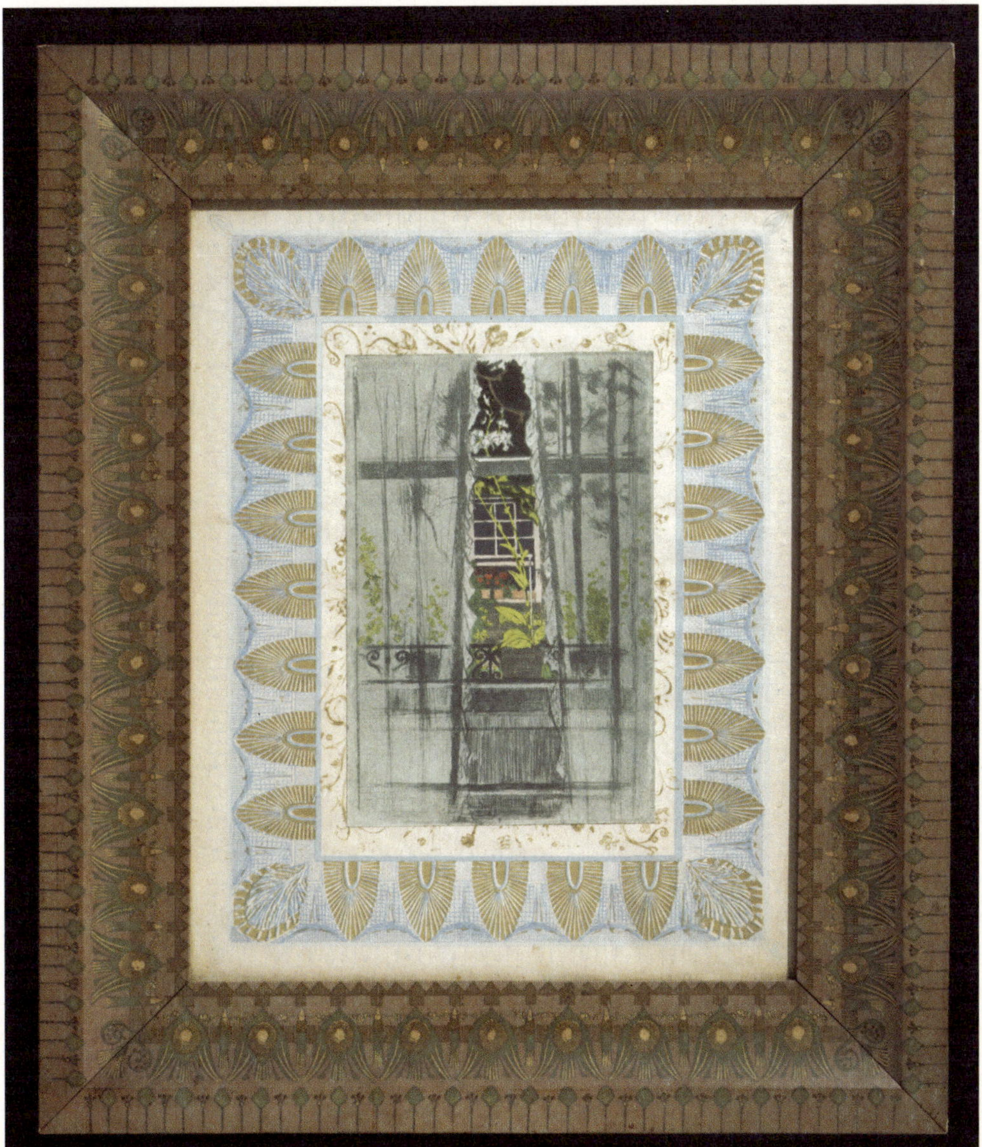

Theodore Roussel,
A Window Seen Through a Window,
London, 1897.

The window is an element of domestic architecture often designed to go unnoticed. Like other things we see every day, windows become invisible through familiarity as much as through transparency. Occupying the boundary of the home, they are a crucial portal beyond it – a function that became pronounced during the pandemic. As well as a source of natural light and fresh air, windows became a place to gaze out at trees, track the weather and reflect upon the world beyond the cramped confines of one's home. Perhaps for the first time, people took note of their neighbours through the window pane, witnessing the intimate theatre of the everyday in spaces that mirrored their own. The ability to glimpse others from behind their walls transformed the pandemic into a shared experience, despite individual isolation.

The relationship between windows and good health has long been understood. A window tax was introduced in England in 1696: houses with more than ten windows were charged for every additional one. It was intended to fall upon the wealthy, who were more likely to live in lavish homes, but it impacted the urban poor, many of whom lived in large tenement buildings. Regardless of how these had been subdivided for tenants, they were treated as single structures and taxed heavily. Landlords bricked up many of the windows to avoid the payments – a legacy still visible on façades today.

From the early 18th century, the negative impact of the tax on public health was being decried in pamphlets and popular songs, as those in homes without proper light and ventilation suffered disproportionately from disease. In the battle against Covid-19, the German government encouraged the all-seasons practice of *Lüften* – regularly opening windows to let fresh air circulate through a building – arguing that it was a cheap and effective way of limiting the spread of coronavirus.

Thanks to a popular campaign, the window tax was finally scrapped in 1851, its repeal coinciding with the popularisation of the window box. Window boxes made of terracotta or metal took off in the 19th century in England, and were used to grow vegetables, herbs and flowers, just as we do today. As spring arrived during the first lockdown in 2020, demand for window boxes surged, and the window was embraced as an active extension of indoor space, modest access to nature and a zone where the private space of the home meets the public space of the street. People pinned rainbow paintings (see Rainbows p18) and messages

Aftermath of the Port of Beirut explosions on 4 August 2020.

of support for the NHS in their windows and leaned over their sills on Thursday evenings to applaud key workers (see Hands p338). The window became an active site for the public expression of solidarity and community.

In Beirut, Lebanon, windows entered into public consciousness for a different reason. On 4 August 2020, 2,750 tonnes of ammonium nitrate exploded at the Port of Beirut, where it had been improperly stored for several years. The explosion killed 218 people, injured thousands and left many homeless. The blast was a chilling reflection of the Lebanese government's criminal negligence and corruption, its effects compounded by multiple pre-existing crises: economic collapse, hyperinflation, poverty and the pandemic. One immediate material effect of the explosion was the shattering of glass. Every window within several kilometres of the explosion was blown out of its frame; the reach of the shockwaves was measurable by broken panes in villages miles from the capital. In the hours and days that followed, the grating sound of glass being swept from balconies and into the curb roared across the city. Months on, glass still crunches underfoot like shards of ice, lurks in the corners of people's homes, and piles up in vast mounds for collection, recycling and disposal.

Windows are both mundane and powerful things, thresholds and portals. We take them for granted until they are gone, and it is hard to live safely without them. Think of all the glass from all the windows in Beirut's diverse architecture – its Ottoman mansions, 1970s apartments, Starchitect-designed high-rises and the iconic stained glass of the Sursock Museum – all now half-returned to dust. It makes you thankful for the quiet, familiar presence of the windows in your home.

Text by Rachel Dedman

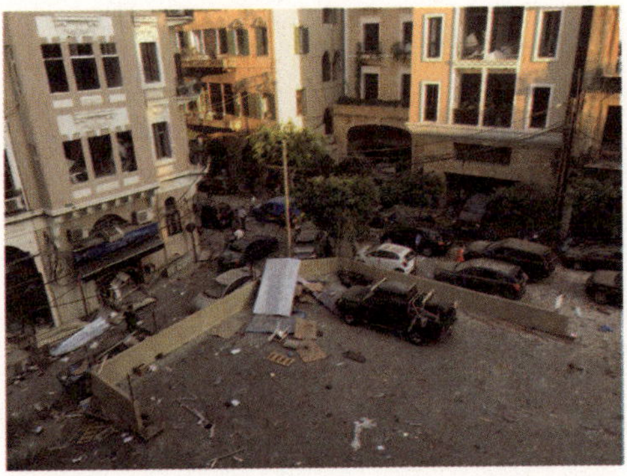

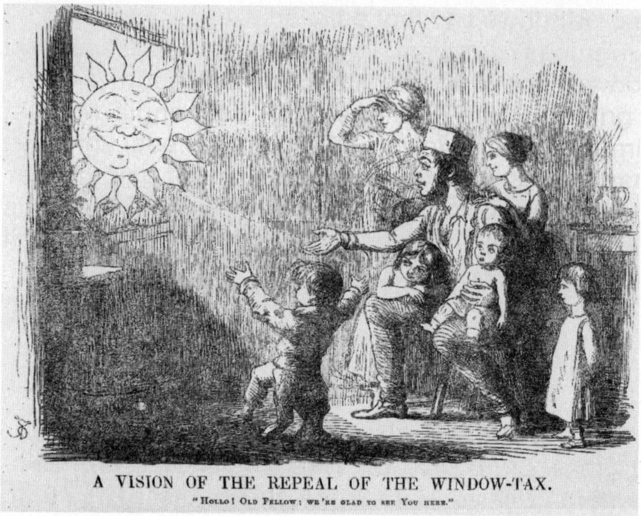
A VISION OF THE REPEAL OF THE WINDOW-TAX.
"Hollo! Old Fellow; we're glad to see You here."

Richard Doyle, 'A Vision of the Repeal of the Window Tax' in *Punch*, Great Britain, 1850.

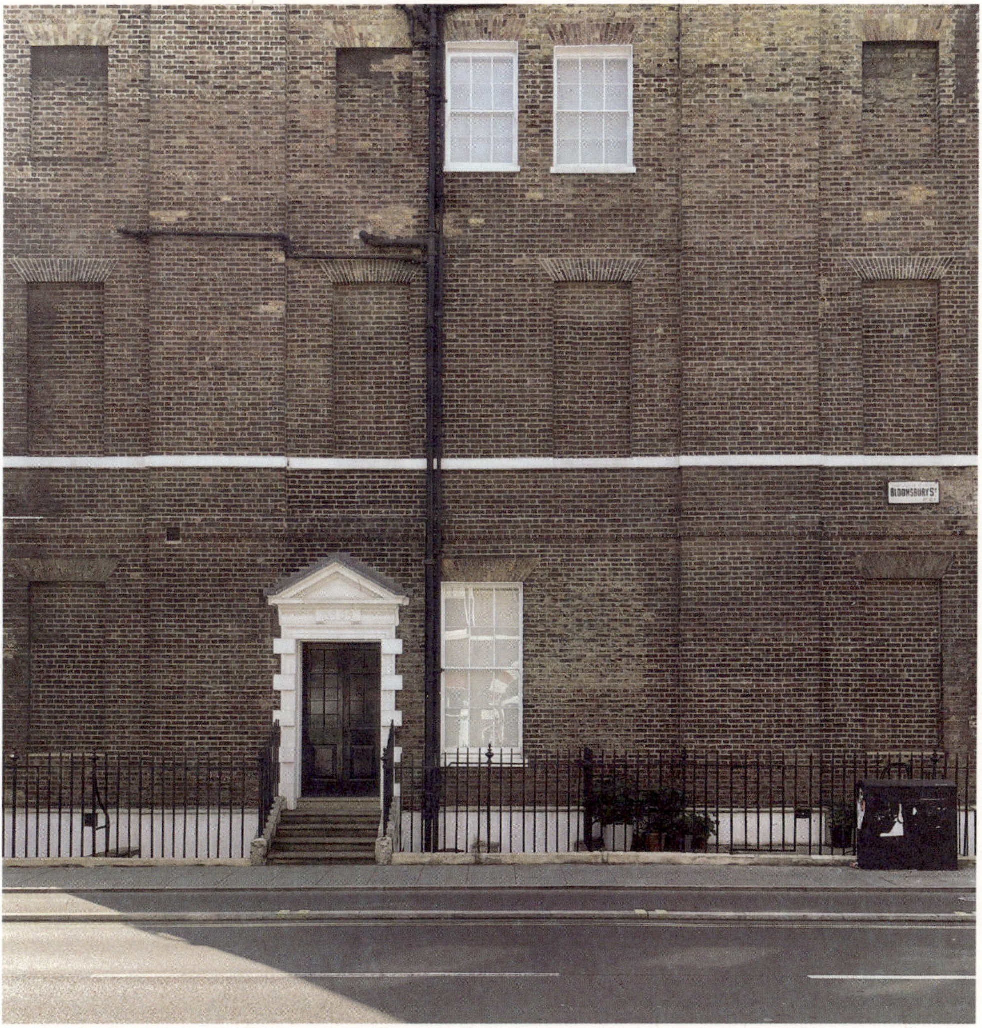

Corner of Bedford Square and
Bloomsbury Street, London.

CEMETERIES

How the cemetery proved to be a space of reflection as well as mourning, providing surprising solace

PANDEMIC OBJECTS

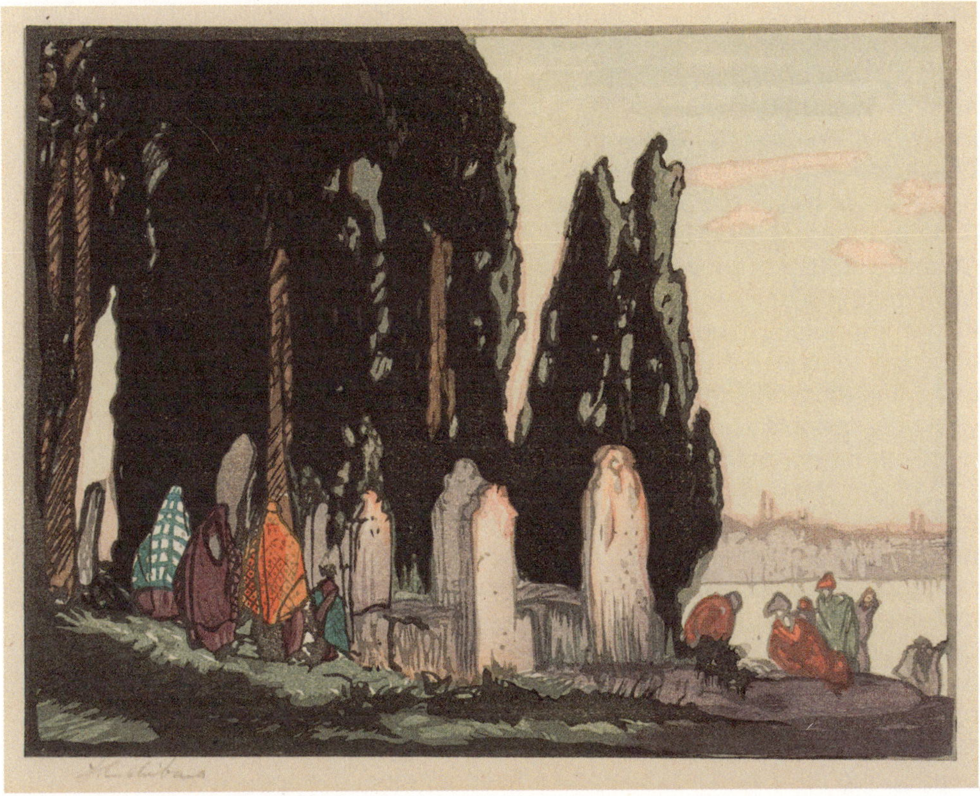

Yoshijiro Urushibara,
The Resting Place, Scutari,
Turkey, 1924.

Our local cemetery in Bristol was established in 1871. This followed a national movement to improve health conditions by moving burials out of church crypts and into the suburbs. Resembling an arboretum or nature reserve, it is bucolic, leafy and utterly charming. When I walked there before the pandemic, the Victorian and Edwardian-era tombs struck me as maudlin, their cult-like relish for death at best odd, at worst creepy and macabre. During the first dreadful lockdown in the UK, the cemeteries were closed. The Covid-19 statistics showed the world that we were not beyond the overwhelming epidemics of the past. We scrolled, daily, through lists of increasing sorrow. Life at home felt as if it was unravelling: how to explain to a five-year-old that an invisible illness was sweeping the world, that she could not go to school or do anything with other people at all? Our small home became smaller, louder, more claustrophobic.

It was the end of April, in glorious weather, when cemeteries were finally allowed to reopen with limited hours. The persistent and unlikely sunshine was a balm, and the cemetery became a place for daily walks. Somehow the importance of the place had shifted. I became oddly immersed in other lives; spent time with the names; wondered about little Ernest (fell asleep, five months), beloved daughter Florence May (eight years, eight months), the only and dearly beloved Lillian 'Lily' (six years). There was a new reality to the lives that had come to rest there, as if the past had been brought forward into the present. I could feel the anguish of the loved ones left behind in my fear for those currently living, so easily also taken away.

There is a certain solace in looking to the past, in reading gravestones from more than a century ago, placed there before an understanding of germs, hygiene or dental care. One grave, found under a beautiful pine tree, caught and held my attention more than any other. It marks the resting spot of two sisters, both eleven years old, who died two years apart. They had botanical names, Violet and Ivy, as was popular at the turn of the century. 'Darling Vi': such a simple epitaph holding such sadness. My daughter and I began to look after 'the girls', as we took to calling them. She collected stray artificial flowers blown from other graves and reverently arranged them at the base of their stone. We cleared away the weeds and kept the grass in order. The girls died so long ago that there is no one alive any longer who would have known

Leonardo Bistolfi's sculpture *Death and Life*, in a cemetery in Zurich.

them. So, we poured out all our worry and care, let it mingle with their past sorrow, and found a sort of peace there. The cemetery was transformed from a morbid place, in which to be reminded of the inevitable end, into rather a calming space, filled with the love people have for one another.

When spoken with my American-accented voice, the word cemetery has four syllables and sounds like it contains an 'a' towards the end. But in the UK, where I now live, it is pronounced like the word 'symmetry', at least so it sounds to my ears. There is something very apt in this. The cemetery is a mirror of our living community, creating, if not a city of the dead, perhaps a neighbourhood of the dead; symmetric, separated from us by only a road and some fancy gates. This pandemic and the isolation of lockdown taught me a new appreciation of these spaces – that regardless of our imposed isolation, we are connected to others, and always have been.

Text by Alison Moffett

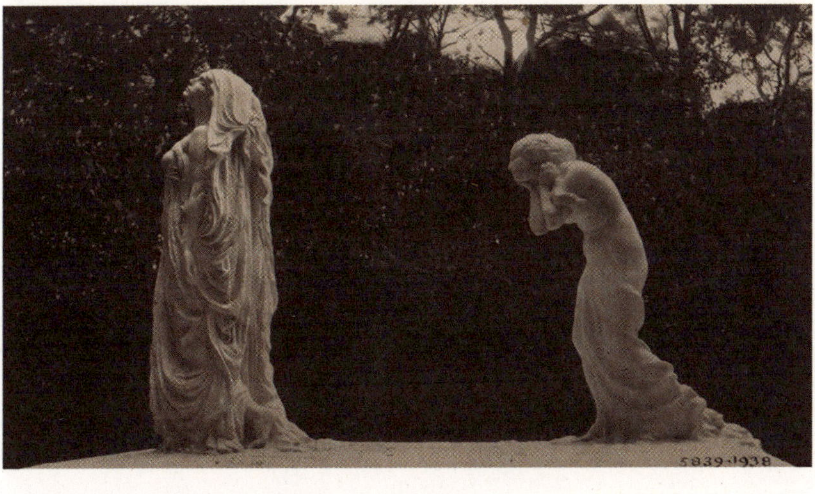

04

ABSTAIN

A large part of pandemic life entailed living without certain spaces and things. The classic hallmarks of convivial civic life were shut: pubs, performance venues, cafés, clothing shops and hair salons. Public transport remained only for essential workers to keep the city functioning, but ridership plummeted. Even certain objects, most notably cash, became vilified, with many supermarkets and off-licenses refusing to accept physical money, as it was believed to be a vector for disease.

This time of being without was an opportunity for reflection. Did we really need these things? Alternatives arose: online shopping thrived, parks became the pre-eminent drinking spot, the living room transformed into a concert venue and people grew their hair long with pride.

Many of these spaces were already under threat prior to the pandemic. A period of forced abstinence allowed us to see these typologies through a renewed lens, revealing previously hidden benefits and providing important clues as to how they should re-emerge in a post-pandemic world. Clothing shops can instil drama and flair that a website cannot, pubs elicit spontaneity that prearranged park meetups lack, and cash – particularly in the form of community currencies – can help support a neighbourhood. To lack something, to feel its absence, has proved to be a useful tool during the pandemic, revealing not only how objects may be used differently but also how we yearn for spaces we once overlooked.

CASH

How the pandemic hastened the shift towards a cashless society, and why physical money must be equitably reimagined

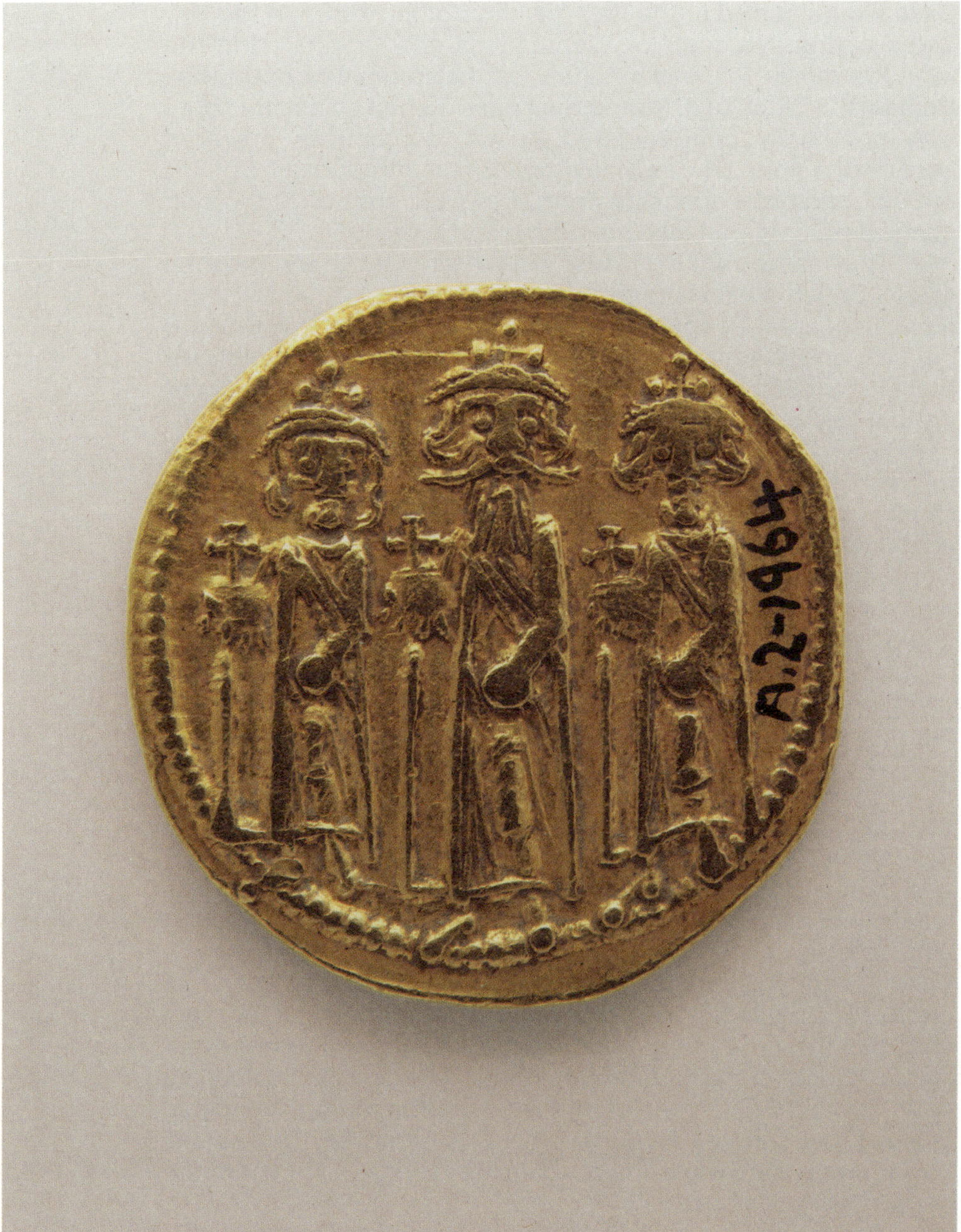

Coin from the Byzantine Empire, depicting Emperor Heraclius with his sons Heraclius Constantine and Heraclonas, Constantinople, c630.

Cash usage halved in the first few days of lockdown in the UK. Signs saying 'No cash' or 'Contactless only' appeared in the windows of the few essential shops that remained open (see Homemade Signs p12). Rather than pass around coins and notes with potentially contaminated hands, contactless payment became the norm. The technology was first introduced in the UK in 2007, and grew apace; in February 2020, around 723 million contactless card transactions were made in the UK.

That same month, it was estimated that there were 1.2 million British adults who were 'unbanked' – individuals without a bank account. People who earn a salary of less than £10,000 per year are 14 times more likely to depend on cash than those earning more than £30,000. Many who do have a bank account are still hesitant to use internet banking due to a distrust of technology, and therefore regularly rely on ATMs or the Post Office to pay bills, or to collect benefits and pensions in cash. Many cannot afford the cost of internet or mobile data to access their accounts, or live in areas where broadband and mobile phone signal are not available.

Contactless technology, and the ability to make payments and shop online, undoubtedly made many people safer and happier during lockdown. However, as with many aspects of the pandemic's impact in the UK, this transition shifted the burden onto the most vulnerable in society while enriching the wealthiest. Generational and class divides, exacerbated by digital poverty, are growing a bifurcation in currencies in the UK, and the demise of cash is a threat to the diversity and independence of our communities.

Money is an act of faith. Its value is not the sum of the materials that constitute it. Instead, people are brought to believe that either a physical object or a virtual signifier represent an agreed worth – a transaction in symbols. Throughout history, cash has created political identities, designed to affirm both the borders and identity of nations; coins from the Byzantine Empire, for instance, were distributed to homogenise trade within colonised countries. While currencies are a way of providing economic stability, their physical forms also act as a reminder of who holds power, emblazoned with images of the sovereign or stamped with emblems of the state.

This flow of power can, however, be reversed: launched in 2008, the Brixton Pound (B£) harnessed the power of cash as a catalyst to create belonging and identity with its introduction as the UK's first local urban currency. Supported by a network of independent businesses and shoppers, the B£ reinforces a strong and diverse local economy by helping money 'stick' to Brixton. The notes are designed to commemorate renowned individuals who called Brixton home – such as musician David Bowie and political activist Olive Morris – whose likenesses are combined with imagery lifted from local landmarks and public sculpture. Localised currencies such as the B£ point to one of the benefits of physical cash: it creates social connections and retains value within a community.

There are examples of activists and artists who have used the symbolic value of currency, such as Walthamstow's Hoe Street Central Bank (HSCB) which opened in March 2018 and operated until the end of 2019. The notes, which were screen-printed by artist Hillary Powell, featured portraits of different local community leaders as well as important causes that were implemented to improve deficiencies within Walthamstow, one of the most deprived boroughs in the country.

Through the initiative, HSCB was able to raise £40,000, half of which went to the causes represented on the notes; the remainder was used to purchase and write off local debt valued at £1.2 million (debts are often sold off at a fraction of their face value in the secondary market). The B£ and HSCB are important templates for how trade and money can be reimagined for a fairer and more economically inclusive society, something made all the more urgent by the unfolding financial consequences of the pandemic.

Text by Georgia Haseldine

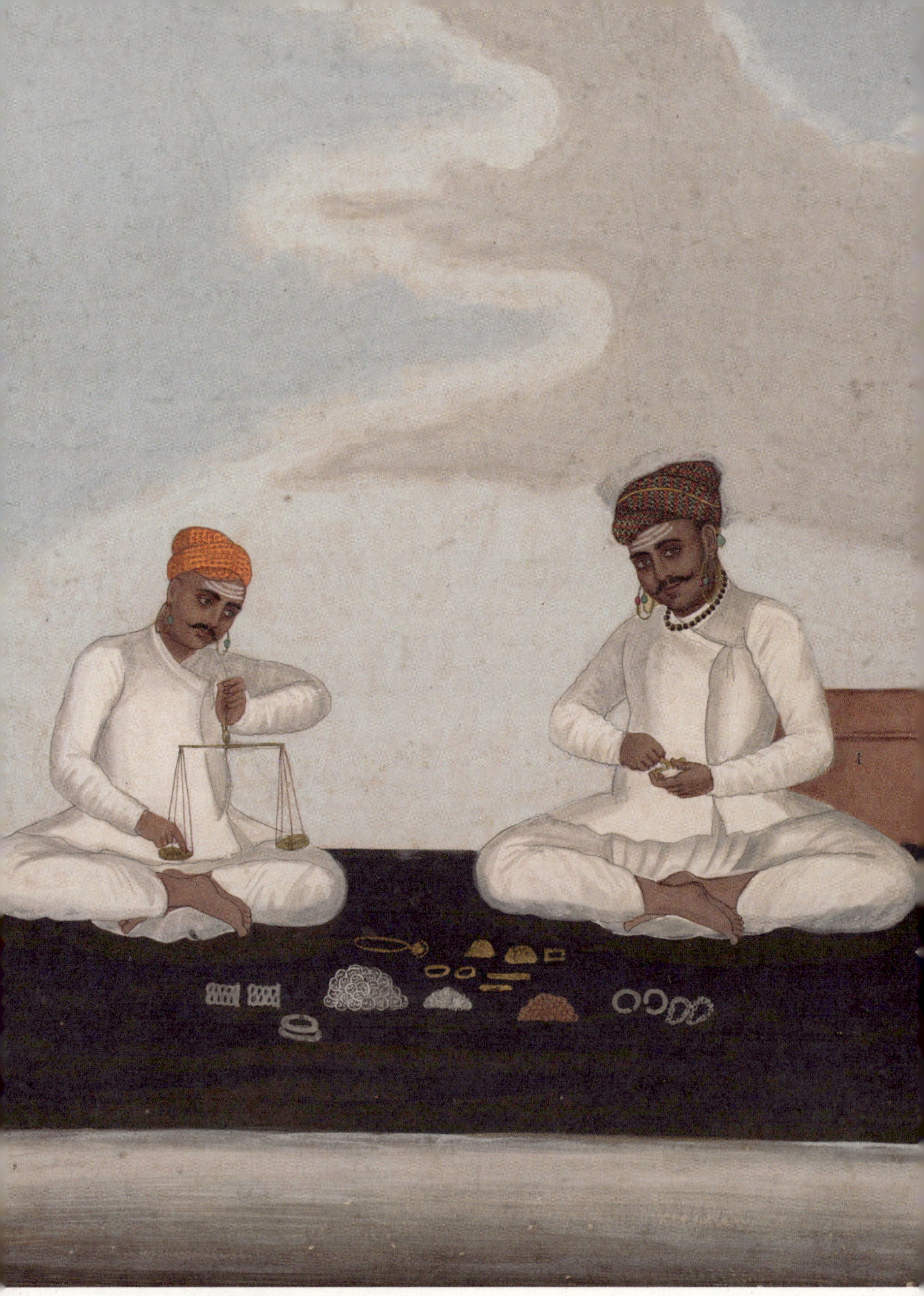

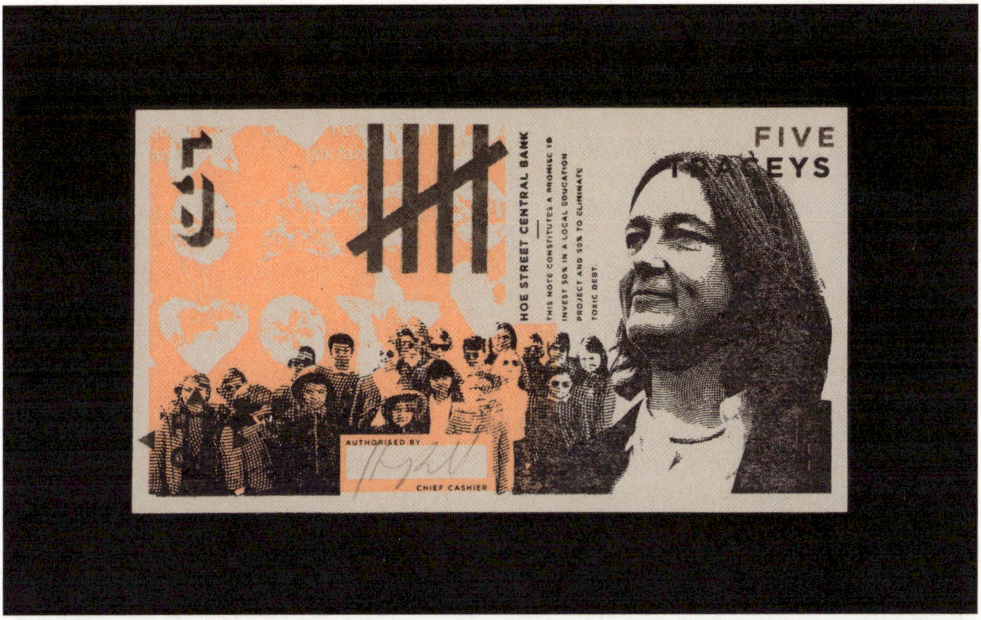

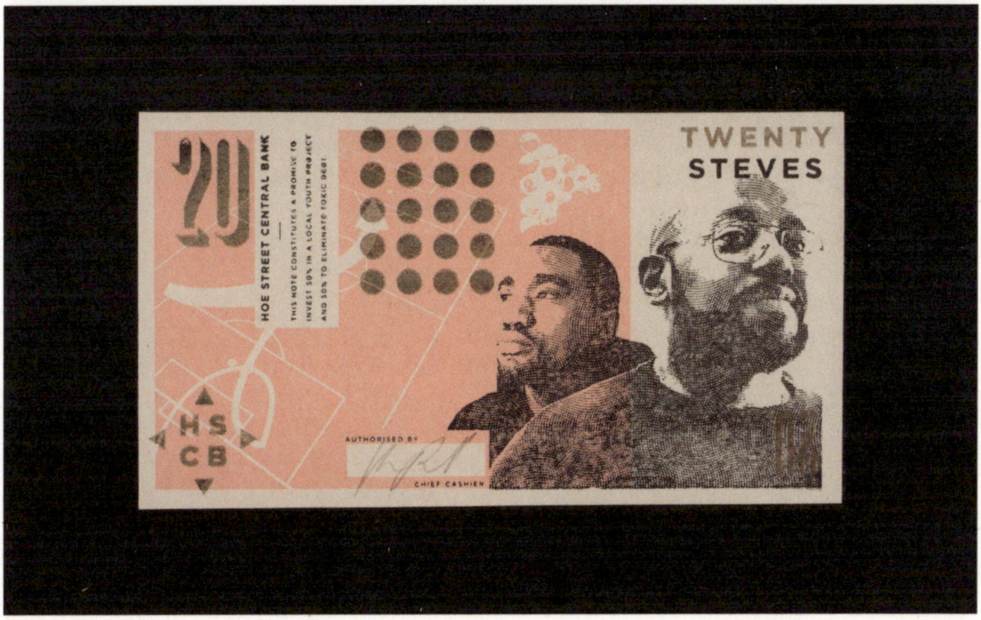

Painting depicting two *shroffs* or cash-keepers, Tanjore (now Thanjavure), c1805.

Five Traceys and Twenty Steves, denominations of two of the currencies produced by Hoe Street Central Bank.

CLOTHING SHOPS

How clothing shops can conjure new spatial experiences as a way of competing with the rise of online shopping in the post-Covid era

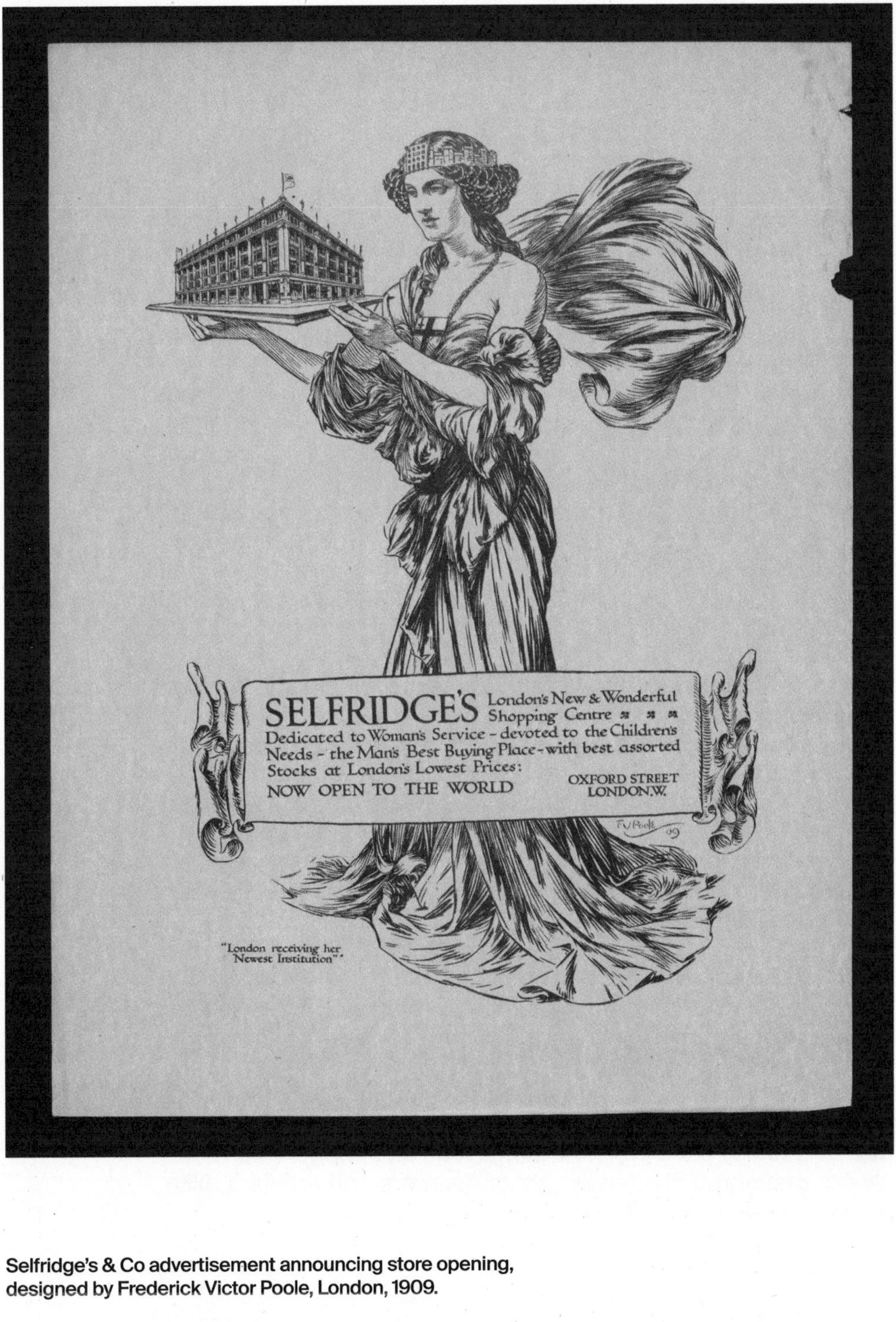

Selfridge's & Co advertisement announcing store opening, designed by Frederick Victor Poole, London, 1909.

ABSTAIN

The clothing sector was one of the worst affected by Covid-19 restrictions in the UK. More than 17,500 stores permanently closed after non-essential shops were forced to shut at the beginning of the first lockdown. The landscape of the British high street has fundamentally changed, with familiar brands including Oasis, Warehouse, and Arcadia Group's Topshop, Topman, Miss Selfridge and Dorothy Perkins all filing for bankruptcy in 2020 and ceasing to exist as brick-and-mortar shops.

Some of Britain's oldest and most established department stores – which had survived multiple recessions and bombing during the Blitz – did not go unscathed; the collapse of Debenhams, which was established in 1778, was a particular blow. In 2020 high-end department store Harrods, established 1849, and Selfridges, of 1908, cut 700 and 450 jobs respectively, due to the pandemic and resulting recession. John Lewis, founded in 1864, permanently closed one third of its stores and converted large parts of its London flagship into office space.

The clothing shop has been under threat for many years, as consumer spending habits have shifted away from in-store purchases and towards e-commerce. With many people confined to their homes, few opportunities to get dressed up for social activities and retail spaces remaining closed for the better part of a year, the pandemic only accelerated that shift. The Office for National Statistics revealed that in the UK, in-store fashion sales plunged 25% in 2020, while online transactions were up 32% for the same period. This stark contrast in fortunes is underlined by online fashion retailer ASOS reportedly tripling its profits in 2020. Alongside fast-fashion peddler Boohoo, ASOS acquired many of the failing high street brands for their digital platforms, closing down stores and making them online-only. Despite this trend, numerous reports highlighted how UK shoppers were keen to return to physical stores.

What was missed in a year of not going clothes shopping? And what aspects of in-person retail cannot be replicated through shopping online? Trying things on before buying is cited as a key reason for customers wanting to return to in-store shopping. Many consumers want to feel the materials, see the finish, and assess if an item suits them sartorially and is a good fit. Being physically separated from the clothes when buying online, and deciding to buy based on how things look on a model's body, has always presented challenges for consumers and retailers alike, resulting in vast amounts of returns.

For brick-and-mortar clothing shops wanting to survive and thrive in a post-pandemic world, innovation and adaptation are key to enticing shoppers back into the physical retail space. As a source of inspiration, it is useful to look back at some of the 20th-century pioneers of fashion retail who would pave the way for a new type of sartorial shopping experience.

Take Selfridges, for instance. At a time when department stores were one of the few public spaces designed for women's pleasure, Harry Gordon Selfridge stated 'A store should be a social centre, not merely a place for shopping'. His visionary approach saw Selfridges become the first department store to install women's toilets in 1909, meaning that women could spend the whole day away from home without causing moral indignation, which led to shopping becoming a leisurely, enjoyable activity. Selfridges emphasised the experiential spectacle of shopping, with an ice rink and shooting range on the roof, and theatrical shop window displays which were the first to be illuminated at night, drawing significant crowds.

Established in 1955, Mary Quant's Bazaar boutique at 138a Kings Road in Chelsea was the forerunner to the explosion of boutique shops which opened in the late 1950s and 1960s in London. Bazaar played music, served drinks, hosted fashion shows and – for a brief time before Quant was caught out by strict trading laws – offered Saturday late-night shopping. Quant's irreverent approach to window displays, forward-thinking visual branding and marketing, and constantly changing stock ensured a steady stream of repeat customers. The inclusion of Alexander's restaurant below the shop cemented Bazaar's reputation as a cultural hub – a place to 'see and be seen'.

Barbara Hulanicki's Biba began as a mail order business in 1963 but it quickly became a retail phenomenon. Its ultimate success was its affordability, which set it apart from other boutiques and swiftly fostered mass-market appeal and celebrity endorsement. Each successive boutique offered the unique Biba sensorial experience: moody and dimly lit, filled with antiques and Victorian furniture, and featuring a communal changing room.

Penneys flagship store in Dublin prepares for its reopening in June 2020.

Big Biba, which opened in 1973, was the epitome of immersive, experiential shopping: seven floors of opulent, palm-filled departments – each with a unique Biba logo – where you could buy everything from Biba baked beans to wallpaper and curtains. It attracted up to a million visitors a week, making it one of London's most-visited tourist attractions. Other features included a flamingo-filled roof garden, which lived on as Kensington Roof Gardens until 2018, and the Rainbow Room restaurant which doubled as a venue for bands including the New York Dolls and the Ronettes, and later featured in David Bowie's 1984 'Blue Jean' music video.Finally, Vivienne Westwood and Malcolm McLaren's iconic boutique at 430 Kings Road, Chelsea is a great example of brand reinvention and creativity. Between 1971 and 1979, the pair changed the shop's name and décor to suit the clothing, operating as Let it Rock, Too Fast to Live Too Young to Die, Sex, and Seditionaries before finally becoming Worlds End. Of these, Sex was perhaps the most notorious incarnation, decked out in spongy rubber and featuring pink rubberised letters spelling out 'SEX' above the door. The boutique quickly gained a cult following by selling fetish wear to sex workers, those with 'underground' sexual tastes and young punks brave enough to wear the look.

These visionary fashion retailers all underline the many possibilities granted by physical retail space, going far beyond simple sites of transaction to conjure immersive social spaces in which to connect, explore and dream.

Text by Stephanie Wood

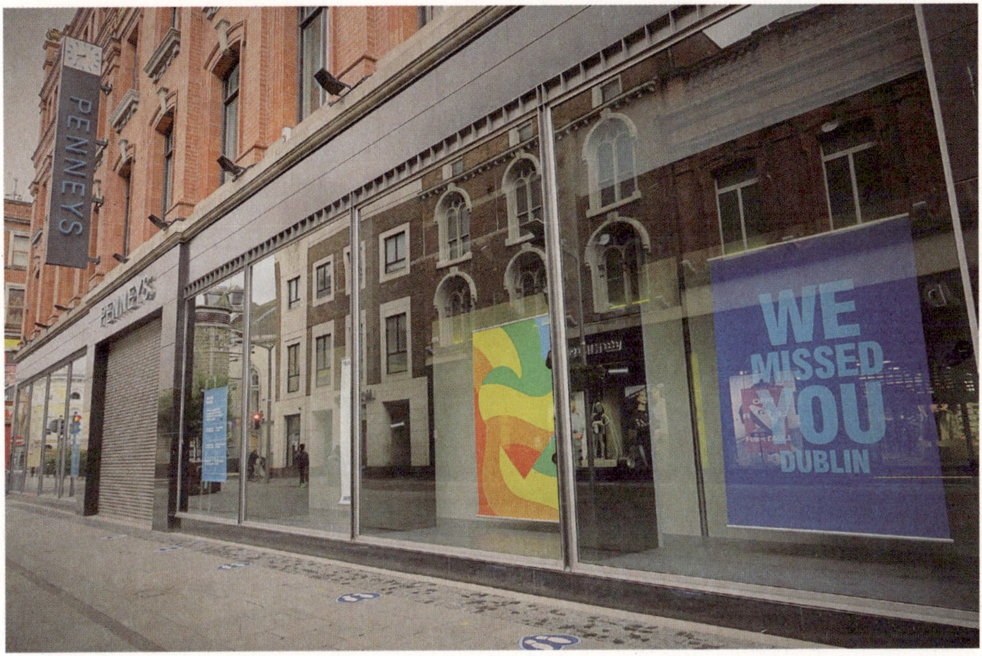
PENNEYS
PENNEYS
WE
MISSED
YOU
DUBLIN

HANDBAGS

N'hpye, a Burmese shoulder bag,
Burma, 1900–35.

How the resilience of the handbag's popularity showed the symbolic significance of fashion through lockdown

PANDEMIC OBJECTS

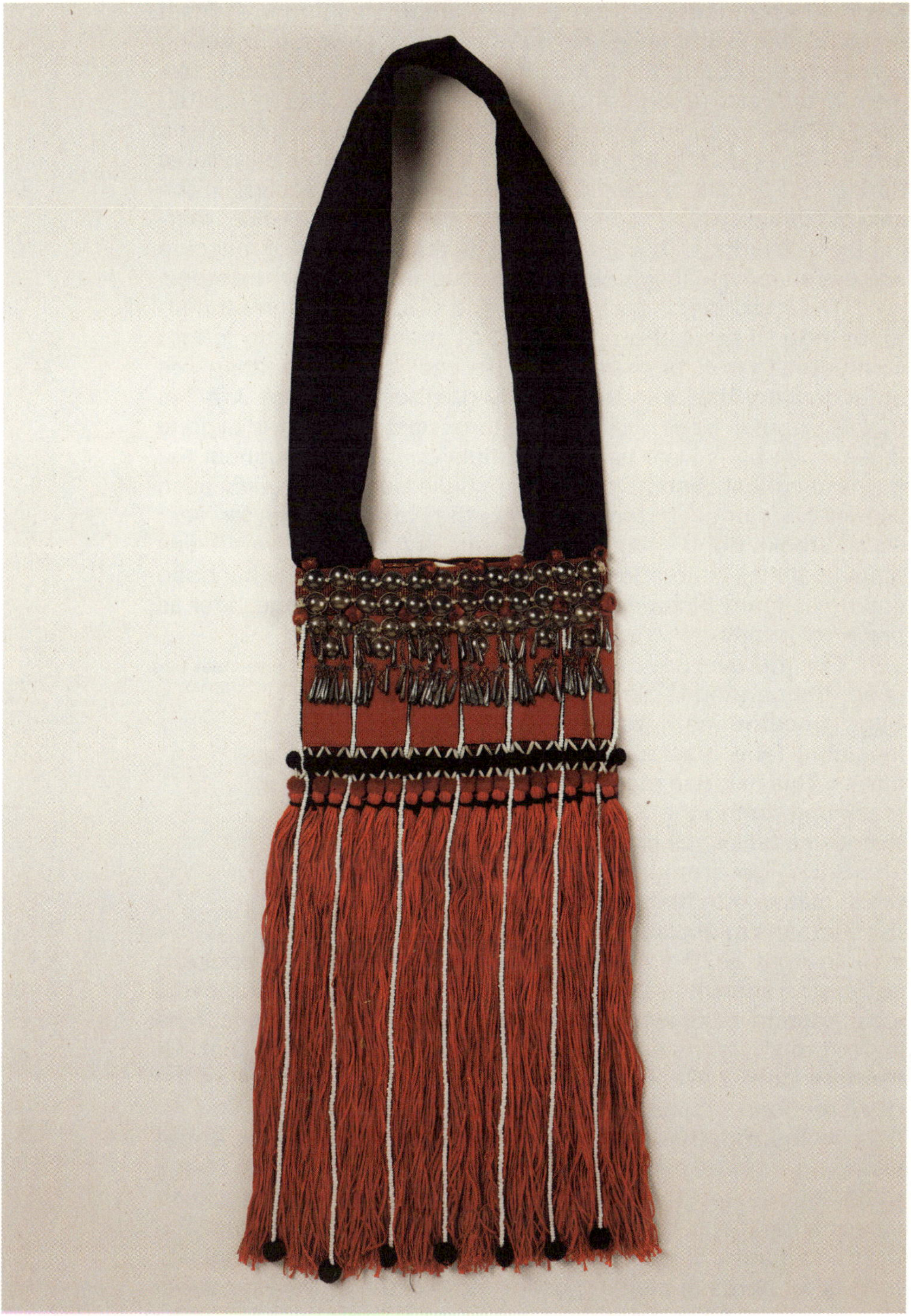

ABSTAIN

Covid-19 changed the way we think about fashion – at least momentarily. Exuberance was out, functionality was in. Dressing up was gone, comfort was king. Many months of lockdown saw the rise of 'waist-up dressing', with some brands cleverly capitalising on new working patterns – Prada, for instance, introduced items with logos placed just under the collar, an area still visible during video calls. Make-up brands saw a sharp decline in the sale of lipstick, which had become impossible to use while wearing face coverings. By contrast, the increased sales of mascara and eye shadow highlighted how the eyes had taken centre stage.

The handbag offers a useful case study in fashion's tumultuous ride through the pandemic. As many people no longer commuted to work or socialised in the evening, the handbag was an accessory that was temporarily deemed obsolete. Articles that focused on bags had a double tone: nostalgic for the bygone times when bags were used in multiple contexts throughout the day, and critical of some of the more ludicrous past trends, such as mini bags or oversized bags. Was the handbag gone forever? Or, as Brooke Bobb suggested in *Vogue* in April 2020, was it now more useful as a storage container at home? Would the handbag end up as many historical trunks have – first as luggage, later as pieces of furniture?

For the everyday bags that were still being used, the pandemic also changed their contents. Bags became carriers of personal protection, including face masks, hand sanitiser (p341) and gloves. This new use recalled the British civilian gas mask bag during the Second World War, designed to house a bulky gas mask elegantly and efficiently. The British government advised that people carry these masks with them at all times, out of fear that the Germans might launch a chemical attack.

Gas mask bag, UK, 1940–43.

In April 2020, while many had resorted to using pockets, backpacks and cross-body bags that left hands free when moving locally during lockdown, something unexpected happened. China started to lift its restrictions and news arrived reporting that the Hermès store in Guangzhou recorded $2.7 million sales on the day it reopened. Luxury fashion had returned.

In the months that followed, while retail and high street shopping suffered in many parts of the world (see Clothing Shops p166), vintage websites and online auction houses increased their sales of handbags. With more time available to spend online and the bag's mantra of 'one size fits all', it was easier to buy handbags than other items of clothing online, as no fittings were required.

Christies even sold its most expensive handbag ever, at 4 million Hong Kong dollars (around £370,000), in an auction in 2021. Some luxury brands even raised their prices on handbags during 2020 to recuperate the loss of income from other lines.

Bags had a double meaning during the pandemic: not only practical, but also deeply symbolic. While the handbag's usefulness was limited throughout lockdown, their enduring popularity shows us how apparel and accessories still fundamentally form many of our aspirational desires – even when isolating. The act of buying these statement accessories provided a certain sliver of hope for the consumer that one day soon an appearance – of both bag and owner – may enter the public realm again.

Text by Lucia Savi

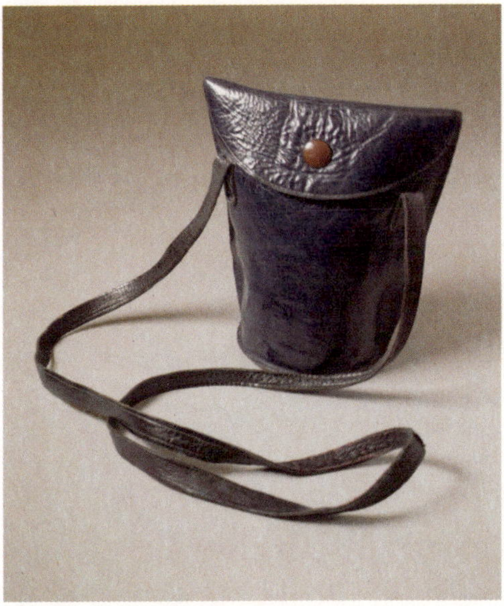

ABSTAIN

HAIR SALONS

How the absence of hair care services under lockdown revealed the hidden value of salons as a social experience

PANDEMIC OBJECTS

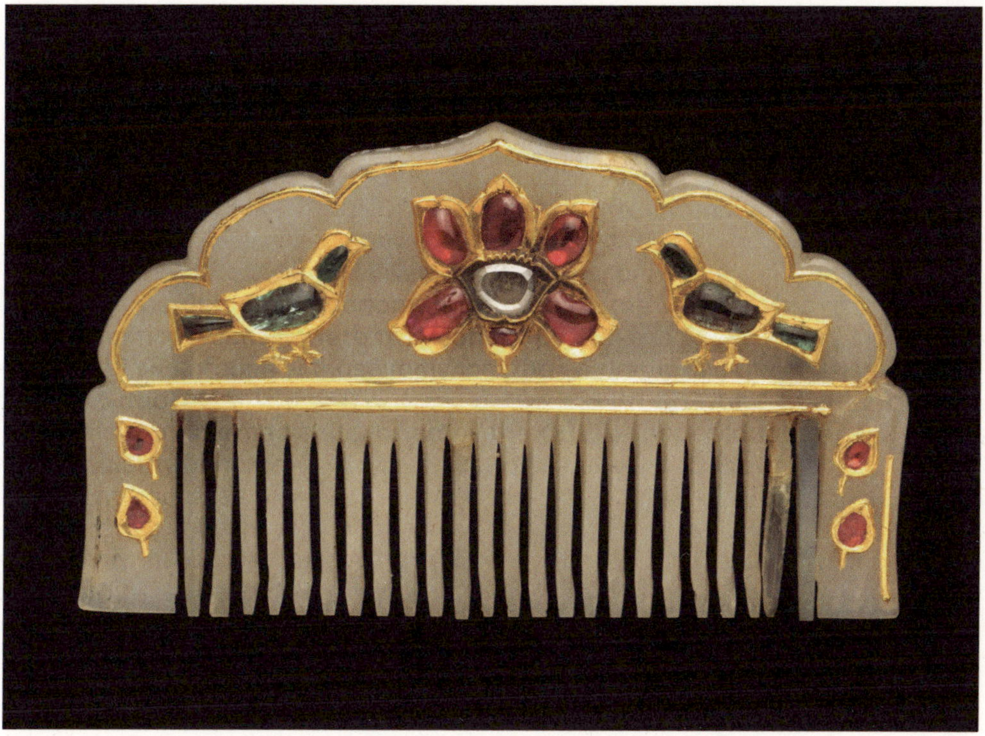

Comb from the Mughal Empire, 18th century.

ABSTAIN

Throughout the lockdowns, access to professional hair care was cut off. As this separation lengthened, anxiety began to grow among those who regularly visited hair care professionals for a variety of treatments, and an assortment of videos began to appear on social media and news sites offering advice on how to cut or dye hair at home. In response, participants who attempted to follow these instructions posted photos and videos of their unsuccessful or unflattering attempts with hashtags such as #LockdownHair and #CoronaCuts. Politicians, journalists or anyone appearing on television via video link had to do so without access to the usual hairstyling services. For example, former Scottish First Minister Nicola Sturgeon cheerfully posted her attempts to cut and colour her hair on Instagram, as she was talked through the process in a live FaceTime session with her regular hairdresser and makeup artist, Julie McGuire. While these inventive and comical responses to a lack of professional hair care kept us largely presentable, social engagement within the spaces of the salon and barbershop was compromised.

At the turn of the 20th century, few women would have visited hairdressers, a profession which, until the outbreak of the First World War, had mostly been made up of men. When long hair was in fashion, there was no need to regularly cut it, and women would dress their own hair – or, in the case of the affluent, had it styled by a maid. The popularity of marcelled (waved) hair and short hair styles, along with a growing number of female hairdressers saw immense growth in visits to salons and professional hair care became integral to everyday life.

With the introduction of new mass produced equipment and tools, such as the Gillette safety razor in the early 20th century, barbers lost a large portion of their regular male clientele, and by the mid-century the evolution of the salon became apparent. Weekly visits to these spaces for a 'shampoo and set' became a part of many women's lives. By the 1960s, it was common for both men and women to attend salons for haircuts and colour services and today, many people book regular appointments at hairdressers and barbers for an assortment of services, including beard trimming, bleaching, highlights and braiding.

Upon the lifting of lockdown, UK government guidelines required hairdressers to change the way they worked. Clients were staggered and the traditional chat between hair professional and client was muted, either with both wearing masks or, in the case of the stylist, a full-face shield. Screens and barriers separated customers from one another. There

Eugène Atget, *Coiffeur, Palais Royal*, Paris, 1926–27.

were no waiting areas, and clients were expected to book in advance to reduce the flow and interaction of patrons. No magazines or reading material were offered, nor refreshments. The experience was turned into one fraught with hidden danger, changing the social value of the salon to a purely functional one. This stark contrast only serves to highlight the enduring value of the hair salon or barbershop not simply as a service, but as a social experience, one which is cherished by clients – some of whom may return to the same salon for decades, seeing it not just as a saviour of their locks but also as a friend.

Text by Kathleen Walker-Meikle

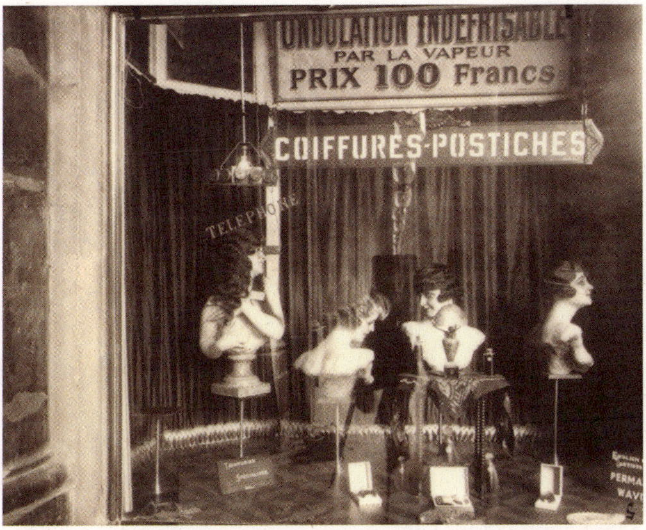

MUSIC VENUES

How the prohibition of public gatherings revealed the importance of live music, leading musicians to embrace the possibilities of the internet

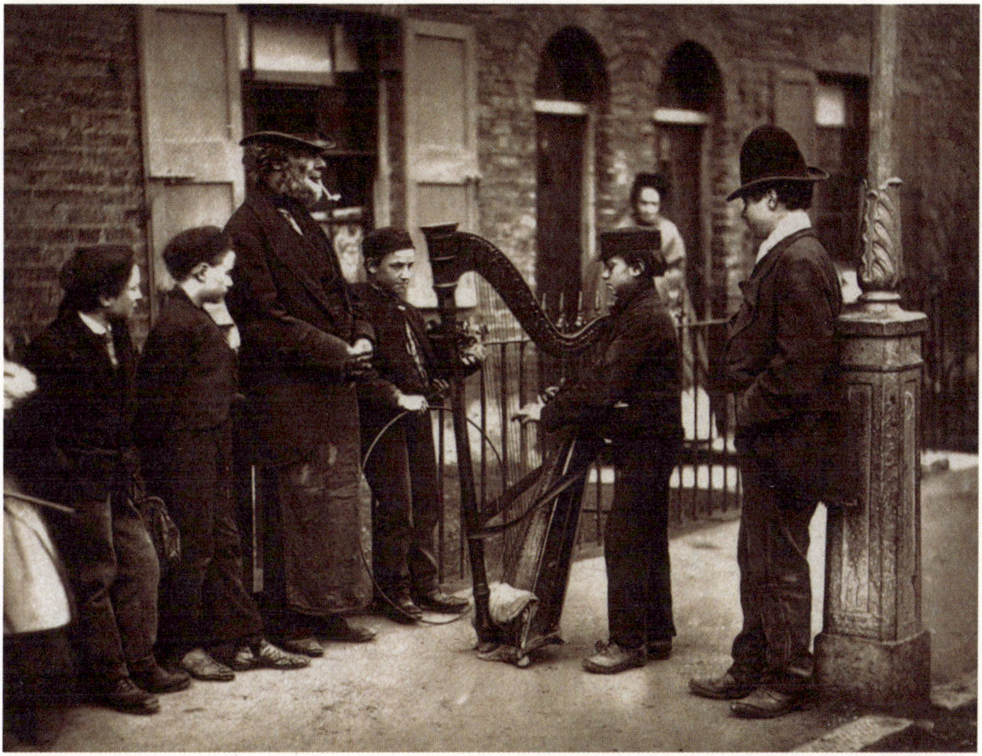

John Thomson, *Italian Street Musicians*, London, 1877–78.

ABSTAIN

On 18 March 2020, the announcement came that the upcoming Glastonbury Festival – the 50th anniversary of the event – would be cancelled. For many, come rain or shine, via the BBC or at Worthy Farm, 'Glasto' was an important expression of summer, of Britishness – a place to find kindred spirits, creative freedom and connection. In their statement, co-organisers Emily and Michael Eavis said: 'Clearly this was not a course of action we hoped to take for our 50th anniversary event, but following the new government measures announced this week – and in times of such unprecedented uncertainty – this is now our only viable option'.

In the following days, music lovers across the world had to come to terms with the fact that all live performances in the near future were cancelled. It was shocking to see cultural life being put on hold as the virus took its grip on society. The economic and emotional effect was felt almost immediately: the grave impact of pulling the plug on this booming industry – worth £5.2 billion to the UK economy in 2018 – trickled down beyond promoters and audiences to the fragile creative world that supports it, from freelance conductors to costume makers, from sound engineers to stage managers.

A glimmer of hope was seen in the work of the Musician's Union, which quickly established a £1 million Hardship Fund for members who were suffering loss of work due to the pandemic. On 25 March 2020, Help Musicians launched a £5 million Coronavirus Financial Hardship Fund, the funds for which were exhausted by 2 April after the charity received in excess of 17,000 applications. The streaming platform Bandcamp temporarily waived its revenue shares for one day, with $4.3 million going directly to artists and small labels. Eventually, government schemes and furlough programmes were launched to help networks of creative professionals.

Articles optimistically looked to a Covid-free future where culture could again thrive. Writing in *The Times* in late March, Caitlin Moran anticipated that 'next summer the world will explode with joy – there will be street parties and raves and hugging will come back'. However, as lockdowns continued throughout 2021, the real explosion of a summer of live music had to wait another year.

While 2020 will be remembered as the year of being physically distant, it was also a moment of great exploration and experimentation with how virtual audiences could become part of fulfilling live events and experiences online. Much of this change had already been underway before the pandemic; the growth of services like Spotify through the 2000s and 2010s has made most of the world's music accessible online (see Streaming Services p142) and the Met Opera has streamed live performances across the internet and the planet.

But Covid-19 precipitated further change. Through various forms of social media and video conferencing platforms, there was an outpouring of generosity and openness from artists willing to stream from behind closed doors. Andrew Lloyd Webber had a 'composers in quarantine' play-off with Lin-Manuel Miranda and Nile Rodgers; Skepta ran a producing challenge on Instagram Live; and Tim Burgess held listening parties on Twitter. In the classical world, the BBC's Katie Derham broadcast *In Tune* from a makeshift studio, bringing together artists to perform 'home sessions'. Derham observed that the situation had 'finally made classical music more accessible as we all do everything remotely without fear or expense of going to venues'.

Online audiences were able to explore live performance in newfound ways, from rising interest in institutions that allowed online visitors backstage and into their archives, like the Vienna Staatsoper with its 360° virtual tour and free daily broadcasts of performance recordings, to Russian ballet dancers practising in their kitchens. The UK's opera houses and festivals gave free access to a rich repertoire of past performances. Musicians from Rotterdam Philharmonic Orchestra live-streamed Beethoven's 9th Symphony from their bedrooms. The English National Opera's costume designers made personal protective equipment (PPE) for the NHS. Across the world people joined virtual choirs and found new ways to share performances. Lady Gaga's *One World: Together at Home* concert brought more than 100 artists from their own living rooms to those of their audience in a fundraising benefit gig that echoed the spirit and scale of Live Aid in 1985.

Processes that had been slowly underway for the past decade suddenly accelerated; audiences increasingly met new performers online before they had the opportunity to see them on stage. High-quality music was created in small, often domestic spaces outside conventional studios and artists found ways to generate income from digital performances while rethinking how to charge for their work, where to host and what to do with their recordings afterwards.

ABSTAIN

After two further years of uncertainty triggered by subsequent lockdowns and Covid-19 variants, the sting in the tail of this digital optimism has been the direct impact of the pandemic on the live performance industry, with cancellations due to Covid-19 restrictions affecting income generation, job security and business confidence. Despite an explosion of creativity and a demand by audiences to return to live music shows, the situation for venues, crew and musicians has remained precarious even as the musical landscape is rebuilt. The ecosystem that feeds this creative economy is now also at greater risk in the UK, with cuts to arts funding announced in November 2022 alongside spiralling operating costs, soaring energy bills and a cost-of-living crisis. With creativity, innovation and resilience, the live music industry can overcome these new challenges, but in the meantime, it's useful to remember, respect and value the contribution that culture and music gave us during the darkest times of the pandemic.

Text by Kate Bailey

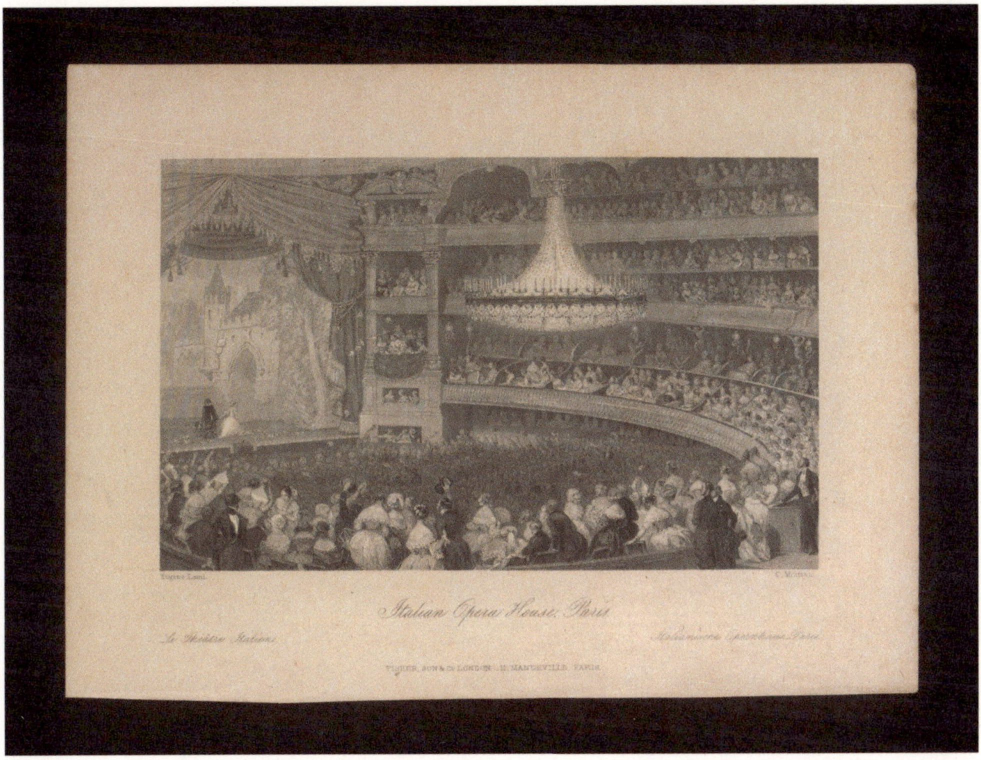

Print depicting the Italian Opera House in Paris, c19th century, drawn by Charles Mottram and engraved by Eugène Lami.

PUBS

How lockdown highlighted the need for spaces of leisure and socialising in the city, away from work and home

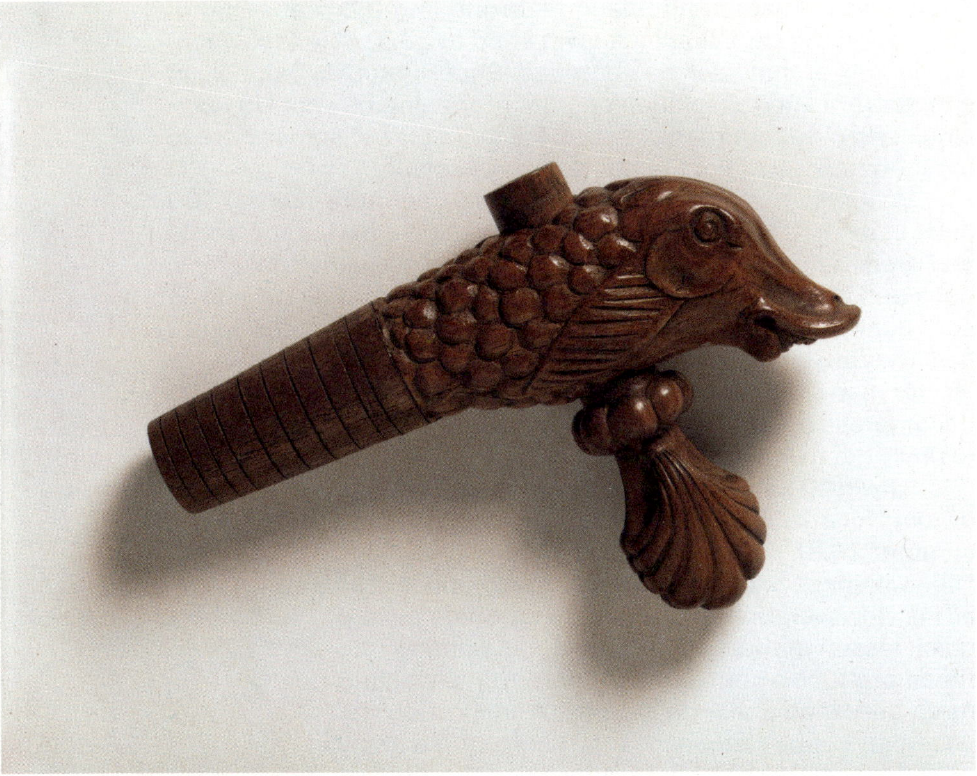

Barrel tap, France, 1700–30.

There was palpable anticipation surrounding the reopening of pubs when the UK's first lockdown lifted in 2020. The first weekend in July of that year was branded 'Super Saturday', signalling a temporary end to isolation and the reopening of what US sociologist Ray Oldenburg refers to as the 'third place': somewhere to meet others outside of the home or a workplace.

A survey from November 2019 recorded more than 47,000 pubs in the UK. For centuries, they have been a part of the social and architectural fabric of Britain. In large post-industrial cities, pubs and former pubs are everywhere, reflecting their origins as community hubs in densely populated working-class communities. They are still a very active part of modern social and economic life; for many, a post-work drink or a 'swift half' offers a chance to decompress and reflect after a day at the grindstone, and a place to really get to know your colleagues.

Covid-19 altered the fundamental experience of going for a drink with some friends in a pub. In early summer 2020, some pubs sold large milk cartons filled with beer, to drink in the park (see Public Parks p214). However, the textured plastic bottles gave a quick lesson in material properties as pouring into these produced considerably more foam, wasting more beer than a standard glass. When lockdowns eased and pubs reopened, they came with a litany of new rules and protocols. As well as the ubiquitous social distancing, there was mandatory table service, mask wearing and limits on group size, measures which transformed the experience of enjoying a pint poured straight from the keg.

Print by George Cruikshank, c1820, depicting revelers crowding outside the Mother Red Cap and ignoring the King's Head, satirising the popularity of Queen Caroline over King George IV.

Pubs have two clearly essential elements: a bar to order drinks, and somewhere to sit and consume them. However, another important but largely intangible factor is 'atmosphere': the look and feel, the general 'pubbyness' of the establishment. This is the thing that is impossible to recreate at home. Pubs are inherently social spaces, designed to facilitate spending time with others. The pandemic revealed how the design of many pub buildings clashed with public health ideals, squeezed into historical footprints with cramped customer seating and toilets that are too small. Landlords and managers did their best to direct queues and one-way systems around their tumbledown saloons. In late 2020, kitchen facilities offering a 'substantial meal' – following new government rules – became absolutely essential. More than ever, a generous garden or outside space was a key asset, even in cold weather. The fact that so many were willing to endure the cold spring of 2021 speaks strongly to the desire for a 'third place' among the socially isolated. If anything, the pandemic reinforced the place of the pub in the British psyche as a symbol of company, friendliness and normality.

Pubs in the UK were already in decline before Covid-19 struck. Increasing costs, higher expectations from customers and competition from supermarkets have caused many to close. Expanding corporatisation has depreciated must-have cosy and inviting atmospheres. Most pubs have been forced to diversify their offers beyond the imbibing of alcohol, becoming increasingly reliant on good food and entertainment. The pandemic did reveal the true extent of the role pubs play in British social culture; in a country with some of the longest working hours and smallest houses in Europe, there is a clear need to preserve pubs as 'third spaces' located close to workplaces and homes. The cost of a pint has inevitably gone up due to the converging issues of pandemic fallout and rising costs, but the desire to have a social drink has not diminished.

For the time being, while passion for pubs remains strong, they are in a precarious position. Some estimates suggest that pubs in England and Wales are closing at a rate of 50 per month. As the cost of living has risen, enthusiasm may not be enough to keep the doors of the local boozer open.

Text by William Newton

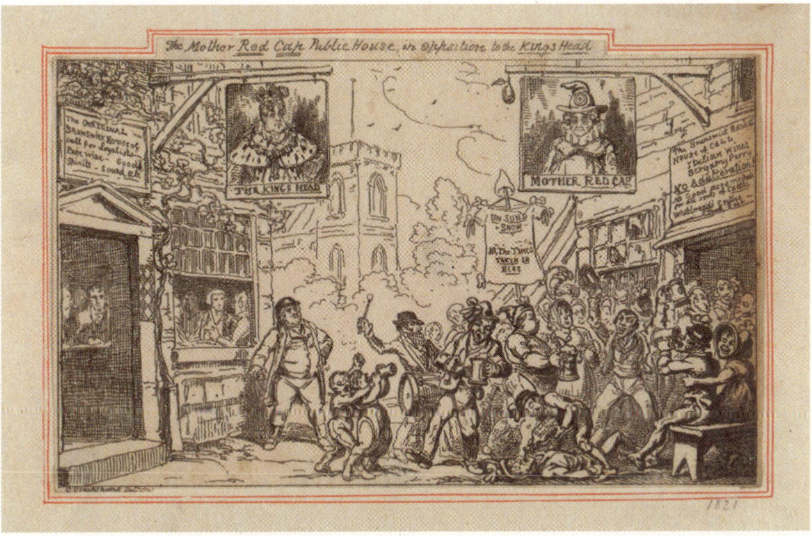
The Mother Red Cap Public House, in opposition to the Kings Head
THE KINGS HEAD
MOTHER RED CAP
1821

THE UNDERGROUND

Poster advertising the London Underground designed by Taylor Horace, UK, 1924–26.

How the pandemic prompted reflection on what travel infrastructure means to a city

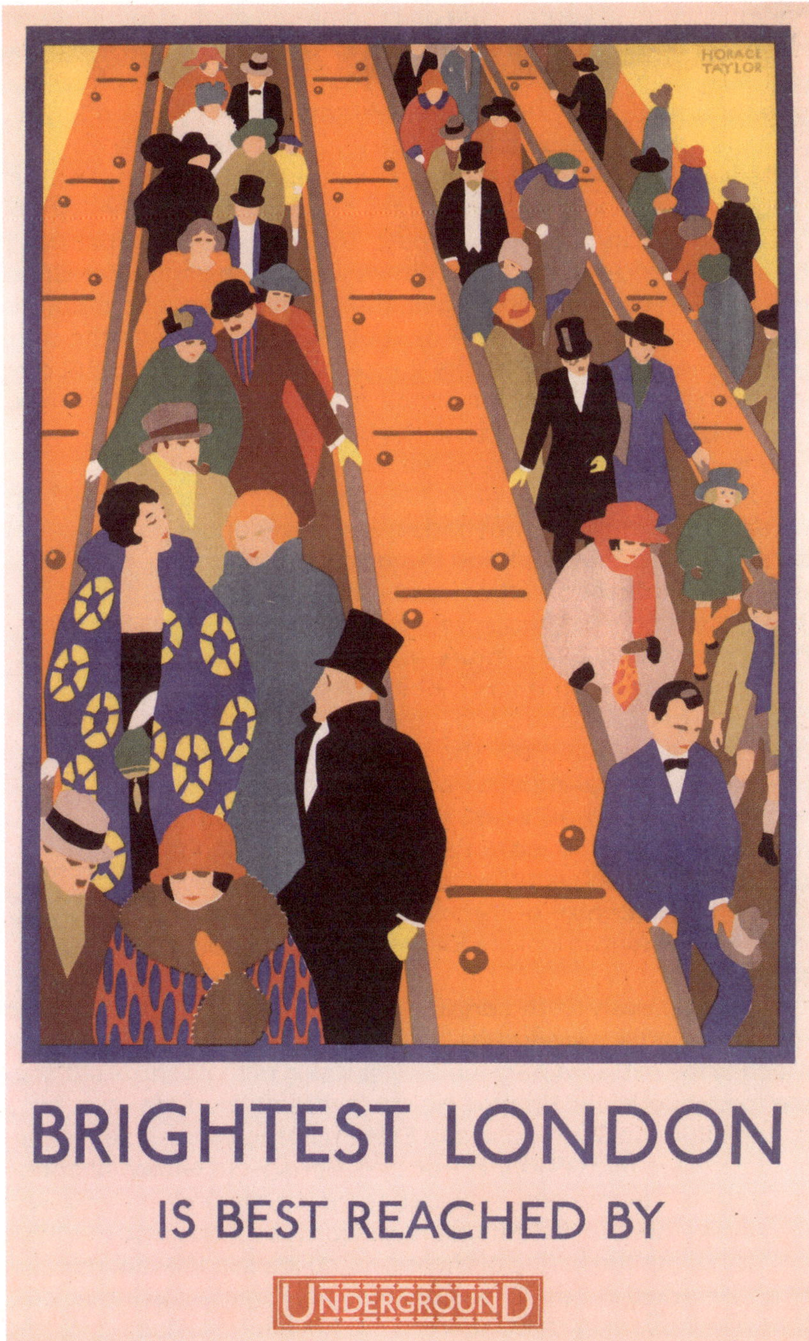
HORACE TAYLOR
BRIGHTEST LONDON
IS BEST REACHED BY
UNDERGROUND

For most living in London, the daily commute on the Underground has never been a highlight of the day. Wedged into a rush hour tube carriage while pressed up against a stranger, standing cheek-to-sweaty-armpit with someone else's smartphone jabbed in your shoulder blade, the experience can feel as hellish as any mythical underworld. Yet, as the weeks and months went by during the first stage of the pandemic, it was easy to miss some of the subtler qualities of riding public transport. The opportunity to put one's brain in idle and indulge in people-watching; the panoply of different faces, styles and languages; the peculiar peace that comes from being anonymous; the rush of air in the face as the train approaches in the tunnel; the sense of immersion into the city; and perhaps most of all, the simple feeling of being on the move.

Whether you love or hate the Underground (or love to hate it), it has always felt like a certainty of London life. The images of deserted platforms and carriages during lockdown had an unnerving effect, as they called into question the understanding of the city as many Londoners had come to know it. The construction of underground train lines, which began in the mid-19th century, transformed London into a city based on mass mobility. As a relatively cheap form of transport available to all classes (at one point advertised as 'The way for all'), it had a far-reaching social impact. People had more choice of where to live and work, and those with fewer means were able to leave the squalor of the inner city for better housing further out. Suburbs were born and the centre of the city opened up (especially for women) as a place for recreation, shopping and culture.

Poster showing the font designed by Edward Johnston for the London Underground, UK, 1916.

By the early 20th century, the Underground embodied an ideal of people moving freely and seamlessly through the city. Much of the extraordinary modernist vision of that time is still visible today: consider Charles Holden's streamlined stations, such as the futuristic Southgate, and Edward Johnston's elegant sans-serif typeface from 1916, inspired by the crisp-cut letters inscribed on Trajan's Column and designed to be legible on the move. And of course, there is the famous map drawn by Harry Beck in 1933, which laid out the tangle of Underground lines in the rational form of an electrical circuit. A less tangible heritage lies in behaviours that many users of the Underground have internalised: minding the gap, standing to the right on escalators, and so on. These keep everything flowing as frictionlessly as possible.

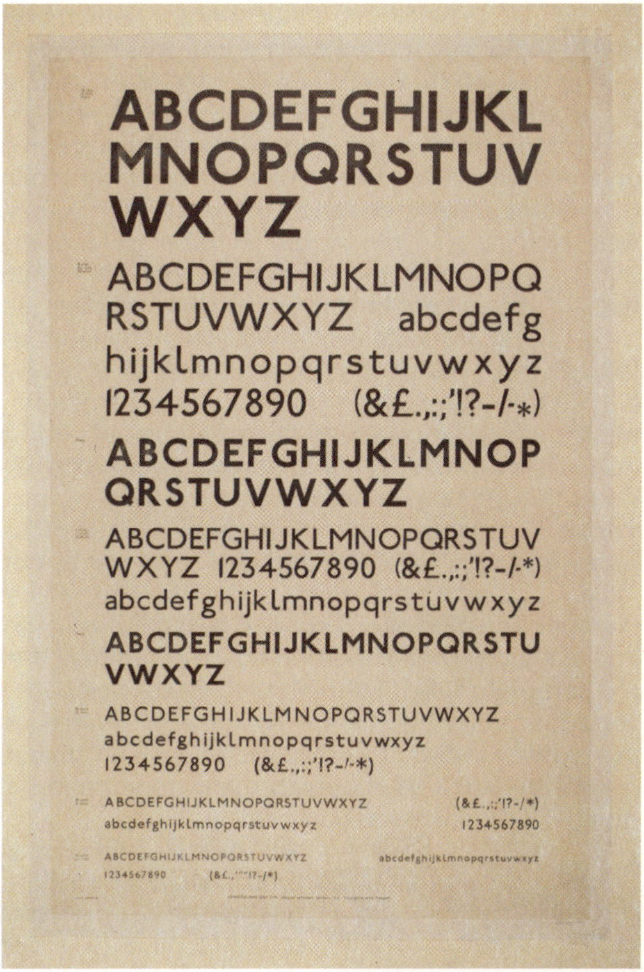

As the urbanist Richard Sennett once pointed out, however, this mobility came at the cost of creating a more disaggregated and ultimately less public city. In his 1994 book *Flesh and Stone*, Sennett described how the London Underground established a new time geography for the urban centre. It acted as the 'veins and arteries' through which the 'human blood' flowed into the heart of the city by day and drained away at night. Nor did people mixing together during the daytime result in strong human connections. 'People worked and shopped and then left for home,' noted Sennett. Cocooned in carriages speeding across the city, passengers travelled like ships passing in the night.

The pandemic highlighted this paradox at the heart of mass transport. In terms of coronavirus transmission, a packed tube carriage was the antithesis of social distancing; an environment where travellers' sense of personal space is suspended. But squished up close with fellow passengers, social interaction is minimal. People distance themselves mentally, retreating inwards into individual bubbles; touching but not connecting; sharing germs more easily than making eye contact or starting a conversation.

An empty carriage on a morning commute on the Piccadilly line in November 2020.

In 1999, this state of affairs was challenged by a group of 'anarchitects' called the Space Hijackers, who held a 'Circle line party' that involved transforming a Circle line train into a pop-up moving disco. Sound systems, refreshments and even coloured gels to fix over the strip lights were smuggled onboard in suitcases. It was the first of many acts of 'tactical frivolity' through which the Space Hijackers pursued their mission to 'oppose the way that public space is being eroded and replaced by corporate profit-making space'. The idea was to creatively repurpose dead, highly controlled public spaces shaped by institutions and corporations, and to challenge the hierarchies they entrench. Why, for example, are corporate advertisers allowed to solicit on the Underground, while homeless people are not? The Underground could in this sense be considered a prototype of the 'non-places' of consumer capitalism, such as shopping malls and airports, that are only a mirage of organic street culture.

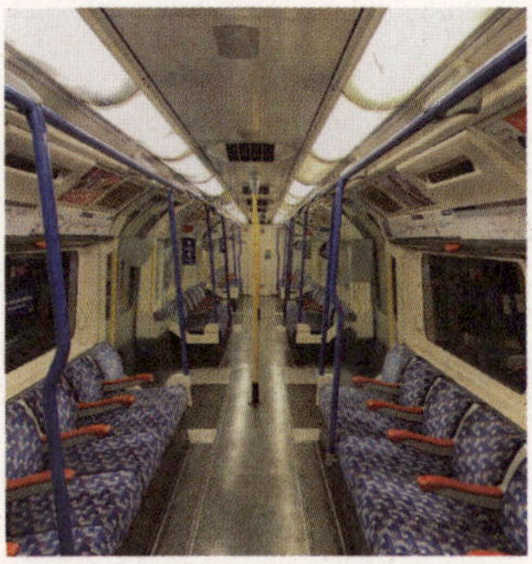

Emergency bailouts and new health and safety protocols kept Underground trains and London buses running throughout the pandemic for those unable to shelter at home. But the crisis exposed the vulnerability of the system. Since 2015, London has been one of the only cities in the world that receives no government grant towards the operating costs of its public transport network, leaving an essential service heavily dependent on revenue from fares. Failure to safeguard the transport system around which London has grown would both exacerbate existing social inequalities and increase the reliance on cars.

In many ways, the pandemic made people question situations that they habitually accept as normal. One idea that gained attention was the '15-minute city'. This is an approach to planning developed by urban scientist Carlos Moreno that re-envisions the city as a series of overlapping neighbourhoods in which most of your needs (work, shopping, healthcare, education, leisure, culture) are met within a 15-minute walk or bike ride from your front door. It is a notion that pushes against more than a hundred years of planning that has favoured centralising infrastructures, such as the Underground, and the zoning of cities according to separate activities.

In an era of post-Covid recovery, reorientating cities around the principle of micro-mobility could have a host of benefits: stronger communities; resilient local economies; less time, stress and carbon emissions expended on daily travel; a more equitable distribution of amenities; increased opportunity for people to cocreate their neighbourhoods at grassroots level. In some places the goal of a 15-minute city is already being boldly embraced – Paris mayor Anne Hidalgo made it central to her successful re-election campaign in 2020.

In November 2022, weekday passenger numbers stood at 78% of pre-pandemic levels as many who had been working from home recommenced their journeys to and from the office. But established work/life patterns do not seem as inevitable as they once did. Whether by experiencing remote working, or engaging differently with one's neighbourhood and community, many commuters have gained new perspectives on how they might inhabit the city. The London Underground underpins a particular 20th-century vision of urbanism. The enforced holiday from it might yet help in imagining different approaches to urban space and mobility that will be better equipped to meet the social, ecological and health challenges of today.

Text by Catherine Flood

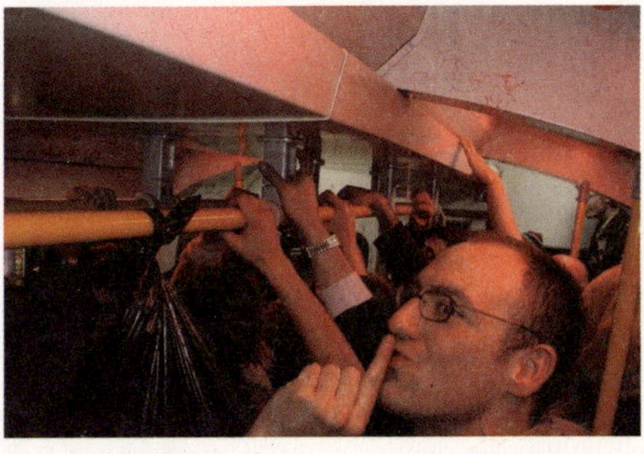

A reveler urges silence on one of the Space Hijacker's Circle line parties on the London Underground on 14 March 2003.

05

PIVOT

The pandemic was an enormous collective pivot. In corporate parlance, the term is often used to suggest that in order to thrive, businesses must remain nimble and open to adaptation. However, demanding such flexibility at a global scale was, to a large extent, unreasonable. Despite short-term government stopgaps to keep enterprises afloat, many were simply unable to navigate the new conditions and succumbed to closure. Likewise, governments, especially those that had pursued neoliberal policies for decades, suddenly found themselves lacking the mechanisms to efficiently deliver the care needed.

Regardless, the imperative to shift tack provided useful test cases for design, manufacturing and service delivery. How could dating apps thrive when in-person dating itself was not possible? What could industries do when demand suddenly plummeted? How could student housing be sold when there was nobody on campus? In some cases, the pivots that occurred have had an enduring impact. Cities around the world have embraced cold-weather outdoor dining. Emergency efforts designed to keep services going revealed hidden possibilities and desires that, once tested, found new acceptance. To pivot, to change direction, can unfortunately lead to closed doors and dead ends. With perseverance, however, new paths reveal themselves, often resulting in unexpected discoveries.

DATING APPS

How dating apps pivoted to accommodate lockdown dating, revealing the quick adaptability of app design

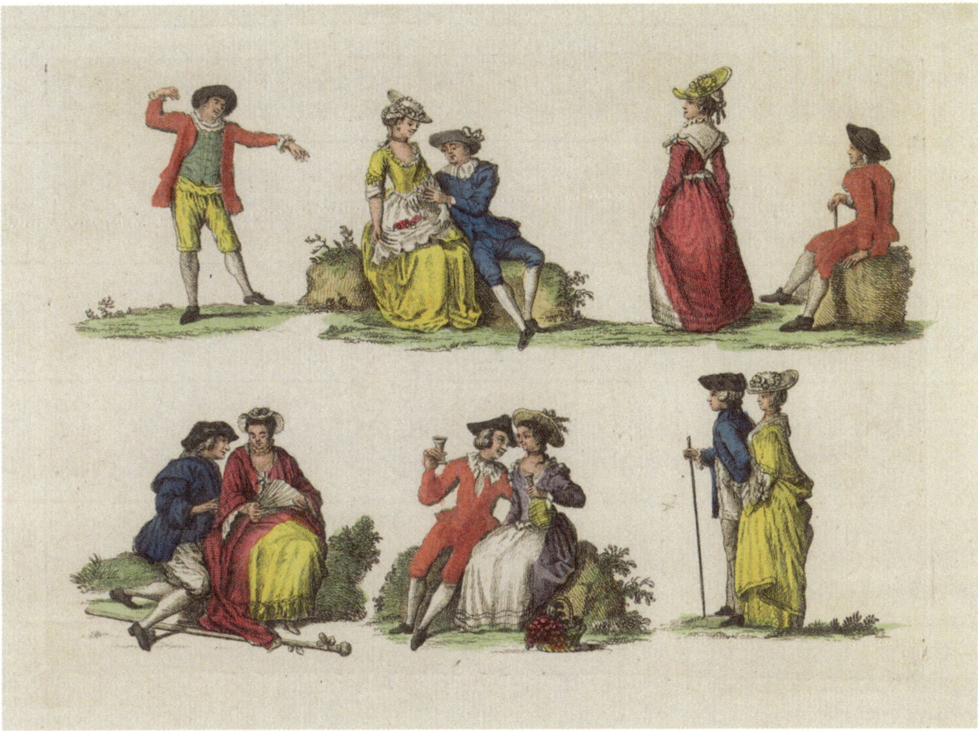

Scenes of courtship, 1756–57.

The start of the pandemic saw a surge in the use of dating apps. On 29 March 2020, Tinder reported the highest ever number of swipes in a single day, at 3 billion; over the following 18 months, that single-day record of 3 billion was broken 130 more times. By the autumn of 2020, one in five UK Bumble users said they had joined the app after ending a committed relationship as a result of the pandemic. Before the pandemic, these platforms were matchmakers used to facilitate face-to-face encounters; they worked as a springboard to IRL experiences. When the UK government advised everyone to stay at home, the rules of the dating game changed, but dating apps were nevertheless quick to adapt.

First, there were prevention messages. On 3 March 2020, when the world death toll was reported at 3,000 (by May 2023 it exceeded 6.9 million), the online dating platform Tinder started showing Covid-19-related pop-ups to its users. The message encouraged users to prioritise safety over 'fun', wash their hands and seek further health information on the WHO website. Once the prevention message was acknowledged, the user could keep using the app to swipe, match and chat as usual. However, as the pandemic continued, the fear of contracting the virus, combined with the monotony of 'walking dates' out in all types of weather, started to deter even the most tenacious dating enthusiasts. As many countries across the world oscillated in and out of lockdowns, dating apps transitioned from just creating interactions and pivoted towards shaping them.

By the end of 2020, platforms such as Tinder, Hinge, Match, Happn and Plenty of Fish had all launched in-app video calls and camera icons appeared in chats, giving users more ways to connect online. The new addition required a behavioural change from daters who had never thought of their phone as a romantic rendezvous venue before, and developers had to rethink user experiences (UX) and modify user interfaces (UI) to ease people in.

The dating app Hinge provides an interesting case study. The market testing of their video calling feature during the first lockdown coincided with the launch of Hinge Labs, the first dating app research programme backed by behavioural data and not based solely on surveys. Hinge Labs helped identify the potential of the new feature – where 70% of users said they would be open to video dates – as well as possible obstacles to its development, such as users' fear of awkwardness or questions about how to start a video date or how long it should last.

With new meeting modes came a new dating etiquette. Tinder's blog, *Swipe Life*, listed 'do's and don'ts' to conquer this new evolution in cyber dating. It advised preparing games and activities, both revealing the platform's awareness of users' Zoom fatigue and highlighting how apps have contributed to the gamification of dating. Another tip encouraged daters to curate their video background, using lighting and props to display their personality and seduce the person on the other side of the screen. This illustrates how virtual dates have modified the geographies of our intimacies, inviting 'strangers' into our homes at a very early stage of a potential relationship. Despite the sudden shift, dating apps found that video dates could stick around: in 2021, 52% of Hinge users who went on video dates said that they would incorporate them into their dating process after Covid-19 restrictions were lifted. After a short absence from some platforms as the UK emerged from lockdown, video features returned for good and are now not only normalised but also promoted as a safety measure to take before meeting face-to-face, quite apart from social distancing recommendations.

In parallel to promoting video calls, some platforms encouraged daters to get ready for 'hot vax summer' – an expression that played with the idea of a dating boom once singles were vaccinated. Vaccination status became a critical new criterion for dating, with a YouGov poll conducted in May 2021 showing that 59% of respondents would either prefer their date to be vaccinated or would not date an unvaccinated person at all. Dating apps partnered with the UK government to boost vaccine uptake: from 7 June 2021, a few days before under-30s would become eligible to get their vaccine, Hinge, Bumble, Match, Badoo, Plenty of Fish, OurTime and Muzz added features to their apps as part of the 'every vaccination gives us hope' campaign. The platforms updated their reward systems by offering free tokens or access to premium features to newly vaccinated users. The campaign also led to a modification of users' profiles and search criteria: on Hinge, daters could add their vaccination status to their profile; Tinder allowed users to add a 'vaccines save lives' badge to pictures; and on OkCupid, vaccinated people became a new category prominently highlighted on the app. With the softening of lockdown measures, dating apps also became a helpful launching pad back into social life. Alongside vaccination status, new features invited users to indicate their preferences regarding masks, social distancing and the type of location they would feel comfortable meeting in – a positive and inclusive endeavour for those who continued to act cautiously.

The way dating apps were able to respond to the pandemic highlighted the adaptable nature of app design: it is quicker to gather and analyse data, tailor a service to an audience, and implement changes to a software, than it is to a redesign a physical object requiring the retooling of a factory. Many apps can be updated in the background, without action from users. Change is effortless. While they mirrored the rollercoaster of our lives as we came in and out of lockdowns, dating apps also highlighted our resilience when it comes to connecting with others.

Text by Maude Willaerts

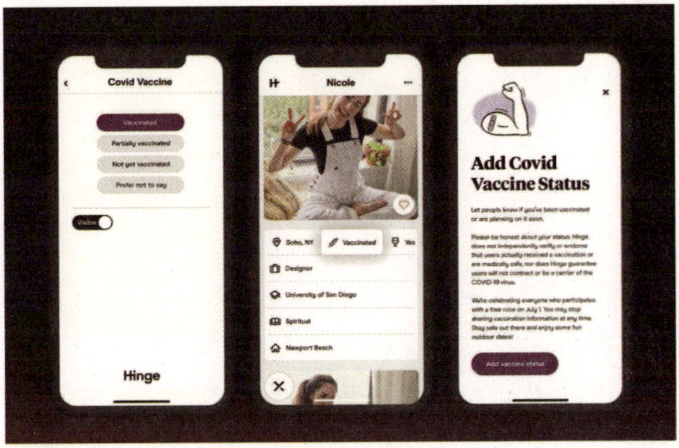

Hinge rapidly produced Vaccine Status (above) and Date from Home (below) as new features, 2020.

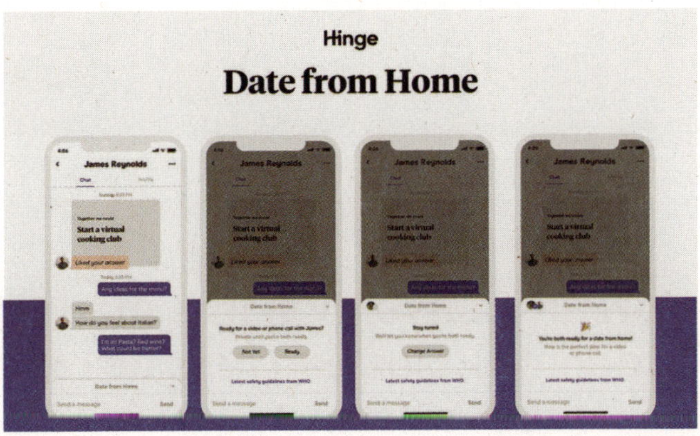

ROSES

Wallpaper designed by Sidney Mawson
and made by Jeffrey & Co, UK, c1907.

How an intervention that made new use of a sudden surplus can help us rethink the design of production systems

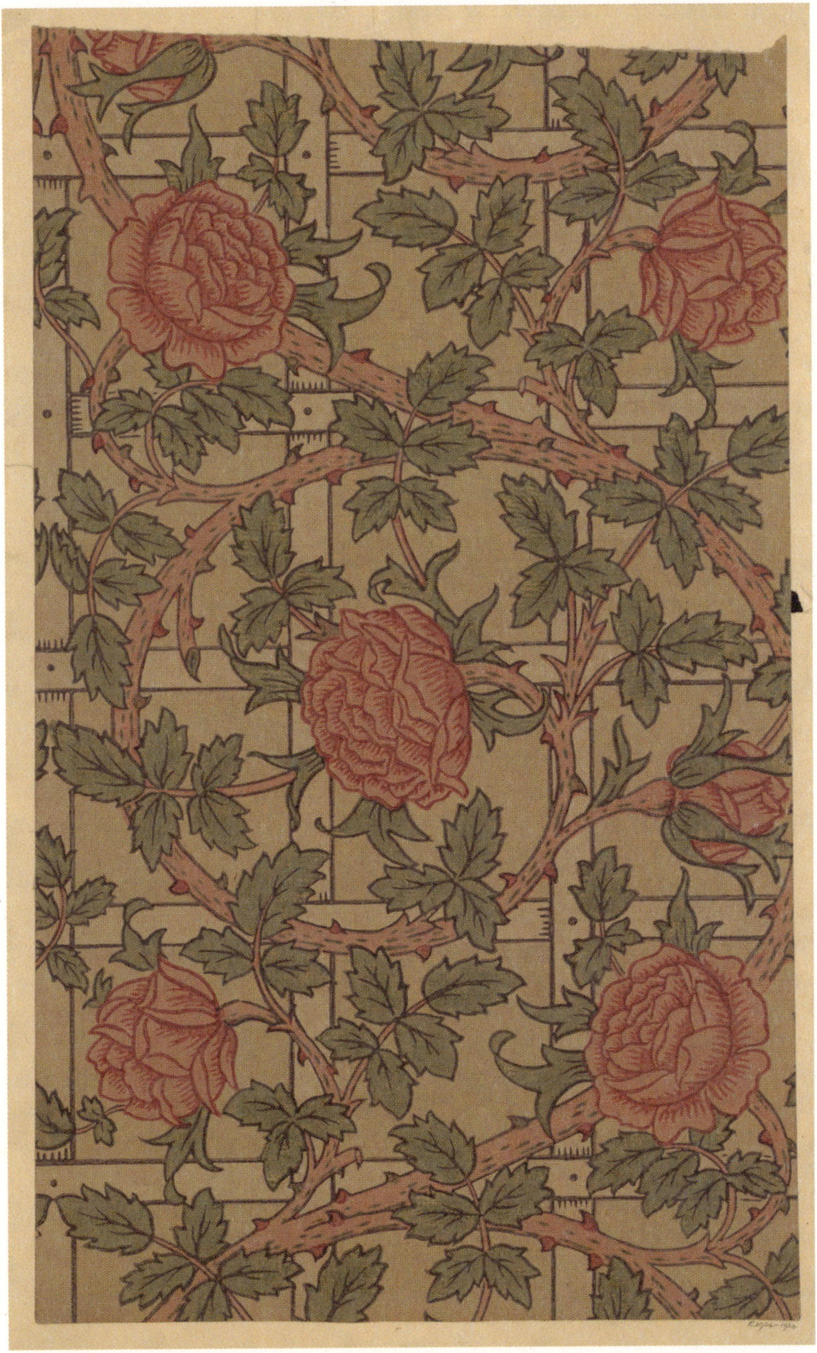

The cut flower industry was hit particularly hard by the Covid-19 pandemic. With weddings, anniversaries and other social events cancelled, the occasion for buying and gifting bouquets and arrangements suddenly vanished. Flowers wilted and decayed; truckloads were dumped in fields or were used for fodder and compost. In the Netherlands, the hashtag #BuyFlowersNotToiletPaper was circulated in a bid to rescue their beloved national industry. While in London this particular crisis was felt with the closure of flower shops, there were – as with so many things about Covid-19 – knock-on effects at the other end of the supply chain, out of sight from the average UK consumer.

One of those places is Kenya, where a huge rose industry has developed over the past few decades. Tens of thousands of flower workers were sent home without pay because of the pandemic – workers who were already leading precarious lives due to low earnings from their jobs. At the same time, massive crops of roses were left to die in their plasticulture rows, haunting scenes that were captured by Coltrane McDowell in his 2020 short film *The Scent of Economic Loss*. A student in the Social Design programme at the Design Academy Eindhoven, McDowell spent several months on the Tambuzi rose farm in Kenya using his iPhone and a GoPro to document the changes unleashed on the land by the pandemic. Throughout this period, he also worked with the farm owner to set up a system for distilling the flowers into rose oil, rescuing some of the production from oblivion. The narrative of the film poetically explores the nature of global supply chains, using the rose as a fragile carrier of symbolic value.

The problem of sudden surplus and plummeting demand hit several industries at once during the pandemic. The crisis inflicted dire challenges and anguish everywhere, with layoffs and so-called 'zombie jobs' that might never return. But in McDowell's effort to save some of the surplus flowers, a powerful story is revealed. The film begins to uncover the role design can play in helping industries think about managing change, helping them to creatively reconsider how existing infrastructure, labour and materials might be preserved and reconfigured to continue adding value. What new forms can a production site take, which both preserve the knowledge and expertise of its staff, and also produce something entirely new?

Text by Brendan Cormier

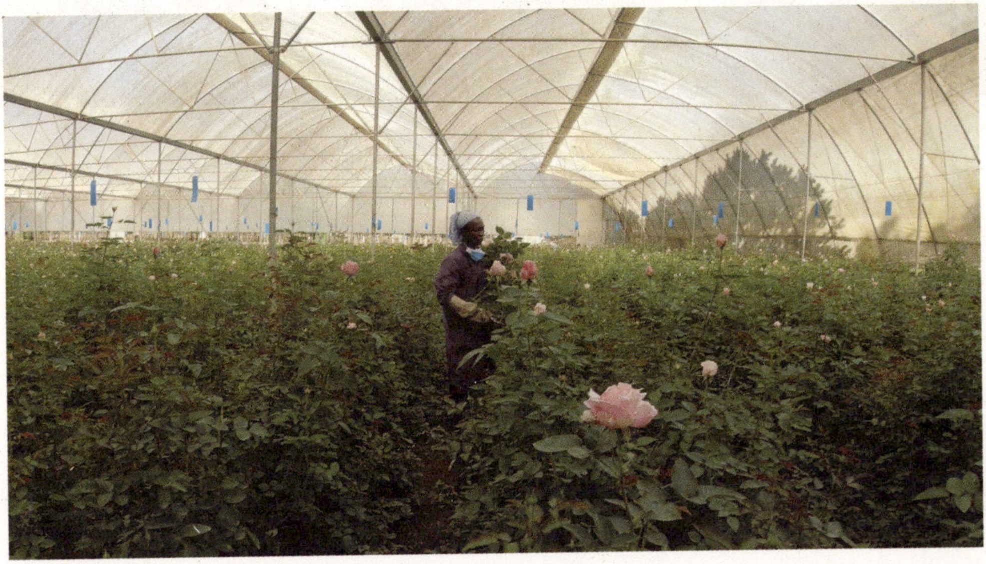

Still from *The Scent of Economic Loss* by Coltrane McDowell.

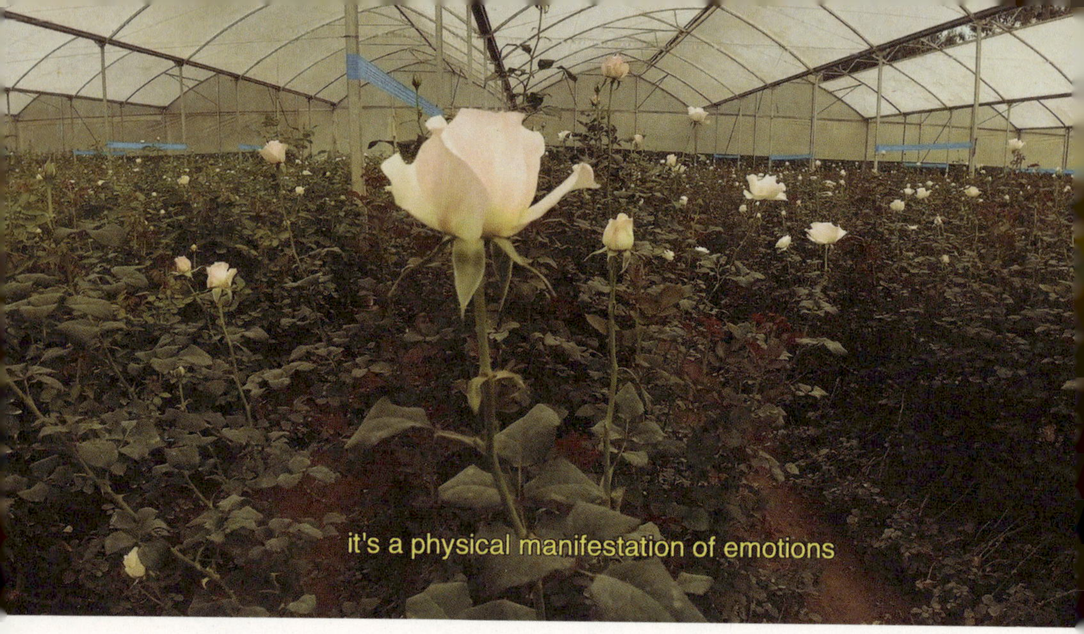

Stills from *The Scent of Economic Loss* by Coltrane McDowell.

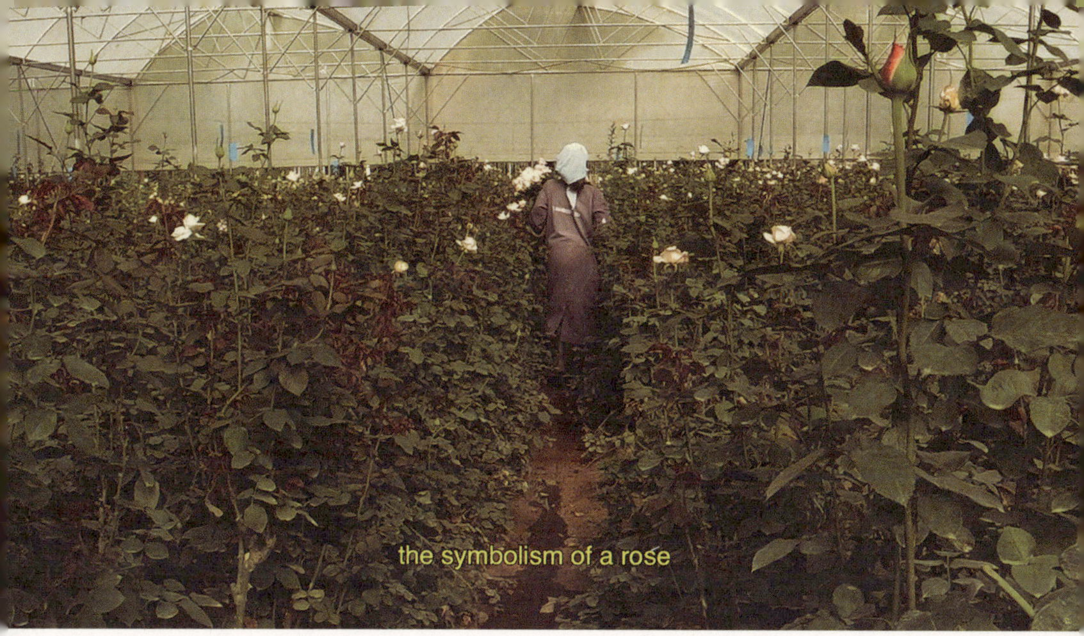

PIVOT

AL FRESCO

How al fresco dining transformed spaces within the city into new outdoor areas for social interaction and casual eating

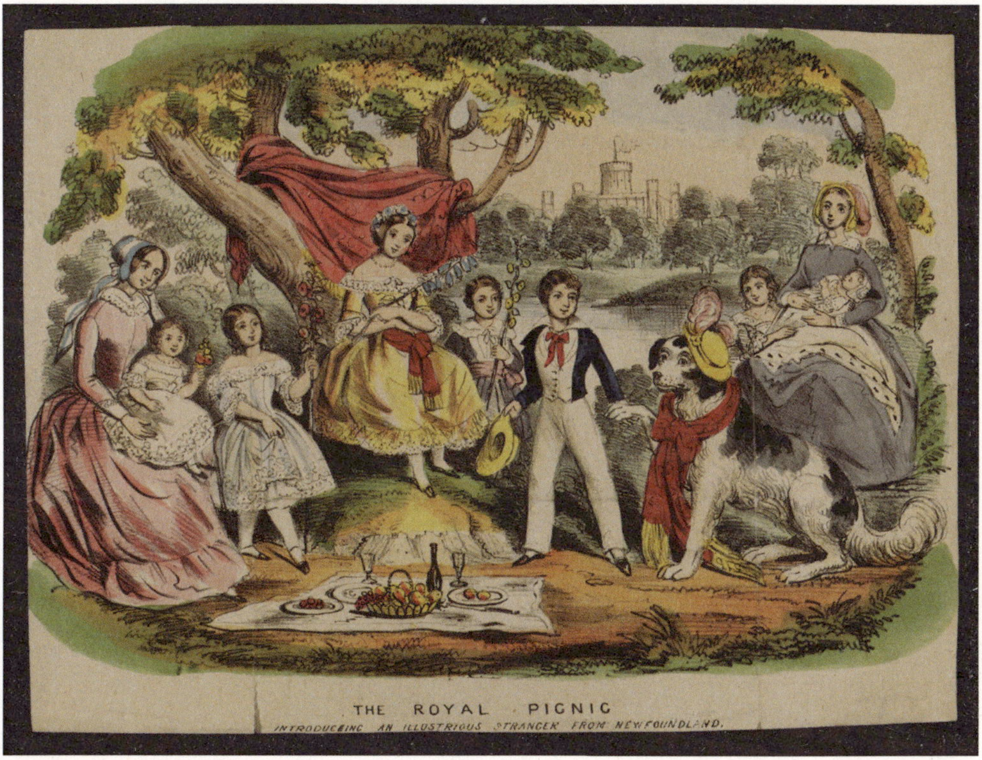

The Royal Picnic introducing an illustrious stranger from Newfoundland, Great Britain, c1850.

In October 2020, my sister and I used a room at the back of our Toronto home as a staging area for an outdoor Thanksgiving meal. Though public health officials had advised hosting no more than 25 people outside, our group was cautiously capped at ten. Guests sporting masks and woolly layers arrived in the garden bearing elaborate salads, steaming roast vegetables and freshly baked sweet and savoury pies. Potluck contributions were arranged on a table inside, with guests invited to identify their preferred dishes and then receive their plates one-by-one through an opened window – a delivery method not unlike the reactivation of 16th-century Florentine wine windows, small apertures for the sale of wine that have proved particularly useful as a social distancing measure, first during the plague of 1630 and again in 2020.

Eating outside – in gardens and parks; on porches, sidewalks and patios – became increasingly normalised in 2020 as numerous regions clamped down on indoor gatherings in response to the pandemic. While eating 'al fresco' was once one of several options for communal dining, Covid-19 made noshing *en plein air* the new default. Technically speaking, the term 'al fresco' derives from the Italian words for 'fresh air' and can refer to myriad outdoor dining scenarios, many of which were explored and innovated during the pandemic. One example, picnicking, an activity hitherto associated with mild temperatures, bucolic settings and unfussy foods, became a popular cold weather pastime.

Francis Frith, *Group at a Spanish café*, c1850–70.

In some cities, swift amendments were made to municipal rules to expand al fresco dining infrastructures. According to David Rider, writing in the *Toronto Star*, the CafeTO programme led to 801 new, temporary patios across Toronto, 'including more than 200 in curb lanes closed to vehicle traffic'. Restaurants and bars hustled to adapt and build comfortable outdoor spaces: in a BBC News piece from October 2020, Sophie Williams gives examples of London and Boston establishments buying yurts and tents and enclosing their patios. As a result of surging commercial and personal interest, many stores reported selling out of canopy tents, outdoor heaters and firepit accessories during the 2020–21 winter season.

Prior to the pandemic, al fresco dining may have connoted an outdoor repast that was more refined, intentional and held in pristine settings. During the pandemic the feeling of fresh air and sunlight – or even bundling up to ward off an evening chill – amid the company of friends or strangers felt appealing regardless of the quality of the foodstuffs or the elegance of the backdrop. The pandemic revealed how the delights of al fresco dining can be truly democratic, taking place in a park, on a stoop or on a pop-up restaurant patio in a former bike lane, and appreciation for the social and sensorial pleasures of gathering to eat – wherever possible – has only grown.

By Esmé Hogeveen

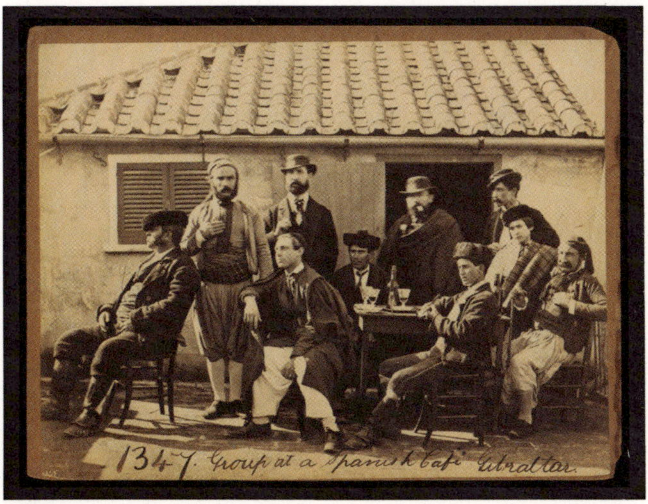

PUBLIC PARKS

How public parks became a vital setting for health, restoration and conviviality during the pandemic, reigniting the fight for better access to green spaces

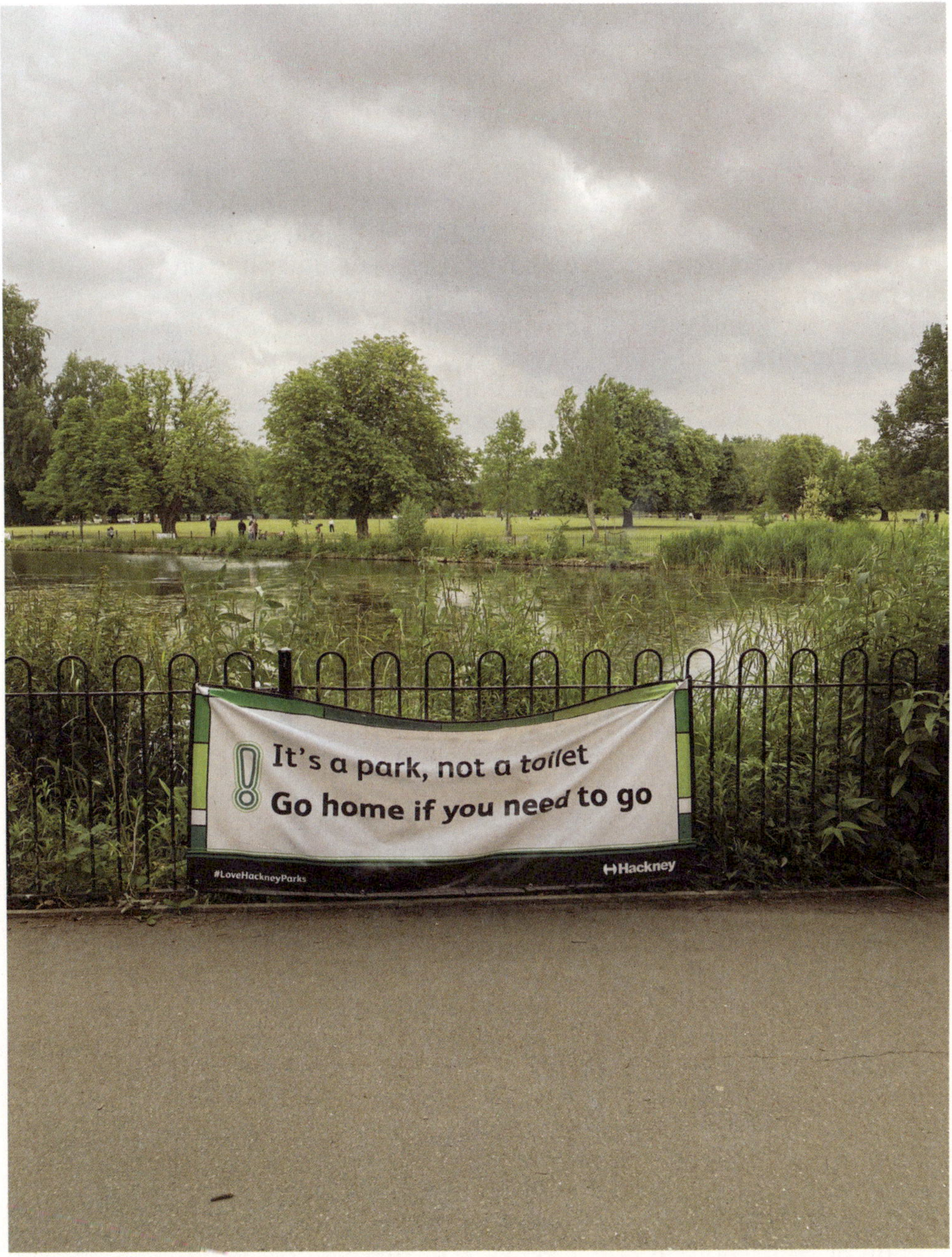

Polite reminder in Clissold Park, London.

The importance of green space for public health has long been known. From the outset of the first lockdown in the UK, outdoor exercise was permitted by the UK government, with restrictions on going outdoors progressively easing from there – from local walks once a day to 'unlimited' outdoor exercise, to permission to have a socially-distanced picnic. For those living in crowded cities, public parks played a vital role in restoring mental and physical wellbeing: a space of collective healing during Covid.

Beliefs in the restorative capacities of the natural world are not new, and indeed 'nature cures' have long been thought to boost immunity and tackle respiratory health in particular – from the healing powers of sunlight, deployed in heliotherapy, to the vital necessity of fresh air, with 'air bathing' treatments implemented in 19th and 20th-century European sanatoria. The more intangible, emotional joys of reconnecting with the natural environment are also powerful. In early lockdown, Instagram feeds marked the arrival of spring with endless documentation of tree blossoms as Londoners walked around more and perhaps spent more time in green spaces than ever before.

However, the use of public parks during the pandemic did not go uncontested. For one, public green space was an arena for confronting the dramatic change in social codes. Park use during the first UK lockdown had the memorable slogan of 'keep moving', where one was quite literally no longer permitted to sit. As parks were recalibrated for Covid-safe use, the traditional objects that furnish the green public realm were also taken out of operation. From police lines cordoning off brightly-coloured playgrounds (p341) to taped-up picnic tables and benches, the warning signs of an ongoing pandemic were constantly visible. New signs entered this sphere too, namely the graphic of two figures separated by an arrow (see The Ground p30), often conflicting with meandering lanes and narrow paths. Venturing off-path and traversing a rolling green expanse became a strategy to avoid others, and the old forms of careless casual strolling seemed no longer applicable.

Parks have a long history as a stage for diverse forms of behaviour on display – from conspicuous promenading in fashionable dress, performed in London's Vauxhall Pleasure Gardens throughout the 18th and 19th centuries, to the unspoken codes around group sport and safely flying frisbees today. German choreographer Pina Bausch created a poignant homage to the parade of behaviours in public parks with *1980*, a now-famed work of her *Tanztheater* (dance theatre) company in Wuppertal. As the realities of Covid-19 set in, public parks became the principal setting for leisure during the pandemic, and a stage for new choreographic practices of collective trust. Instances where such trust and consideration for socially-distanced leisure were reportedly considered lacking saw London park management introduce wardens to monitor behaviour, with structures for issuing fines.

The contested experience of public parks during the pandemic also sparked important debates over equitable access to green space. In the case of London, the UK's most densely populated region, the pressure on public parks was high. Google's Covid-19 response venture of 'Community Mobility Reports' (which was rightly flagged for privacy concerns) mapped global data patterns on park visitation, with London data from the end of May 2020 showing a 67% increase compared to Google's baseline. Successive weeks of lockdown saw surges in park visitor numbers, with many reported cases of overcrowding and threatened closures over public health concerns. The outcry over the temporary closure of Brockwell Park in south London in April 2020 proved a key turning point, throwing into sharp focus the long-existing inequalities of green space experience in London.

For many, in the absence of the luxury of a private garden (p114) or even a balcony (p346), public parks have been the only outdoor green spaces to offer respite from lockdown confinement. Access to parks remains unequal, with a report by *The Guardian* highlighting the city's wealthiest wards having the highest proportion of spaces, at 35%, compared to only 25% in the most deprived. Indeed, the very emergence of public parks, as distinct from commercial pleasure gardens and royal grounds, was part of a 19th-century movement to ensure fairer access to green space. Victoria Park in east London was the city's first purpose-designed public park, and opened in 1845 with a layout by architect James Pennethorne. It is not without significance that the very idea for its creation had its origins in a public health campaign sparked by epidemiologist William Farr, who called for the urgent need for green space and fresh air recreation in densely populated, working class urban zones. Local residents rallied, with more than 30,000 people signing a petition to Queen Victoria to create what became known as 'The People's Park'. During the pandemic, the ever-popular Victoria Park was overwhelmed with daily visitors, resulting in tight regulations for its use.

The pandemic provided a conclusive defence of the fundamental right to public parks, and this should not be forgotten. As shared community assets, public parks will continue to play an important role for public health, and the wider environmental balance of cities, as the living ecosystems and 'green lungs' that sequester carbon, purify air and help slow the dangerous pace of climate change. Across the UK it is estimated there are currently 27,000 parks. However, as the pandemic has shown, green public space is absolutely vital. We may look to other major cities for inspiration on enhancing access to nature in the public realm. For example, San Francisco's bold move to open vast swathes of golf course territory to the public during the pandemic sparked a petition for a similar policy in the UK. Urban design policy and housing developments will also need to safeguard public greenery in planning.

The public's reconnection with parks during the pandemic will hopefully have a lasting and vital benefit, as both a timely rekindling of people's close need for trees and green public spaces and a reappreciation of the crucial role these play in rebalancing polluted urban habitats. Understanding our entanglement with the natural world has never been more important.

Text by Zofia Trafas White

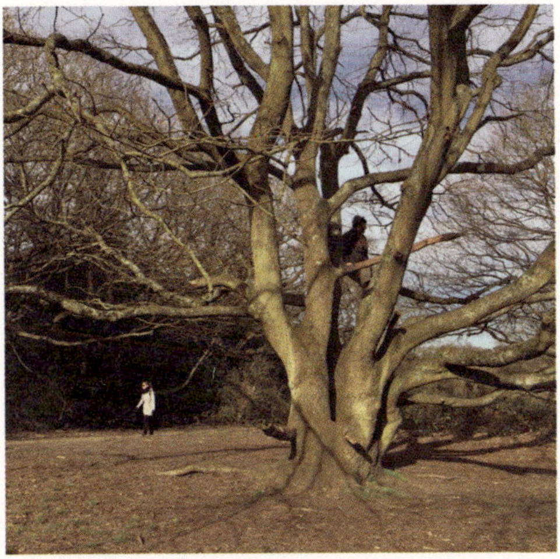

Hampstead Heath, London.

Plan for Victoria Park by James Pennethorne, London, 1841.

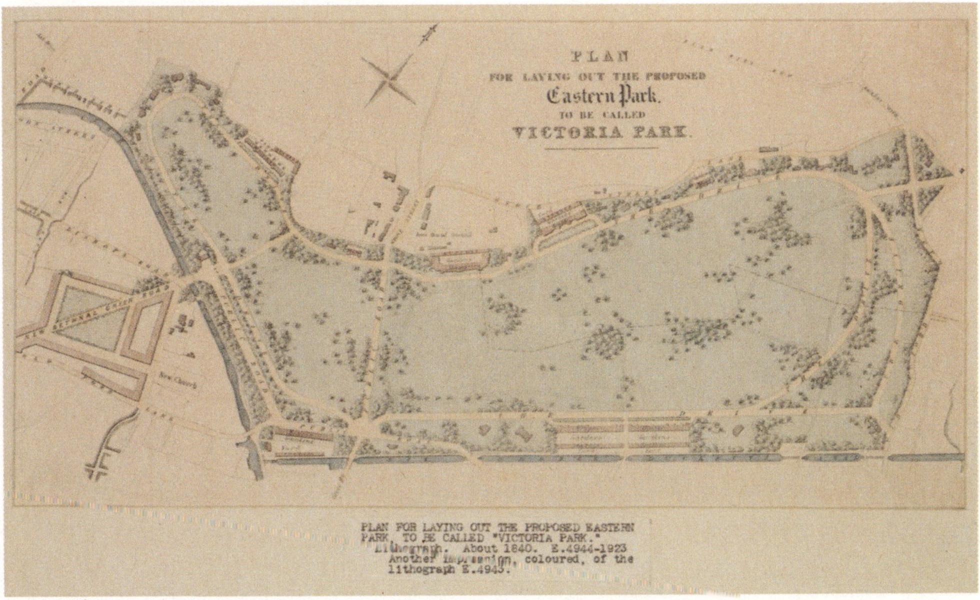

STUDENT HOUSING

How student housing during the pandemic became a flash point in a wider debate about university finances

PANDEMIC OBJECTS

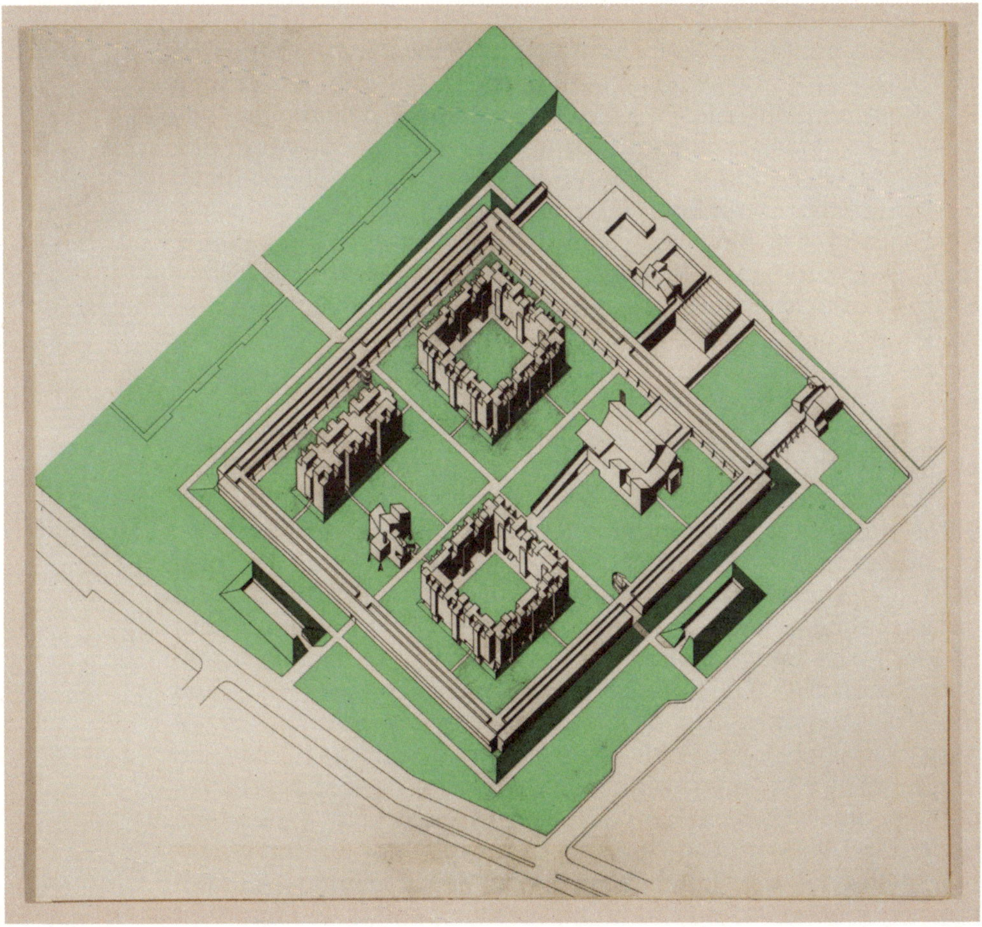

Competition drawing for Churchill College, University of Cambridge by Stirling and Gowan, UK, c1958.

The reopening of UK universities during the pandemic was subject to heated debates in the summer and autumn months of 2020, with approaches to student accommodation among the most contested issues. One prestigious English university made headlines for introducing new student accommodation contracts, which made eviction possible at short notice should new pandemic restrictions come into force. Elsewhere in England, the challenges of social distancing meant significant increases in rent, as twin rooms were turned into singles and students were charged double as a result. In Scotland, meanwhile, new legislation gave students the right to end or cancel their tenancy for coronavirus-related reasons, offering new, better protection to students in uncertain times.

The rush back to campus during a pandemic brought into sharp relief the ideological commitments of the UK higher education sector today. The desire to attract students back to their university-owned and supposedly Covid-19-safe housing, was, of course, an issue of university finance – the university accommodation sector is today worth a staggering £72 billion. But campus accommodation is also an important part of the kind of 'student experience' that many have come to expect. As Carla Yanni, author of *Living on Campus: An Architectural History of the American Dormitory* (2019), puts it, 'residence halls are not mute containers for the temporary storage of youthful bodies and emergent minds. They reveal', she argues, the 'educational ideals of the people who built them'. The idea of the student experience goes hand-in-hand with the rise to prominence of dedicated, often purpose-built student accommodation. Communal student housing embedded within the university space is an important tool of a particularly Anglo-American educational ideology, motivated by a commitment to socialisation through interactions occuring both in and outside of the classroom.

While most of the oldest European universities, including the University of Bologna, Utrecht University and the Sorbonne, did not offer substantial dedicated student accommodation until the 19th century, in the UK and the US living on campus has always been an integral part of university education. At the University of Oxford and the University of Cambridge, medieval monasteries served as the architectural precursors of the characteristic quadrangle model of college accommodation (which in turn became a model for many colleges in the US, including Thomas Jefferson's Academical Village at the University of Virginia, the Radcliffe Quadrangle at Harvard University and the Old Campus at Yale University). Notably, Harvard's first governing board thought that provision of on-campus accommodation, integrated into the college space and separate from the world outside of it, provided a unique advantage to learning. It was believed that cohabitation as part of this scholarly community – which studied, ate, slept and socialised together – was to create America's first class of leaders. In this Anglo-American model, then, university and college accommodation was designed to construct and maintain cultural norms and hierarchies, and to encourage socially acceptable forms of interaction. When University College London (UCL) was first established in 1826, its critics saw the lack of a student accommodation provision as proof that this new institution was no real university at all.

In the years following the Second World War, as access to university education increased and the higher education sector expanded dramatically, a boom in construction of dedicated student accommodation also followed. The University of California, for example, could house 2,900 students across all of its nine campuses in 1958; by 1970, its capacity had increased to 20,000 residential spaces. In the UK, 67 new on-campus student halls were built across the country between 1944 and 1957, supported by dedicated government funding. Postwar university accommodation became somewhat more democratic, but the integration of housing with the idea of student experience remained central; as the authors of *Which University?*, a UK university guide published in 1964, put it, 'many people now feel that for students to live at home is a negation of the idea of university education'. The 1960s university expansion saw a proliferation of new campuses across the UK, often in modern and brutalist styles, inclusive of comprehensive accommodation provision. Today, in the UK more than 80% of all full-time students leave home for study and around 30% live in purpose-built student halls. In Ireland, on the other hand, one study showed that two thirds of undergraduate students live with their parents and in Australia students are more likely to live in their family home than at the university. Across Europe, only 18% of students live in dedicated accommodation.

The role of student housing in the UK is such a central part of the student experience that *Times Higher Education* – a leading trade publication for the higher education sector – now publishes a league table ranking the top 50 student accommodation halls in the UK. A far cry from the student housing blocks of only 20 years ago – somewhat shabby, a tad smelly, furnished with the least comfortable beds and decorated with compulsory garish curtains – student accommodation today is increasingly designed to impress. The website mystudenthalls.com's ranking list of 'Top

Ten Instagrammable Student Halls' mentions the Stay Club in Colindale, London – which features an in-house nightclub, picturesque roof terrace, cinema room and lounge area lined with vinyl records – and Scotway House in Glasgow, furnished with playful neon art, pink velvet seating and lush green hanging plants.

What has not changed with the arrival of the 'luxury' student accommodation block, however, is the temporary nature of student housing. An exact copy of the other 300 rooms in a purpose-built student accommodation block, a student room is a space of transition into the freedom and independence of adulthood (with few of the associated responsibilities). It is never designed to feel like home. During the pandemic, when home came to represent a new kind of intense and enforced domesticity, this unhomelike space posed unanticipated challenges. While some student accommodation halls have replaced communal bathrooms with individual en-suite showers and swapped communal dining halls for modern kitchens in self-catered flats, these residences remain set up for communal living; shared spaces designed to enable and encourage interaction. That is, they constitute a model of living which makes social distancing difficult at best.

As universities prepared to welcome their students at the start of the academic year in 2020, assurances of Covid-19-related safety provisions for accommodation were aplenty. But reports of Covid-19 cases among students started proliferating almost as soon as they returned to universities. According to data collated by UniCovidUK, on 2 November 2020 there were 34,555 reported student cases across 119 UK universities. Student accommodation blocks became the new Covid-19 hotspots – 'the care homes of the second wave of the pandemic,' as *The Guardian*'s Jonathan Wolff put it – and heavily contested spaces of living. Monitored by private security firms implementing strict lockdown rules, the student accommodation block became one of the most heavily policed spaces of the pandemic. This transformation of the ways in which bodies in these spaces were monitored and controlled made visible the disciplinary function of educational institutions in new and unexpected ways. And while, as Michel Foucault reminds us, discipline is always a characteristic feature of education, the new restrictions imposed on student housing proved controversial not as a means of controlling Covid-19 outbreaks but because they simultaneously encouraged and prohibited the very approach to student experience that has made communal accommodation such a significant component of university education.

The restrictions placed on students living in accommodation blocks where outbreaks were recorded proved particularly strict, far surpassing those imposed on people self-isolating elsewhere. As a result, grassroots activist groups emerged on campuses across the UK. The introduction of fencing around halls of residence in Manchester as a Covid-19 control measure led to a wave of student protests in the city. The 'Cut the Rent' campaign called for rent strikes in a number of major university cities (with 1,000 students pledging to join the rent strike in Bristol alone). Others, including the 'Students Before Profit' group, campaigned for better conditions for students experiencing lockdown in halls. Demands from different groups varied, but pressure to release students from their accommodation contracts was a prominent feature of the campaigns. As a second lockdown was announced in the UK on 31 October 2020, and speculation grew of a pre-Christmas university lockdown, growing numbers of students chose to, quite unsurprisingly, defy the guidance, leave their student accommodation and get back home before new restrictions came into force. This unseasonal exodus of students was a telling manifestation of the changing function, meaning and perception of student halls during Covid-19. No longer hubs of activity and hardly essential to the student experience – which, during the lockdowns, was socially distanced and predominantly lived online – student halls became a poignant symbol of the commercialisation of the higher education sector and a stark expression of the broader impact of economic pressures during the pandemic.

Text by Kaja Marczewska

Norfolk Terrace Student Accommodation at the University of East Anglia, designed by Denys Lasdun, UK, 1962-68.

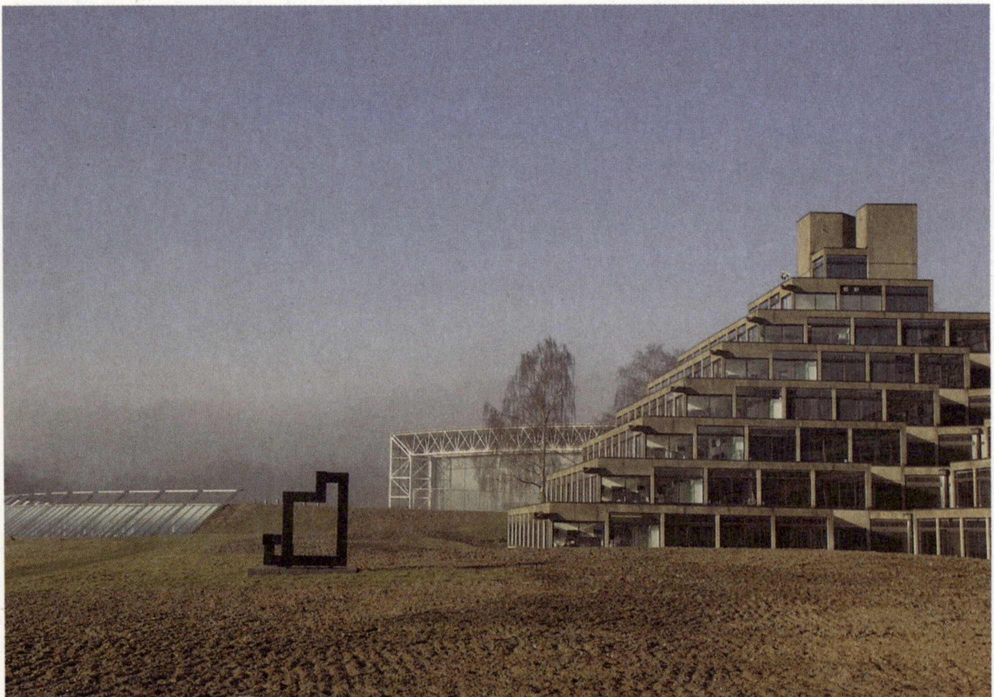

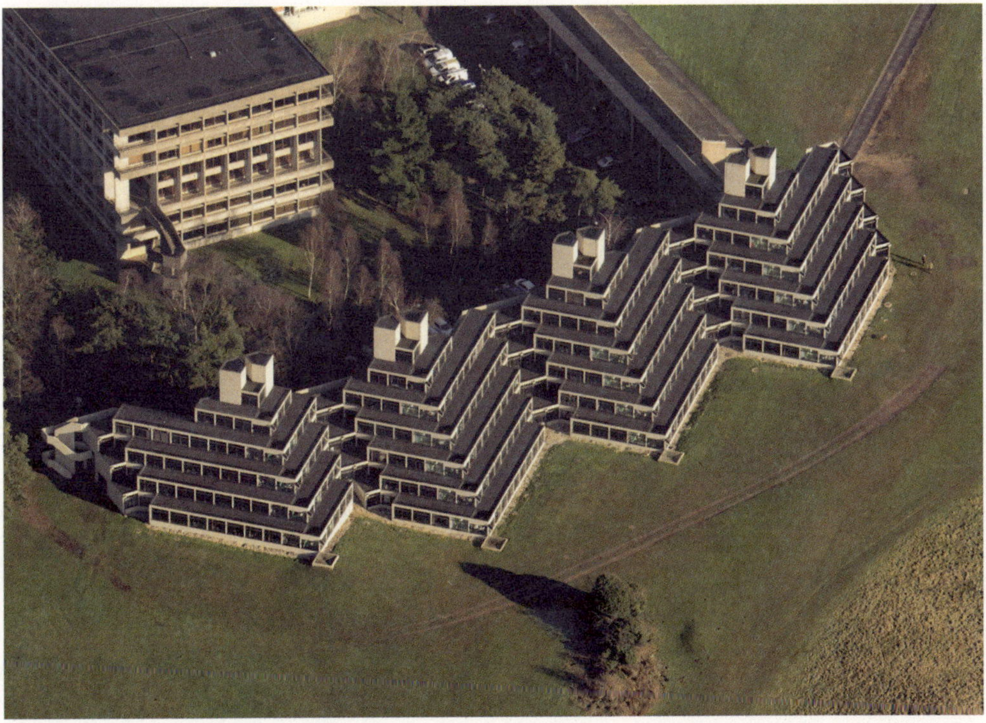

PIVOT

BEDS

Aubrey Beardsley, *Self-Portrait in Bed*,
Great Britain, 1894.

How the bed became a workspace, both as an ersatz desk and as an arena for self-promotion online

PANDEMIC OBJECTS

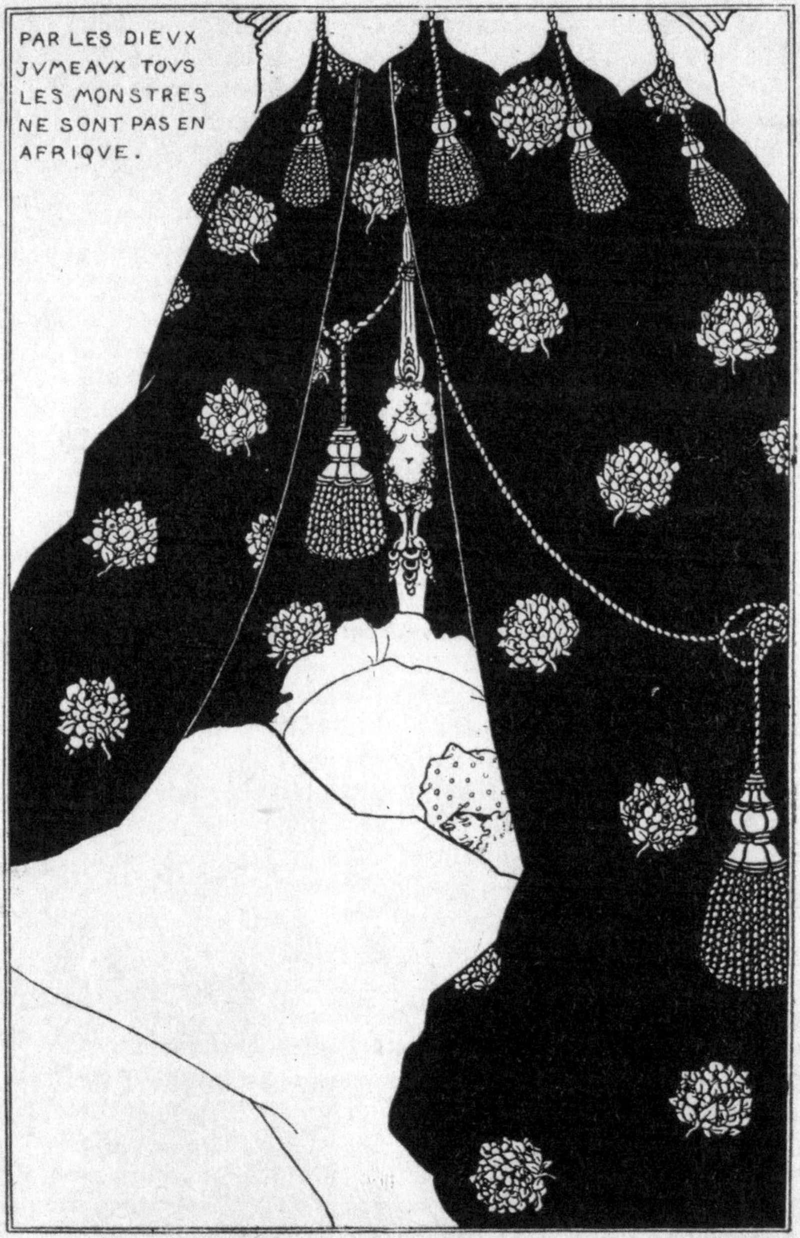
PAR LES DIEVX
JVMEAVX TOVS
LES MONSTRES
NE SONT PAS EN
AFRIQVE.

PIVOT

When the first lockdown in 2020 saw office workers suddenly compelled to work from home, for many that meant work from bed. By the end of that year, the BBC reported a study showing that 72% of those surveyed sometimes worked from bed, with as many as one in ten spending 'most or all of their workweek' in bed. Much of this phenomenon may have been down to the sudden availability of repose; a welcome collapse in the face of overwhelming uncertainty and exhausting news cycles. For many, however, working from bed was the best, or only, real option. Small bedrooms in shared flats may have afforded enough space when the city could accommodate almost all of our wakeful functions, but in lockdown these collapsed back into the home – and into the bed.

This had a disproportionate effect on young workers, more likely to live in major cities on starter salaries, with UK workers aged 18–34 twice as likely to work from bed as their older counterparts. By early 2021, articles had begun to appear that warned about the 'ergonomic nightmare' being inflicted upon spines everywhere, as well as the importance of 'sleep hygiene' – in which all the associations of work and wakefulness must be kept off clean bedsheets in order to preserve rest.

The working bed is not new: both Pliny the Elder and Younger wrote from bed, as did John Milton, Jean-Jacques Rousseau and Truman Capote, who in 1957 told *Paris Review* that 'I am a completely horizontal author. I can't think unless I'm lying down'. In an August 1942 entry for *Esquire*, Salvador Dalí declared his proudest symbol to be 'The sign on my sleeping chamber, "POET WORKING"', while in 1960, Hugh Hefner relocated his office to his bed when he moved into the first Playboy Mansion in Chicago. But the widespread encroachment of work into our most intimate spaces during a pandemic does not reflect the languorous working lives implied with the figures of Hefner, Dalí and Capote. The news sites and wellness blogs that decried the state of our sleep hygiene generally posed this as a failure of personal discipline, a matter of individual choice and individual fault, rather than the result of broader forces. But this latest advancement is just another sign of the global creep towards perpetual productivity, with late capitalism finding sleep as its final frontier.

As Jonathan Crary noted in *24/7: Late Capitalism and the Ends of Sleep*, published in 2013, the US Defense Department had spent the past few years researching a particularly sleepless type of sparrow, hoping to push back against the human soldier's as-yet unconquerable need for rest. 'As history has shown,' he commented, 'war-related innovations are inevitably assimilated into a border social sphere'. The sleepless soldier would be the forerunner of the sleepless worker or consumer, and the 'expanding, non-stop life-world of 21st-century capitalism' would come to be 'characterised as a generalised inscription of human life into duration without breaks, defined by a principle of continuous functioning'. This interminable condition is what he called '24/7'; 'a time of indifference, against which the fragility of human life is increasingly inadequate and within which sleep has no necessity or inevitability'.

The working bed of the present is the manifestation of this condition. While the beds of the Renaissance were rooms unto themselves, with posts to carry a roof above them and curtains that held the world at bay, the 24/7 bed is far from contained – it is globally networked, infinite, continuous. More than a piece of furniture, it is the world: obtuse to archaic distinctions between life and work, private and public, interior and exterior, self and other. As Beatriz Colomina wrote in *The Architectural Review* in 2020, 'post-industrialisation collapses work back into the home and takes it further into the bedroom and into the bed itself. The whole universe is concentrated on a small screen with the bed floating in an infinite sea of information. To lie down is not to rest but to move. The bed is now a site of action'.

These actions are, of course, largely sedentary, performed propped up on a slope of pillows and surrounded by the debris of the day – mugs, chargers, books, plates or packets of snacks. These auxiliary objects are just satellites to a gravitational centre defined by the twin pulls of the laptop and the mobile phone. These devices are portals to Colomina's 'infinite sea'; they bring colleagues into bed with us through video calls, providing ever-growing glimpses into one another's lives and granting new intimacies. They also provide permanent, unceasing exchange with the endless social-commercial sea of social media sites, venues for the production of a self that is increasingly for sale.

Eugène Atget, *Intérieur de Monsieur T, négociant, rue Montaigne*, Paris, 1910.

This was another condition accelerated by the pandemic. As so many workers were laid off or casualised amid a global economic recession, social media sites became increasingly populated by small businesses – often individuals running a solo operation – eking out a living by marketing themselves through platforms like TikTok and Instagram. Meanwhile, media workers turned to individualised subscription-model endeavours through Substack and Patreon – the latter of which saw 30,000 'creators' registering on the site during the first three weeks of March 2020, the fastest rate in the site's history. This growing individualisation of work – in which every worker is their own complete enterprise; in which the product they are marketing is a representation or fantasy of themself – was perhaps epitomised in the pandemic success of OnlyFans. Simply put, OnlyFans is Patreon for pornography; creators can post content, gather followers and charge subscription fees. The site blossomed dramatically during the pandemic, going from 7.5 million users in November 2019 to 85 million by the end of December 2020 – with transactions rising seven-fold by April 2021, to £1.7 billion. Part of OnlyFans' success, as well as what differentiates its operating model from other adult sites, is that it takes the kind of parasocial relationships that develop on social media and monetises them; the idolisation that happens on Instagram is met with the interactivity of a cam site, with all the seediness stripped out. OnlyFans drew in new customers who had never paid for pornography before, as well as performers making their first adult content – most of it put together in private bedrooms. As with TikTok, on OnlyFans any person can be a performer and any bed is a stage: hundreds of thousands of beds working overtime as atomised arenas for the elaboration of any manner of fantasy.

Text by Max Zarzycki

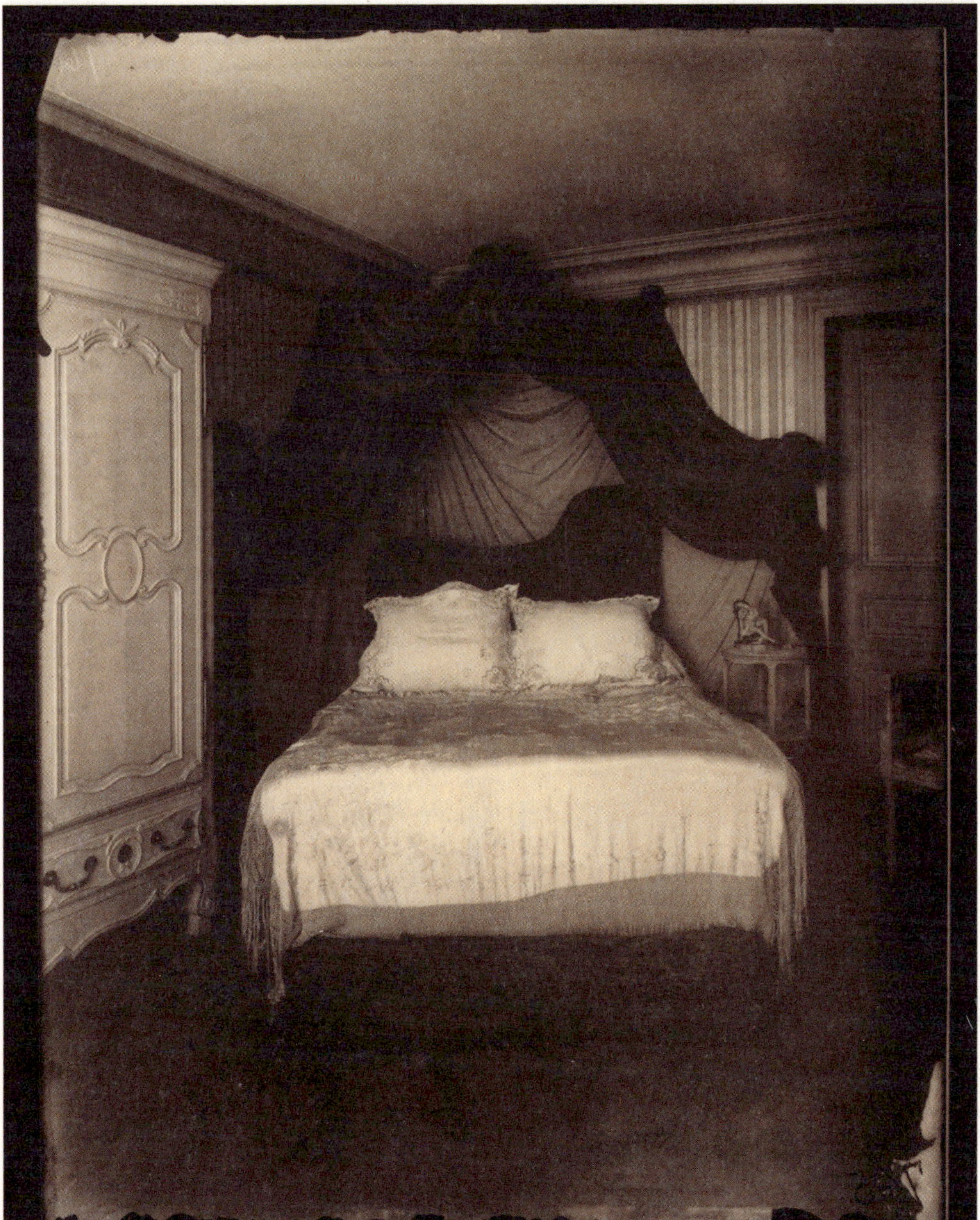

PIVOT

06

REAPPROPRIATE

Objects are defined by their uses – a chair to sit on, a ladder to climb, a book to read. These uses quickly become conventions, dulling our imagination to what else they might do. The truth is, objects can be deployed for myriad functions – a chair props up a houseplant, a ladder becomes a towel rack, a book becomes a doorstop. With limited access to goods at the beginning of the pandemic, an opportunity arose to break free from the conventional uses of things, to hack new ways of getting things done in the absence of other more specialised tools. Sometimes these hacks revealed a deeper meaning to things – a chair is just as much a tool for sitting as it is a symbol for conviviality, while a convention centre is an architectural free space, designed for maximum flexibility. What the pandemic revealed in this instance was both our creativity in adapting objects to new needs, but also the infinite capacity of objects to take on new meaning.

CONVENTION CENTRES

How the inherent flexibility of convention centres led to their reappropriation as centres for care

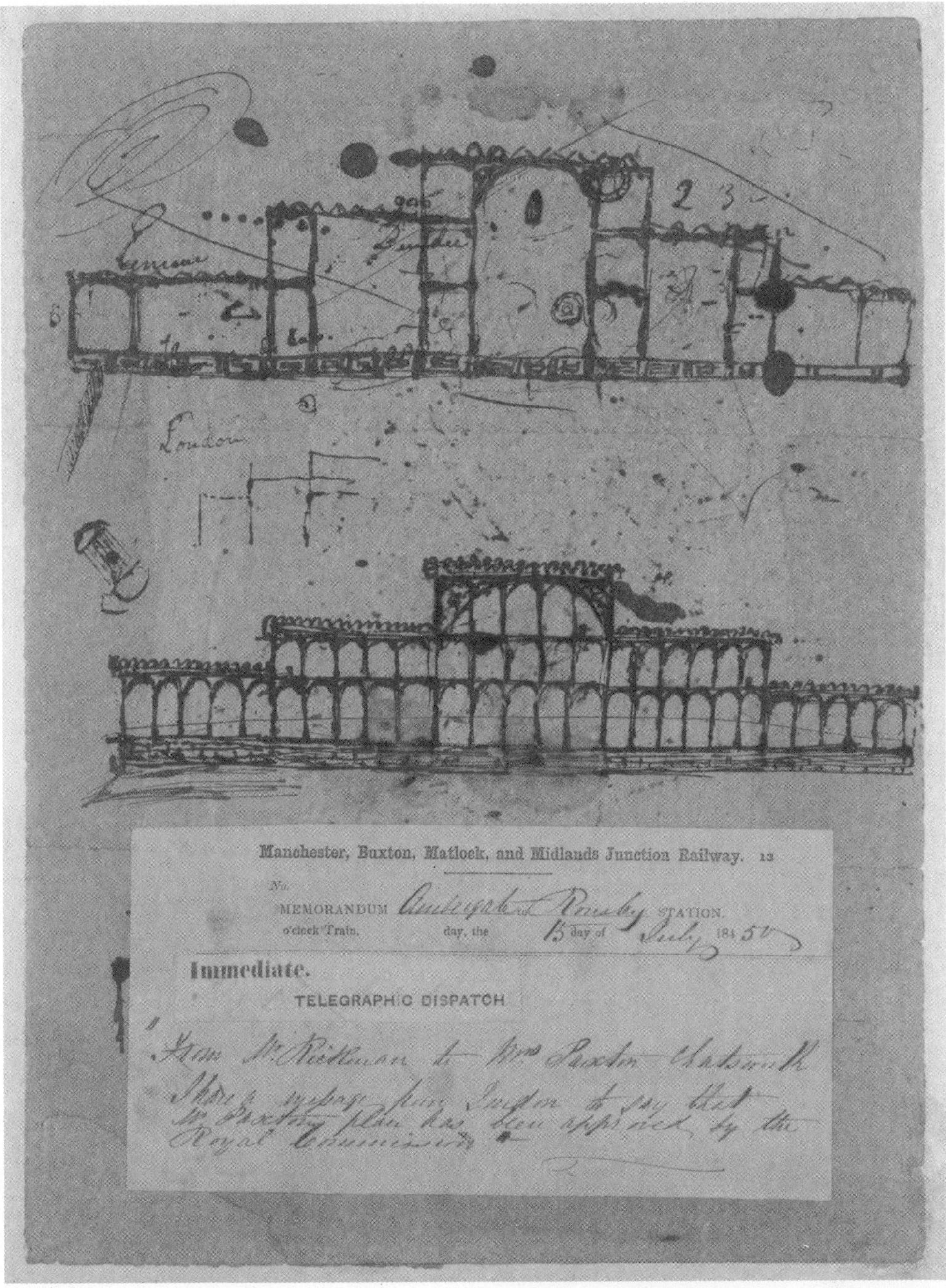

Joseph Paxton, architectural sketch for Crystal Palace, Derby, 1850.

In the spring of 2020, the events planned for London's ExCeL Centre – one of the UK's largest trade show venues – included Intelligent Building Europe, The Call & Contact Centre Expo, Oceanology International, The European Pizza & Pasta Show and, of course, a Comic Con. None of these went ahead – instead, the centre was temporarily converted into an emergency hospital, one of seven NHS Nightingale facilities that were created around the country to respond to the Covid-19 pandemic.

The convention centre typology was surprisingly suited for this. While there are some exceptions, most modern exhibition centres consist of windowless sheds which serve as stage sets for exhibitors' stands. They are typically navigated by vast alphanumeric grids, which have visitors trotting endlessly without the general vista changing all that much. A73 in Hall B looks exactly like F26 in Hall A, only with a different type of pasta on show, or a new tool for oceanographic exploration. This is the point of such spaces. They are highly serviced and highly adaptable.

The convention centre is so embedded into its ancillary infrastructure that it's sometimes difficult to understand as a single complex. Venues often have their own train stations (the Köln Messe stop for Cologne's main halls; the Rho Fieramilano station for Milan's enormous expo complex) which help shuttle visitors in the tens of thousands from nearby airports directly into the venue. ExCeL sits right next to London City Airport. In Las Vegas, one of the US's trade show capitals (the Strip alone boasts 10.5 million square feet of exhibition space), halls are attached to resorts, casinos and public transit systems, with distinctions between any of these spaces thoroughly obscured.

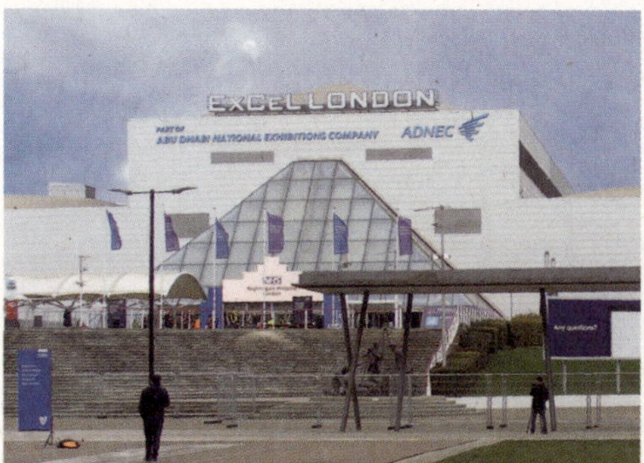

The ExCeL Centre transformed into NHS Nightingale London, March 2020.

It is nonetheless a recognisable building typology with roots in the earliest World Expositions of the mid-to-late 19th century. London's Crystal Palace, which was built in Hyde Park to host the first such event, the Great Exhibition of 1851, was a precursor to the ExCeLs of today. The technologies used to construct it – notably cast iron and sheet glass – were part of the display of the British Empire's industrial prowess at the time. Crystal Palace accommodated more than 14,000 exhibitors and welcomed some 6 million people during its five-month run. Today's convention centres have a quicker turnaround of trade shows (often weekly) and have adapted their infrastructure accordingly. The 1980s and 1990s in particular, as stated by Heywood Sanders in his 2014 book *Convention Center Follies*, was a time when many new purpose-built convention centres were erected. This occured, in part, by accelerating globalised trade, cheap international travel and local governments eager to invest in venues promising a boost in commercial activity.

The ExCeL's transformation was far from unique. In the early days of the pandemic, the China Optics Valley Convention and Exhibition Center in Wuhan was reportedly turned into a 1,000-bed hospital in just 24 hours. Other countries followed suit: the Bashundhara Convention Centre in Dhaka, Bangladesh; the Centro de Convenciones Bicentenario in Quito, Ecuador; and the Javits Center in New York City were only some of the venues transformed into makeshift medical facilities at breakneck speed. In England, seven NHS Nightingale Hospitals were adapted from existing venues into critical care hospitals in March and April. The two largest ones, in Birmingham and London, prepared temporary hospitals with the planned capacity of 4,000–5,000 beds within the National Exhibition Centre (NEC) and the ExCeL respectively.

Nightingale London in the ExCeL was built in just nine days with the help of the Royal Anglian Regiment and Royal Gurkha Rifles alongside NHS staff and contractors, officially opening on 3 April 2020. Nightingale Birmingham in the NEC followed a fortnight later. The speed at which this happened is testament to the enormous effort put in by all involved, but also to the sheer malleability of the convention centre space. BDP, the architecture firm tasked with designing the Nightingale Hospitals, published an instruction manual setting out some of the main principles of converting exhibition centres (or any 'large barn type spaces') into hospitals. Venue requirements, the manual says, include a 'clear

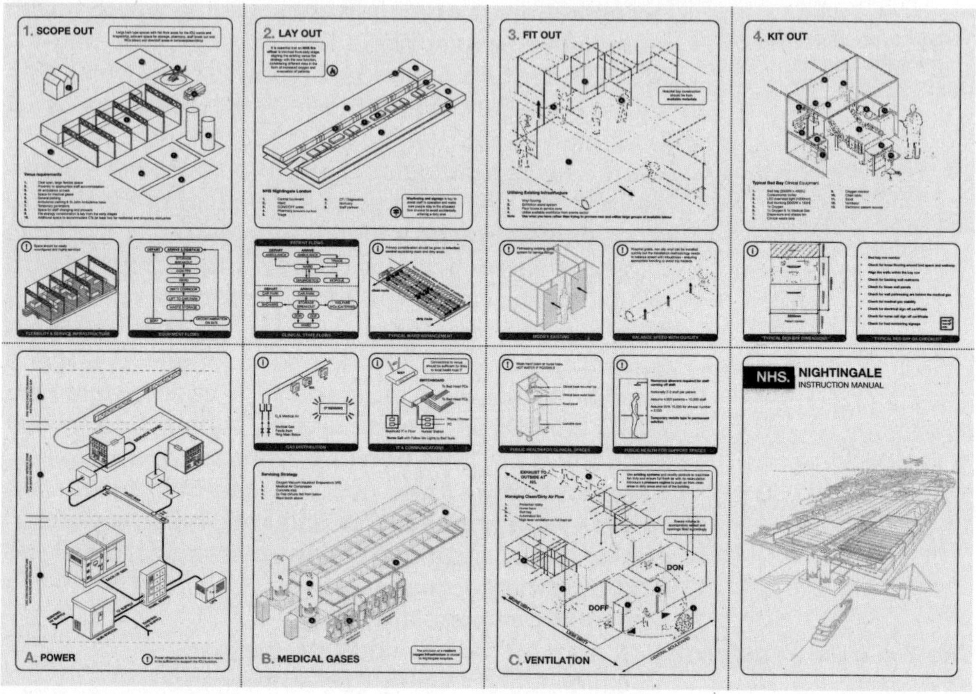

NHS Nightingale Instruction manual produced by BDP, UK, 2020.

span, large flexible space', 'proximity to appropriate staff accommodation', 'space for medical gases', and 'general parking', all of which were at hand at the ExCeL and NEC. It stressed the importance of using existing infrastructure, including exhibition stand systems for building bed bays, and seeking assistance from 'available workforce from the events sector'.

'Both the NEC and the ExCeL used exhibition stand systems,' explained Max Martin, an architect and Principal at BDP who worked on the Nightingale project. 'Those systems were quite simple because they're rectilinear, they clip and click together, and we could make them work for the sizes of the bays.' Ventilation, at least at the NEC, was also deemed to be sufficient for a temporary hospital. 'Because they're large, voluminous spaces that are typically used to having large numbers of people in them, they do have quite high air change rates,' he said.

Other aspects were more challenging. Exhibition centres generally have high electrical capacity, given the events they support, yet hospitals require not only capacity but 'electrical resilience'. Backup generators needed to be put in place to make the spaces more compliant. In addition, the delivery of medical gases – oxygen in particular – proved to be an especially difficult problem. The plumbing for oxygen supplies comes with its own specific fire risks and would normally take many weeks to lay out. 'You also need enough space to put up big gas tanks,' said Martin. Finally, there was the issue of delivering hot water to an unprecedented number of individual points. 'One of the big things with Covid-19, and with hospitals generally, is that you've got to wash your hands a lot. With thousands of beds, that involves lots of hand-wash basins.'

Nightingale London housed a small number of patients in its first weeks, but the demand was not as high as originally anticipated. At the beginning of May 2020, it was announced that most of the facilities would be mothballed and effectively put on standby. The ExCeL was eventually used as a vaccination centre, and closed in April 2021 – in the end, only 54 Covid-19 patients were treated there.

The official line, explained Martin, was that 'the purpose of all these buildings was to provide capacity should it be needed, and it's a positive thing that they've not been needed in quite the way it was thought'. But reports from within the Nightingales suggested that staffing shortages were at least partly to blame for the underuse of the facilities. The 4,000 beds of the London Nightingale would have required 16,000 staff to run at full capacity, an impossible ask for a health service that already had 100,000 vacancies going into the pandemic, and understaffing has only worsened since.

Convention centres converted into hospitals: it was a powerful image of many sectors of the global economy grinding to a halt in the wake of the virus. The significance of the Nightingales lay mostly in just that – their optics of capacity, regardless of the fact that there were not enough staff to fill them. Whether this hollow reassurance was worth the £530 million they cost is still up for debate.

Text by Kristina Rapacki

DISABLED PARKING SPACES

Poster campaign to shift attitudes towards disability, UK, c1980–85.

How changing uses of disabled parking spaces laid bare the ways in which the built environment fails to make space for everyone on equal terms

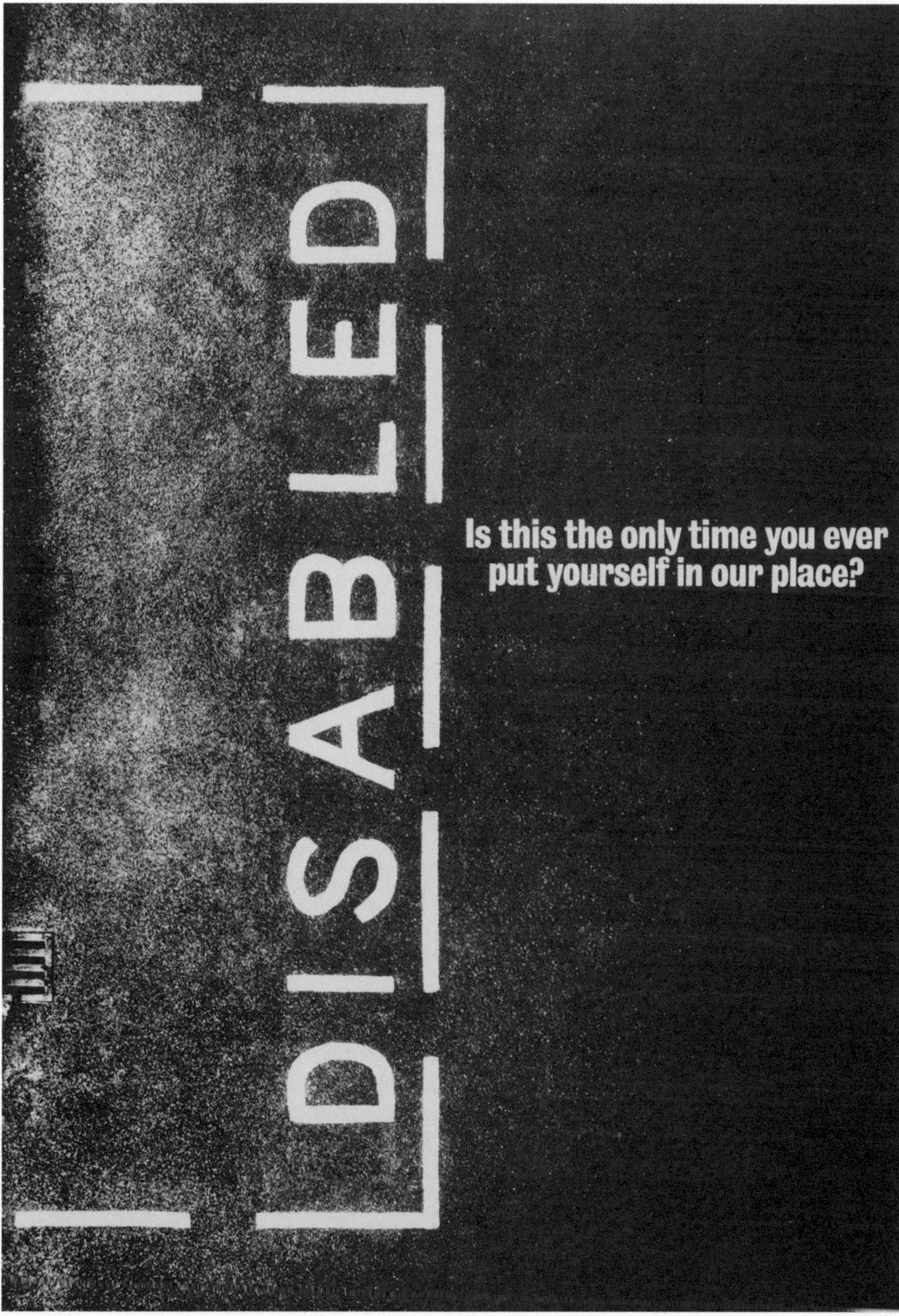
DISABLED
Is this the only time you ever put yourself in our place?

During the Covid-19 pandemic, public spaces across the UK were reconfigured to encourage social distancing. Restrictions on gathering indoors meant that long queues formed outside shops and supermarkets, snaking through car parks as shoppers maintained a two-metre distance between one another. In the summer of 2020, encouraged by Rishi Sunak's 'Eat Out to Help Out' scheme, many members of the British public made an enthusiastic return to pubs, bars and restaurants – often within newly created outdoor dining spaces that spilled onto roads (see Pubs p186 and Al Fresco p210). Additional cycle lanes were carved out of city streets to accommodate those who had chosen two wheels as an alternative to crowded trains and buses. For some, this was a welcome change from the de facto dominance of motorised transport, especially considering the escalating climate crisis; it felt as though people, rather than cars, were able to reclaim ownership of urban centres.

However, these reconfigurations resulted in many disabled parking spaces being decommissioned to make space for wider footways, queues, 'al fresco' dining areas, cycle lanes and car-free zones. Many disabled people consequently found that their ability to complete everyday tasks and participate in society was impeded. The repercussions were significant for a group already disproportionately affected by the pandemic. In turn, this highlighted the fragility of provisions made for disabled people in the built environment and raised important questions about how we define the concept of 'common good' in a health crisis.

Disabled parking spaces at a supermarket were taken over by barriers put in place to organise a queue system in May 2020.

Disabled parking spaces were formally introduced in England in 1971 through the Orange Badge Parking Scheme (now known as the Blue Badge Scheme), which, according to a UK government briefing paper on the subject, was intended to 'provide a national arrangement of parking concessions for disabled and blind people and [...] give them the ability to park close to the facilities and services they need'. These spaces are typically sited by the entrances to shops and amenities, or where parking is not otherwise permitted; because of this, their misuse is nothing new. Yet the Covid-19 pandemic was the first time that these spaces were so widely appropriated in the UK in favour of the needs of the non-disabled population. This could be the result of a misconception that Jos Boys highlights in her introduction to *Doing Disability Differently*: that disabled people are 'in need of the help of others, are passive consumers of services, [and] constitute a minority of

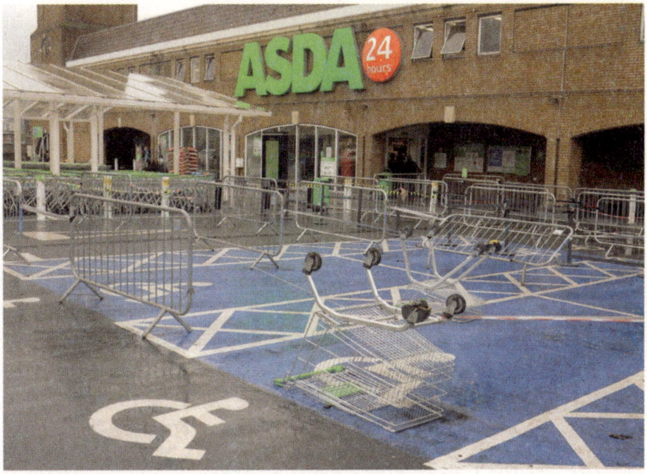

individuals in society who (unfortunately) must bear the brunt of their own medical problems'. The assumption was that disabled people would have to remain isolated as the pandemic wore on, and wouldn't be able to visit these areas; their access needs could therefore be sacrificed to allow others to 'get back to normal'.

This attitude is an example of the medical model of disability, which attributes the limitations faced by disabled people to their own medical issues, and sees accommodations for those issues as extraneous to those required by the non-disabled population. This is at odds with the social model of disability, which suggests that those same limitations are instead caused by the way in which society – and the built environment – is organised. Historically, the medical model has manifested in the provision of 'specialised' buildings, areas or zones; this attitude was fomented in the 19th century with the introduction of asylums which isolated disabled people from the rest of the population. Much has changed in public and institutional attitudes since then, yet the design of accessible infrastructure often still seems compromised. As Ed Warner writes in the *RIBA Journal*, 'Where adjustments have been made for disabled people, the resulting environments can often feel like second class spaces'. In this light, disabled parking spaces are something of an exception, as they impinge minimally on the overall design of urban areas and are sometimes, as Boys notes, 'seen as problematic by abled people as giving an unfair advantage to the disabled'.

Discourse on accessibility often focuses on the binary between those with a disability and those without, yet the pandemic itself created some degree of shared experience, by exposing non-disabled people to elements of many disabled people's everyday reality. In their introduction to 'Crip Pandemic Life: A Tapestry', a special section of *Lateral* journal published in 2022, Theodora Danylevich and Alyson Patsavas wrote that 'the earlier stages of the pandemic brought an eerie sense that the crip spacetime so many of us live in – with its isolations, negotiated vulnerabilities, unique temporalities, and ongoing adaptations – suddenly became commonplace'. The pandemic's supposed role as a great leveller has been widely challenged; while we may have been 'weathering the same storm', social, economic and medical inequality meant that we were definitely not all in the same boat. But by exposing non-disabled people to some of the challenges that disabled people deal with regularly, it threw the iniquity of urban design into sharp relief and emphasised the importance of preparing for, and designing for, a much wider range of needs. As public space undergoes perpetual reconfiguration, how can disabled people claim a right to the city, and how might we ensure that the richness of experience of public space and everyday life is more widely accessible?

Principles for a more equitable and inclusive architectural design process were set out in print in the mid-20th century by Selwyn Goldsmith, an architect and disabilities advocate who himself experienced partial paralysis as the result of a polio infection. Goldsmith's book, *Designing for the Disabled* (1963), was the first manual of accessibility guidance to be published in the UK; he would later develop these ideas into the concept of universal design, which he describes as being 'about making buildings safe and convenient for all their users, including people with disabilities'. Rather than treating disability as an 'other' to be accounted for, universal design caters to all users without the need for adaptation and treats disabled and non-disabled people as equally normal. As Jay Dolmage notes in his essay in *Disability, Space, Architecture*, 'Universal design is not a tailoring of the environment to marginal groups; it is a patterning of engagement and effort. The push towards the "universal" is a push towards seeing spaces as multiple and in-process. The emphasis on "design" allows us to recognise that we are all involved in the continued production of a space'.

The role that people can play in the production of space was emphasised during the pandemic, as behaviours, regulations and needs shifted apace, and the nature and use of the urban environment changed in response. Pavements became cafés, parks became pubs, school playgrounds became vaccination centres and bedrooms became offices. Through the lens of universal design, we can begin to see how these spaces might have been designed to accommodate changing use cases in anticipation of the changing needs of a spectrum of different users and access requirements. This is about basic needs and everyday life, but it goes beyond that, and relates to the pleasures we find in life and our ability to share them with others. Design of the built environment does not need to prioritise the needs of one group at the expense of another; we might instead embrace an approach whose inclusivity allows for shifting contexts, conditions and user needs without reactive or exclusive adaptation.

Text by Anna Lisa Reynolds

GOVERNMENT LETTERS

Poster by Rise, 15, Oxford from *The COVID Letters: A Vital Update by Jonny Banger*, 2020, published by Sports Banger Publishing.

How an official letter turned into a canvas for debate and criticism

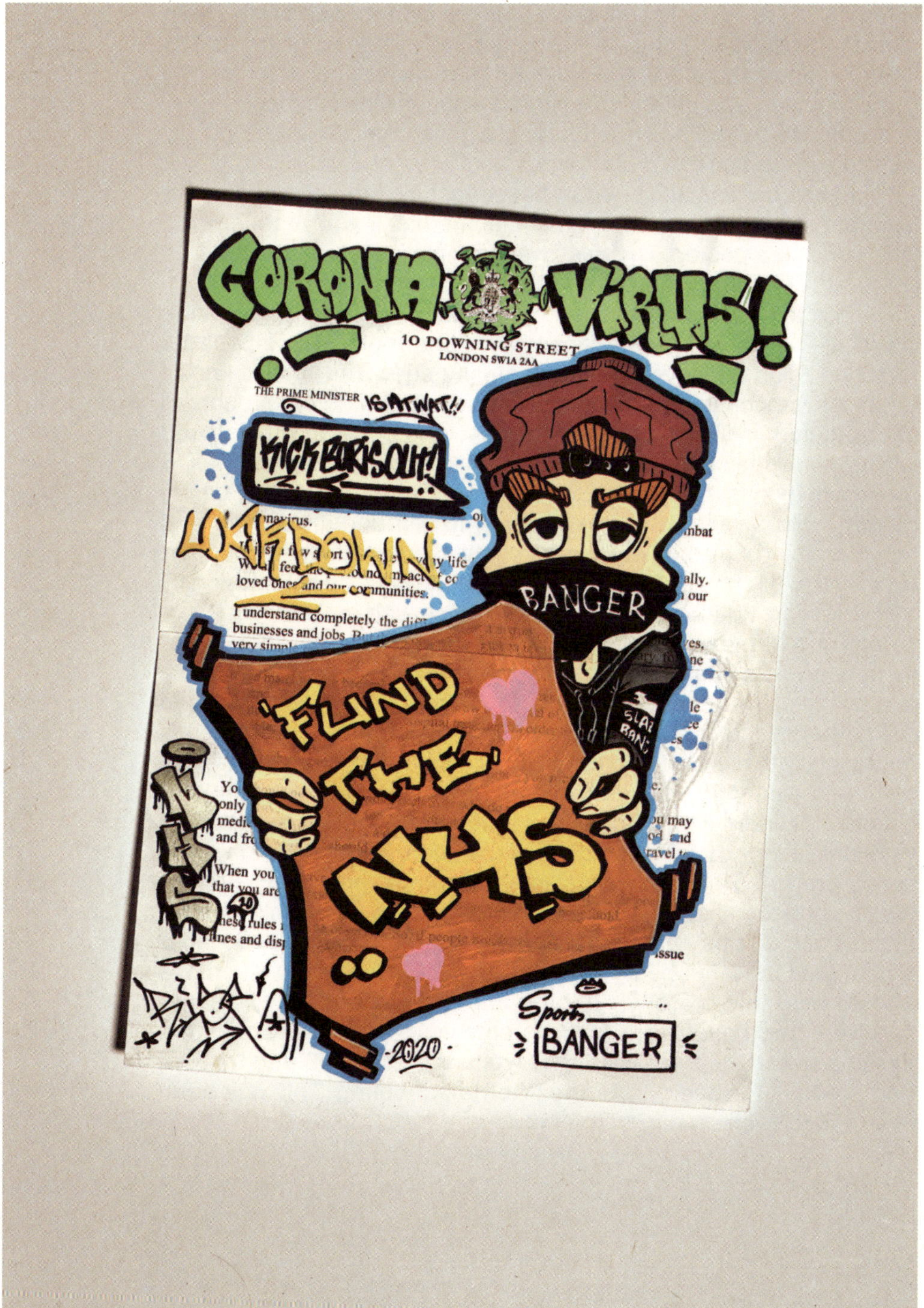
CORONA VIRUS!
10 DOWNING STREET
LONDON SW1A 2AA
THE PRIME MINISTER IS A TWAT!!
KICK BORIS OUT!
LOCKDOWN
BANGER
FUND THE NHS
-2020-
Sports
BANGER

In March 2020, 30 million households in the UK received a letter from then-Prime Minister Boris Johnson about the coronavirus crisis. The letter outlined the steps the government was taking to tackle the surge in cases, and ultimately justified a nationwide lockdown. Many at the time felt anger and frustration at a government that was initially slow to act, leading to a devastating initial wave of deaths.

In this context, the London-based fashion label Sports Banger issued a straightforward call on social media: 'If you've received a letter, design a poster'. The rules were simple: you must be under 16 years old, draw straight onto the letter and use no digital tools.

The tools required for the competition – pencils, pens, paint, crayons – were easily available, and the reappropriation of the letter matched Sports Banger's true bootlegging style. The label is known for its subversion and appropriation of popular branding through an interrogation of British pop culture, class and politics. The defaced letters-cum-posters came flooding in, from toddlers as young as 18 months to teenagers. In total, 203 posters were submitted; the entries ranged from sweet and heartwarming to wonderfully puerile and acerbic. Many of the posters illustrated messages of love and support for the NHS or advice such as 'wash your hands'. One submission by a seven-year-old featured drawings of birds with smiling faces (not beaks) and the text 'I can hear the birds'. Some featured the familiar rainbow that would later be seen in windows of residential streets across the country (see Rainbows p18). Others responded directly to the author of the letter and were more critical of the government's approach, with calls to 'fund the NHS' and for 'more PPE'.

In ordinary times, a government letter is a one-way communication. This intervention subverted that notion through questioning its motive, turning it into a medium of dialogue, criticism and in some cases, protest. 'Little anarchists spreading joy' is how Jonny Banger, the designer behind the label, described the response to his competition. 'I couldn't be happier using my platform to give kids a voice.' Rather than the letter being a top-down mechanism, its function was transformed into a tool for debate and discussion. Jonny Banger received proud messages from parents whose children submitted designs saying they 'discussed the welfare state, NHS and taxes ... and the task formed part of their home schooling. This has been one task they all managed to enjoy'.

Amid the global pandemic, it felt oddly analogue to receive post from 10 Downing Street. Government transmissions are often how important moments in history are recorded, and this letter can be seen as the turning point when the government caught up with the national mood on the pandemic. The modest yet poignant response to the government's actions from the youngest in society was a rare record of their voices in the extreme circumstances of enforced home-schooling and restricted time outdoors.

Text by Meneesha Kellay

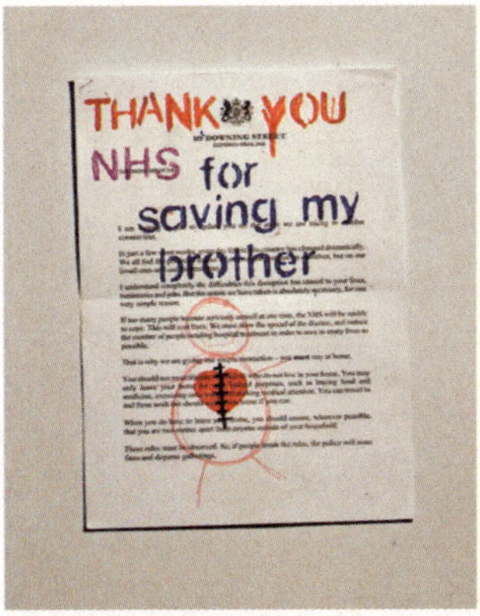

Ozzy, 4, Windsor.

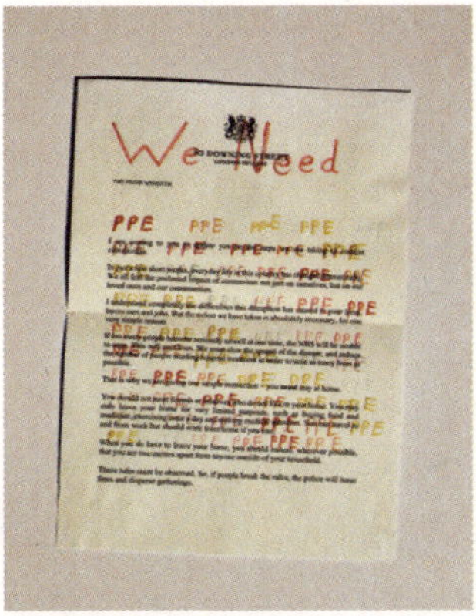

Lorelei, 7, Colchester.

TOTE BAGS

Tote bag by designer Slow and Steady Wins the Race, 2007.

How tote bags became a centre of debate around safety and sustainability, as well as an example of how waste can be reappropriated

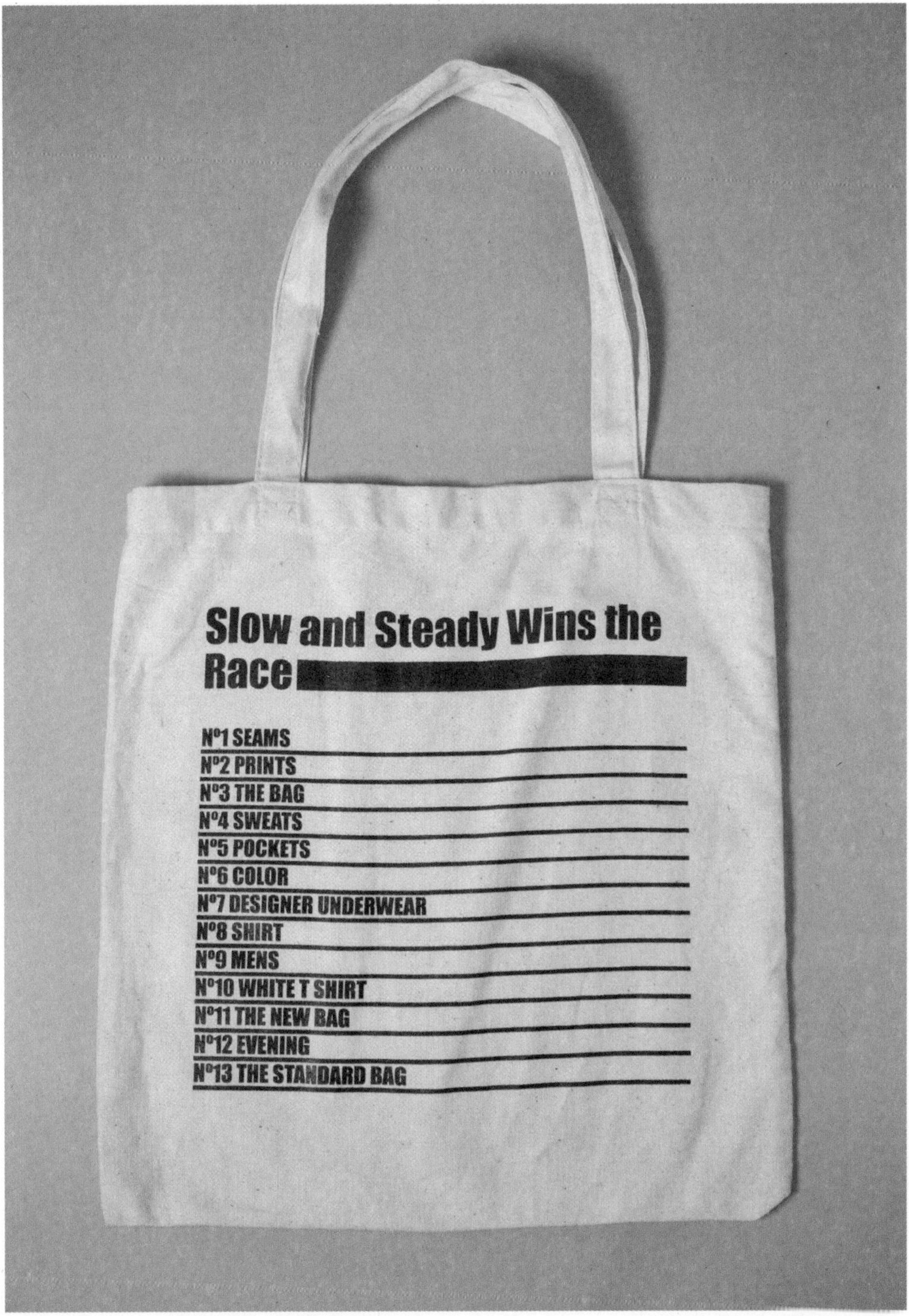

REAPPROPRIATE

Prior to the pandemic, questions about the true sustainability of the ubiquitous tote bag were already circling, due to the environmental impact of their production and distribution. New levels of scepticism were reached during the pandemic, when articles arguing that reusable bags could 'catch' and spread the virus began to appear. US free-market think tanks such as the Manhattan Institute and Competitive Enterprise Institute advocated for a return to plastic shopping bags, and legislation in the US and the UK adopted this to a certain degree; some US states and cities repealed plastic bag bans or banned reusable bags instead, while in the UK, the charge on plastic bags for supermarket home deliveries was removed. These policies were criticised for their inaccuracy; a representative from the British Retail Consortium told *The Independent* that 'there is little evidence to suggest risk associated with the virus being spread via goods'.

The motivations behind the debate surrounding reusable bags were also questioned. Greenpeace USA Oceans Campaign Director John Hocevar expressed concern that articles written by think tanks could be linked to right-wing nonprofits and contain misinformation. Hocevar said that: 'Industry groups have seen this crisis as an opportunity to exploit people's fears around Covid-19 to push their pro-pollution agendas. Even in the short term, plastic does not inherently make something clean and safe, and we should not confuse corporate public relations with factual medical research.'

Just as with many other aspects of the pandemic, scientific fact became a matter of dispute. The tote bag became a symbolic battleground for future approaches towards sustainability, but also an example where the virus sparked efficient repurposing. The tote bag is an annual fixture at Glastonbury Festival, given to attendees as they stagger through the final entry gates of the site. Alongside donations of hand sanitiser, gloves and face masks to the Avon and Somerset Resilience Forum, to be given to emergency workers and NHS staff, the festival team donated surplus tote bags from 2019 to hospitals to be used as wash bags to help prevent contamination from used medical scrubs. As well as being a charitable donation, this was a much-needed positive public relations story for the tote bag, an example where the pandemic prompted sudden redistribution and renewed purpose.

Text by Harriet Reed

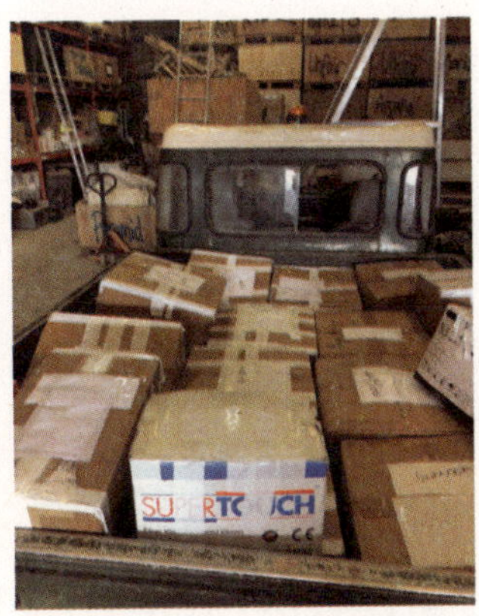

Surplus Glastonbury tote bags from 2019, parcelled up to be delivered to hospitals.

GOOGLE STREET VIEW

How a massive dataset of images enabled virtual travel for those stuck in their homes, providing rich fuel for the imagination

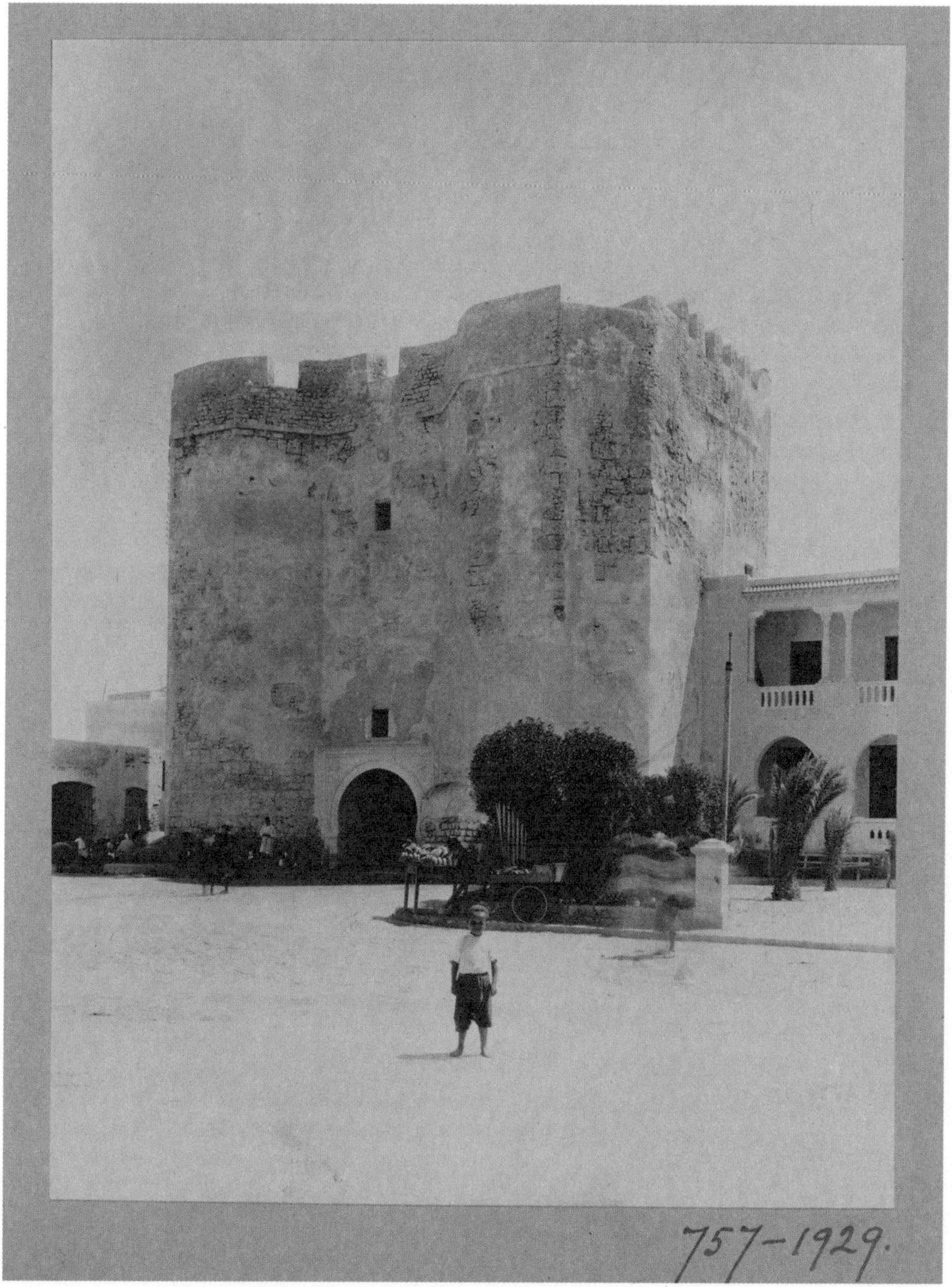

Photograph by KAC Cresswell, Tunisia, 1929.

While imprisoned by the Genoese in 1298, the Venetian merchant Marco Polo dictated memories of his travels to a fellow prisoner and writer, Rustichello of Pisa. Recalling his 24-year adventure across Asia and the Middle East no doubt provided entertainment and solace during their isolation. Published around 1300, Marco Polo's travelogue enjoyed enormous popularity both as inspiration for the so-called European age of 'discovery' and as a guide for the armchair traveller.

On 24 March 2020, a day after lockdown was declared in the UK, the US author Reif Larsen wrote an article for *The New York Times* about his virtual adventures. His recommendation for entertainment during lockdown was Google Street View travel. Unsurprisingly for an author of a digital book told through Google Street View (*Entrances & Exits*, from 2016), Larsen was quick to identify opportunities for exploration. Longing for his cancelled holiday to Charleston, South Carolina, he wrote about how he recreated elements of the trip with his wife and three-year-old son. Rather than dropping down in the centre of Charleston, surveying the buildings and calling it a day, Larsen took his family into a local fish bar, walked along the beach and stumbled across a party. What he added to his trip, of course, was the imagination of an author, the narrative of the journey.

Larsen was not alone in exploiting the benefits of Google Street View to see the world. 'Feast your eyes on these visual treats and be transported,' read the opener of *The Independent*'s list for best virtual travel from 3 April 2020. Among the places listed were the Grand Canyon and Yosemite National Park. Despite their physical closure at the time, a quick trip to Google Street View meant that you too could be hiking up the famous Half Dome or standing on the edge of the canyon. After a few minutes, you might ask yourself how cold it is, how long it took to hike to this point and what the air smells like?

Google Street View was launched in 2007, and by 2017 covered more than 10 million miles of the world's streets, public parks and the occasional building interior. Initiated by Google's cofounder Larry Page, the project first set out to document five US cities at street level. Now Google encourages anyone to add their 360° images, and after 15 years of documenting the 'street' using cars, bikes and hikers, it is a richly layered archive of the world and its curiosities. This unique lens has inspired artists like Jon Rafman, who sees Google Street View as a cultural text that reflects our curious and changing world. For his project *Nine Eyes*, launched in 2008 and revived during quarantine, Rafman collates screen shots from Google Street View that inadvertently capture the strange and the beautiful: a burst fire hydrant, a chaotic flock of angry seagulls, a boy taming a pony on a desolate country road.

It was the bizarre and the unexpected that made medieval travel accounts so intriguing, too. The publication of Marco Polo's *Travels* produced an appetite for tales of voyage – in a period when only a small proportion of society had the means to leave their country, virtual travel was a way to 'see' the world. Another great traveller, Ibn Battūta, a merchant from Tangier, famously wandered across Africa and Asia from 1325–54, recording the details of daily life and local customs. His encounter with the court of Özbeg Khan was one of astonishment: '...we saw a vast city on the move with its inhabitants, with mosques and bazaars in it, the smoke of the kitchen rising in the air (for they cook while on the march), and horse drawn wagons transporting the people'. Not unlike Jon Rafman's *Nine Eyes*, it was the curious details of daily life that stirred the imagination.

In 2020, armchair travel took on a new meaning. While modern travel accounts, like Robert Byron's *The Road to Oxiana* (1937) or Jack Kerouac's *On the Road* (1957), still fuelled a sense of adventure, Google Street View allowed people to 'walk' the streets, returning a sense of self determination and happenstance to the journey. While, ostensibly, the entire reason for the platform's existence is Google's larger mission to collect and monetise data, the side effect of such a large and publicly accessible dataset has been an update to the long tradition of travel guides, enabling virtual wanderlust at a global scale.

Text by Ella Kilgallon

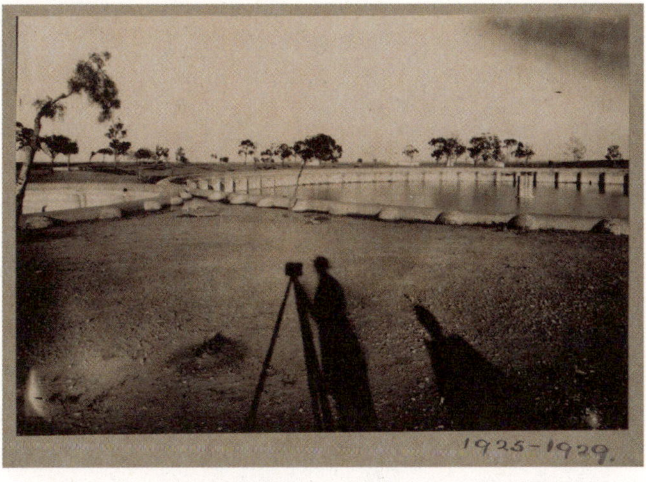

Photograph by KAC Cresswell, Tunisia, 1925–29.

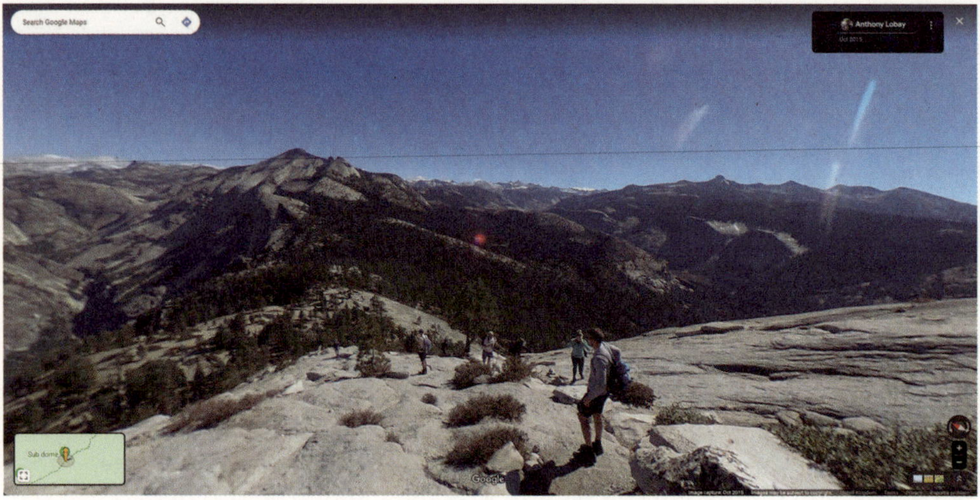

Google Street View image of Half Dome, Yosemite National Park, US, which was closed to the public on 20 March 2020.

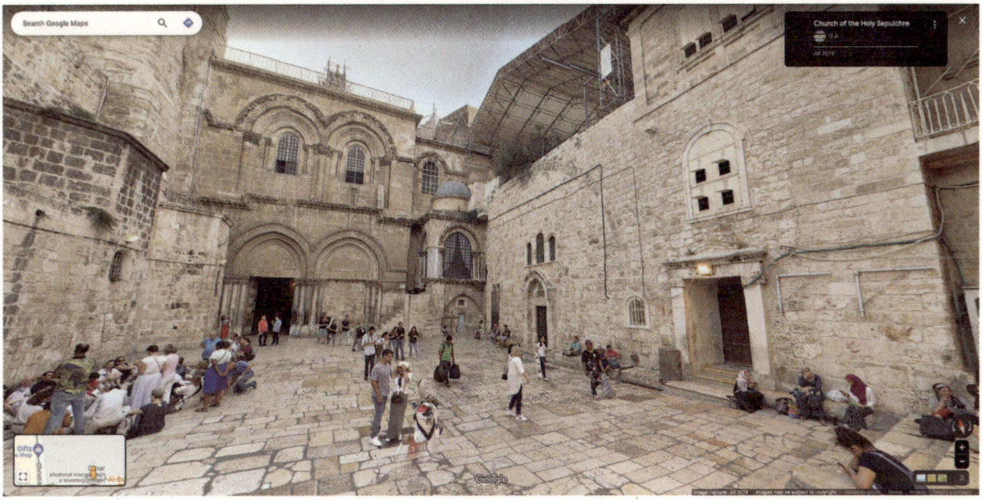

Google Street View image
of the Old City, Jerusalem.

CHAIRS

Chair from China, c1700–80.

How chairs became a tool for organising new social intimacies and a potent symbol of lost civic life

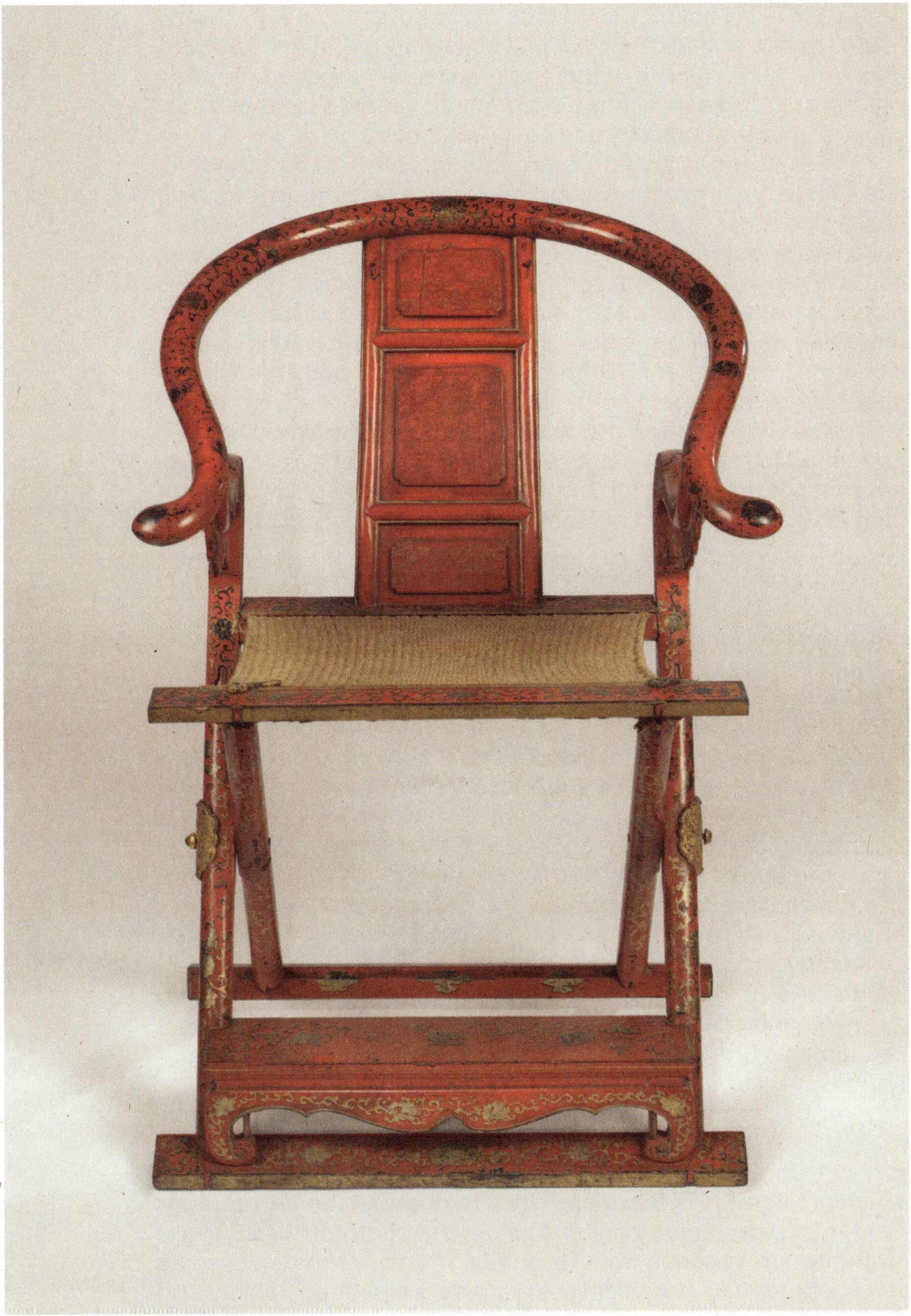

REAPPROPRIATE

Chairs will likely not go down in the history of the pandemic as an object to talk about. Their agency in solving a global crisis was, of course, minimal. But in their own way – as has been the case with so many objects – they played an unexpected symbolic role, connoting both sociability and social distance.

With outdoor social gatherings becoming the standard, and a finite amount of public furniture available, sales in camping chairs and other forms of collapsible lightweight seating soared. Watching people lug their furniture with them, en route to a green patch of grass, became a common sight in London. Chairs never meant for the outdoors also made their way to the sunshine, as they were moved from indoor domestic spaces to stoops, curbsides and front gardens, allowing their owners to participate in the public life of the street.

While carrying a chair with you might have seemed novel, it is steeped in historical practice. Simple folding chairs and stools are some of the oldest furniture designs we know of; evidence of their use dates back to at least the 15th century BCE. The chair was purpose-built for the nomadic life of the time, where one's worldly possessions were fashioned to be able to pick up and go at only a moment's notice. Post-nomadic life, the folding chair has found continued purpose and existence in various military campaigns, exploration missions and film sets.

In the 1970s, when James Hennessey and Victor Papanek published their influential books *Nomadic Furniture* and *Nomadic Furniture 2*, they were looking towards a world that was increasingly mobile. The average American would move every two to three years, they claimed. To emphasise the point, Papanek and Hennessey concluded their preface with the many locations in which the book had been written: Stockholm, Vienna, Copenhagen, Valencia. In reaction to this increased global mobility, they proposed a series of cheap do-it-yourself fixes for furnishing a constantly changing abode. Such jetsetting trends seem antithetical to current ideas about the need for slowing down, reducing air travel and addressing the climate emergency. Yet, remarkably, nomadic furniture flourished under lockdown, in a way I doubt Hennessey and Papanek could have foreseen.

At the same time, chairs demarcate a space of ownership, privacy and distancing, as if to signpost in public that 'this space is mine'. One good historical example can be found in early cafés, which proliferated in European cities throughout the 19th century. Here, mass-produced chairs, such as the enormously successful Bentwood varieties from Gebrüder Thonet, were deployed as a way of carefully organising varying degrees of sociability and

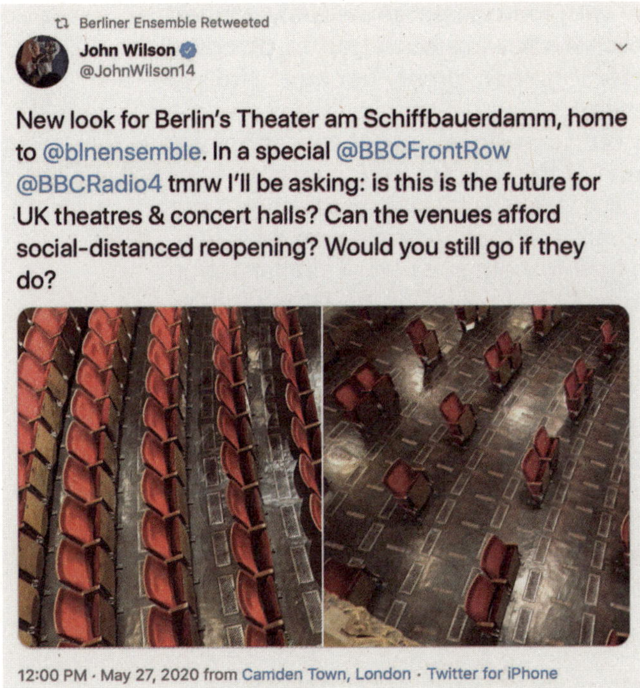
Berliner Ensemble Retweeted
John Wilson
@JohnWilson14
New look for Berlin's Theater am Schiffbauerdamm, home to @blnensemble. In a special @BBCFrontRow @BBCRadio4 tmrw I'll be asking: is this is the future for UK theatres & concert halls? Can the venues afford social-distanced reopening? Would you still go if they do?
12:00 PM · May 27, 2020 from Camden Town, London · Twitter for iPhone

privacy while out in public. In contrast to its predecessor, the 18th-century coffee house, where anyone who entered was meant to engage in open dialogue with others, the 19th-century café was a place to be alone in public. Cheap, lightweight, moveable chairs were a way of quickly marking spaces out into invisible bubbles of privacy, a shield against the hustle and bustle of the increasingly frenetic metropolis.

Chairs further developed this role of demarcating space during the pandemic, as various industries looked to socially-distanced seating arrangements in response to evolving safety requirements. Proposals were sketched by airline industries for instructions on how to rearrange the famously cramped seating of economy class; the unconvincing initial ideas included acrylic shields and a reversed middle seat. The Berliner Ensemble removed 500 of 700 seats in its auditorium to create a new socially-distanced scheme for live performances, revealing a strange and hauntingly fragmented layout.

It was a tricky balancing act; too far apart and the whole point of congregation was lost, while too close together felt like an act of coercion to a public whose trust needed to be won. In May 2020, for example, the White House held press conferences outside in the Rose Garden, with journalists generously spaced out. By 5 June, however, journalists were outraged to discover chairs had been moved closer together, simply because staffers had deemed that it 'looks better'.

The chair, as it turns out, can be a potent metaphor for collective life, producing some of the most uncanny images from the pandemic. On 24 April 2020, 1,000 chairs were placed out on an empty Römerberg Square in Frankfurt as a protest by the restaurant industry for more government support. A similar action took place in Athens on 6 May 2020 in front of the Greek Parliament. This notion of a chair as a stand-in for a person was not quite enough for the fans of the German football team Borussia Mönchengladbach, who paid to have cardboard images of themselves occupy the empty stadium seats during the audience-less matches that took place in May that year.

The image, either of an empty chair or a sea of empty chairs, produced a strange psychological effect. It was an invitation which could not be truly taken up to join again in the crowds of the city; to be together with strangers.

Text by Brendan Cormier

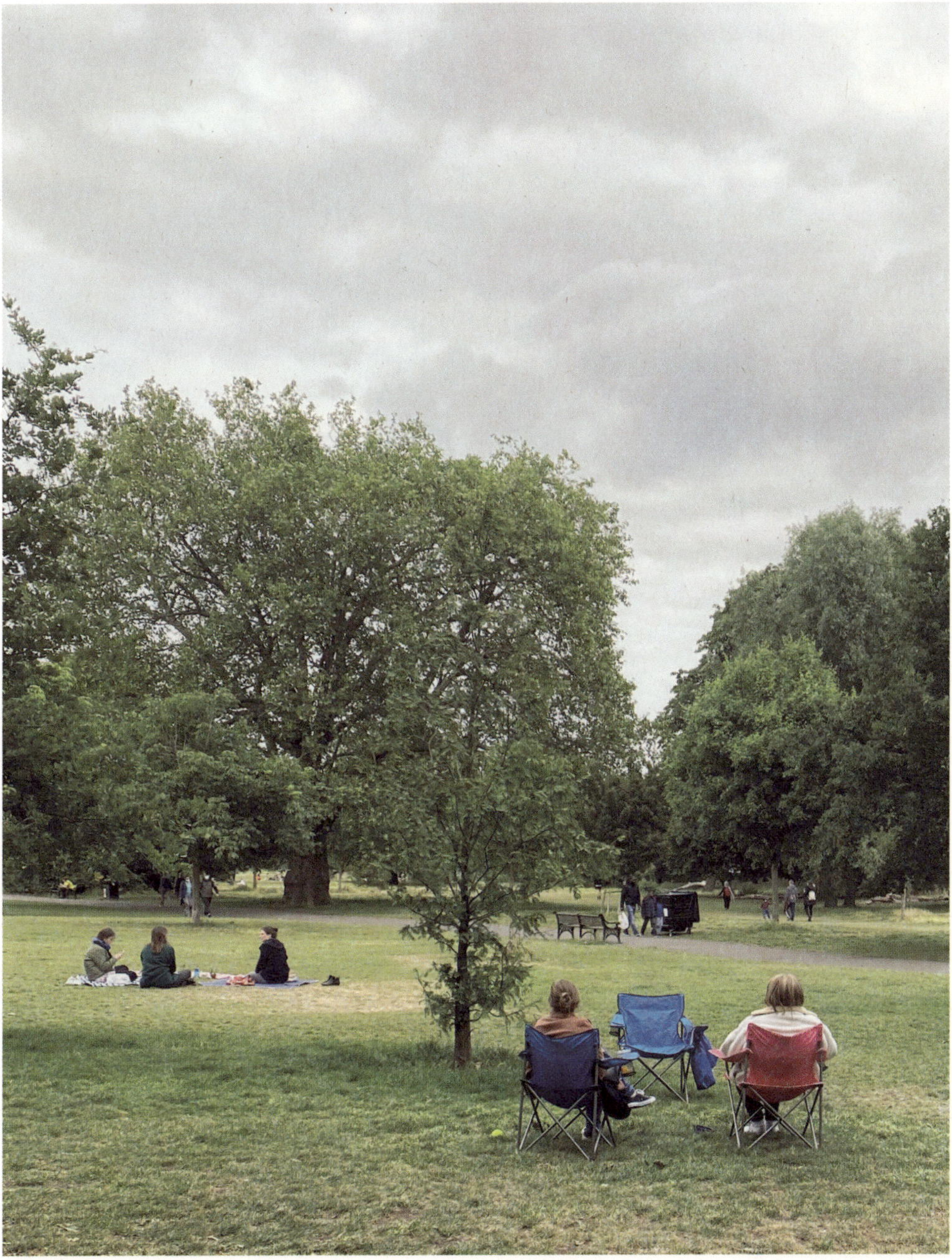

Camping chairs in Clissold Park, London.

07

REVIVE

Objects come and go. A new invention can find incredible currency at the time of its creation, traverse the world and proliferate, before ultimately being surpassed by other technological advances. The bicycle makes way for the automobile, the radio gets an upgrade with the television, and so on. However, most things rarely disappear altogether; rather they slip into the background, still vital to everyday life, yet rarely worthy of any particular attention – the soap we use to stay clean, the sewing machine collecting dust in the corner. The pandemic brought old objects to the fore, not out of nostalgia, but largely because they were ready at hand in a period marked by sudden scarcity. Reverting to old objects for modern times highlighted the incredible resilience of objects to continue to satisfy needs. But it also offered a moment of reflection on notions of progress, and the qualities lost when we move relentlessly from one technological advancement to another.

SOAP

Soap dish made in Bow Porcelain Factory, London, c1755.

How soap and the act of hand-washing shifted the framing of the pandemic as a collective problem to an individual responsibility

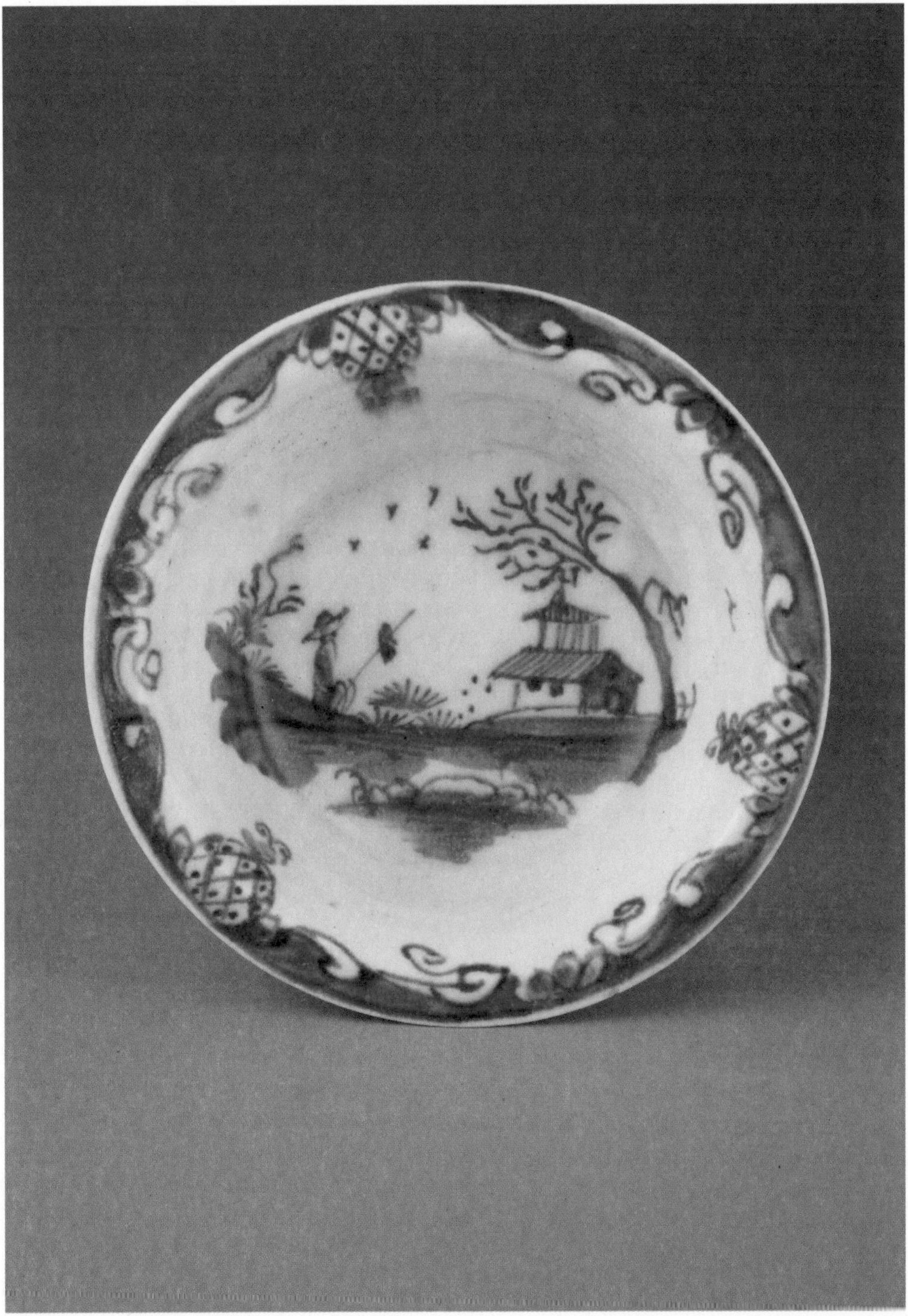

REVIVE

If hands were the problem, then soap was the answer. Around the world, governments implored their citizens to make frequent trips to the sink, asking them to lather and rinse as the first line of defence against the novel coronavirus. But far from having a clean past, the history of soap is loaded with contradictions. And in the case of the Covid-19 pandemic, it became symbolic of a troubling tendency to frame the crisis as one of individual responsibility, rather than collective and co-ordinated action.

During a time of fear and uncertainty, and in an age of advanced medicine, the sudden focus on soap seemed surprising, almost ridiculous. How could this most common of commodities, made from a simple mix of fatty acids and an alkali, possibly be the most effective weapon against a novel and little-understood virus?

And yet, for all its commonality, soap is loaded with significance, as museum collections like the V&A's reveal through the objects that display and contain it. Meticulously crafted from precious materials, soap containers from the 17th and 18th centuries speak to a certain privilege that bodily cleanliness entailed at that time. A late-17th-century spherical soap box, made from silver and engraved with a family crest, would have formed part of a larger toilette set, used by the most fashionable men for their ablutions. In 1712, a tax on soap had been introduced in England, effectively making it a luxury item. Porcelain soap dishes from the 18th century, painted with blue and white flowers imitating Chinese porcelain, could only have been owned by the wealthiest, given the rarity and difficulty of producing porcelain at that time. Soap is present, but associated principally with wealth, with fashion.

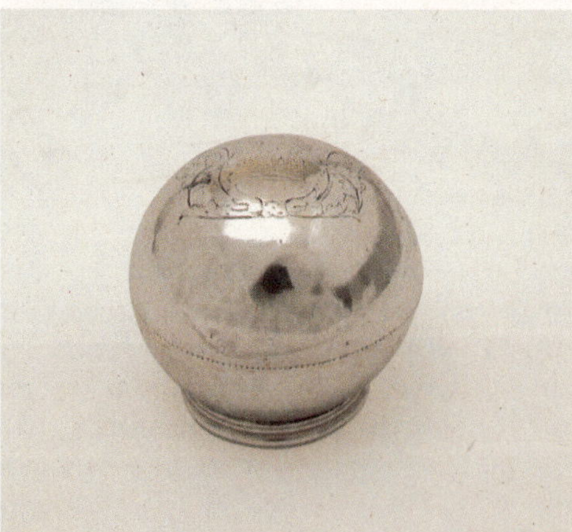

Soap box,
London, 1682–83.

In the mid-19th century, a radical shift took place in the availability, consumption and connotations of soap. Soap duties were halved in 1834 and abolished completely in 1853, meaning that it could be manufactured for mass markets, supported by innovations in industrial production. Tablets of scented soap featured at the Great Exhibition of 1851, appealing to middle-class consumers, and became cheaper and more accessible again to a mass market in the 1920s and 30s. A plethora of posters from the late 19th and early 20th century advertise the benefits and virtues of soaps, produced by companies such as Pears (awarded the prize medal for soap at the Great Exhibition) and Lever Brothers (founded by William Lever, 1st Viscount Leverhulme, later to become Unilever). Pears and Lever Brothers took similar approaches to marketing. Both acquired and adapted paintings by artists of the day to confer artistic connotations and respectability on their products while also commissioning artists to produce boldly coloured graphic designs for posters. These often featured wholesome children, beautiful women with 'blooming' complexions or whiter-than-white laundry accompanied by slogans such as 'Pears soap: Matchless for the Complexion', 'Sunlight! Guarantee of purity' and 'Cleanliness is next to Godliness'.

But these images belie the disturbing undercurrents of the soap industry. Pears, Lever and others aggressively marketed their soaps towards working-class women in particular, seeking to expand their consumer bases by capitalising on growing public awareness of the links between hygiene and disease. By targeting health concerns and through their choice of marketing slogans and imagery, manufacturers persuaded consumers to discard the home- or locally-produced soaps that they had previously used, in favour of these new products that promised to make them healthier and more beautiful, their laundry whiter and easier to clean. But the reality behind those pristine images was rather different. Although public health initiatives were starting to be implemented, many people in Britain still lived in highly unsanitary slum dwellings that lacked proper waste facilities or running water. At the same time, the industries selling these dreams were built on the exploitation of natural resources – such as the mass harvesting of coconut oil in the Solomon Islands and the creation of vast palm oil plantations in the Congo – and the forced labour of colonised peoples. Colonialism overtly informed advertising choices, with posters drawing direct connections between cleanliness and civilisation.

From today's standpoint, one poster seems particularly striking. Issued by the Health and Cleanliness Council around 1925, it reads 'Prevention is better than cure ... Where there's dirt there's danger' but also reminds us, in a pre-NHS age, that 'Soap & water cost less than doctors' fees and medicine'. A century after this poster was made, the guidance that we were issued during the pandemic was startlingly similar. But it also serves as a stark reminder of persisting inequalities that the virus exacerbated in horrifying ways: the responsibility placed squarely on individuals for their own health, while the personal protective equipment (PPE) that was really needed to protect against exposure to the virus was woefully lacking; the scale of poor-quality housing that enabled it to spread; the horrifically disproportionate number of deaths suffered by members of racialised minority communities, including so many healthcare professionals. Suddenly, the bar of soap does not seem so reassuring after all.

Text by Joanna Norman

Print advertising Sunlight soap
by Will Owen, 1919.

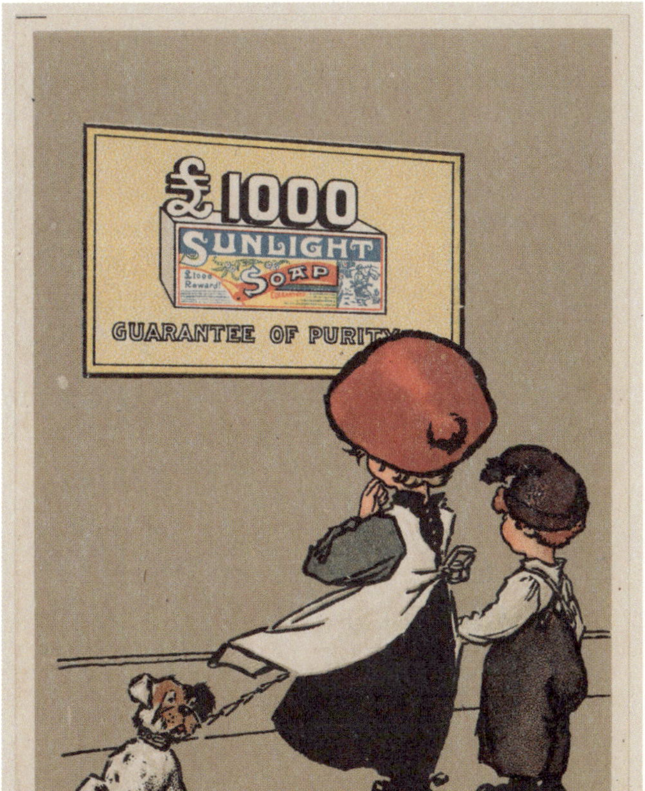
£1000
SUNLIGHT
SOAP
GUARANTEE OF PURITY
WILL OWEN
THAT'S WHAT MOTHER USES
E. 861-1919.

SEWING MACHINES

How a two-hundred-year-old invention saw renewed popularity and filled a production gap for PPE in the early days of the pandemic

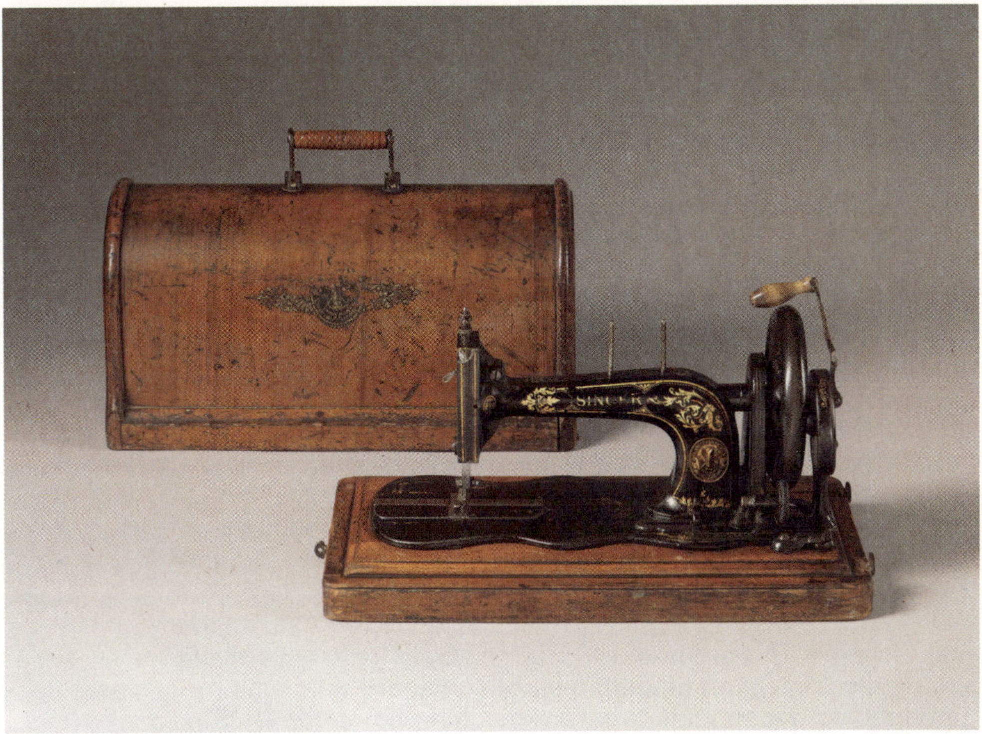

The 'New Family' sewing machine by the Singer Manufacturing Company, first introduced to the market in 1865.

Widely reported supermarket rushes on flour and toilet roll provided a unique snapshot into the consumer psychology playing out during the pandemic (see Flour and Yeast p108 and Toilet Roll p306). Less discussed, however, was the scarcity in beginner's sewing machines, which quickly sold out from most major UK suppliers. The sewing machine has gone in and out of fashion over the course of its two-century existence, and its obstinate survival was what allowed for the incredible boom in home-sewing activity witnessed during lockdown. This unexpected phenomenon sheds some light onto our evolving domestic behaviours while emphasising the social significance of craft and the sense of community that making continues to offer.

Sewing machines were first introduced to households in the US as a mass-produced commodity in the 1850s. It was heralded as both a mechanical wonder and great labour-saving device that would transform the lives of women, who were often responsible for making and remaking family wardrobes and household furnishings. However, the cost of early machines was prohibitive; in 1860, at a price of $50 to $125 (roughly $1,500 to $3,700 today), it represented a significant portion of the average family's yearly income. This prompted IM Singer & Co (later to become the sewing machine giant Singer) to introduce a hire-purchase plan that enabled households to take a machine home for $5 ($154 today). Decades before Henry Ford's 1913 innovation of the moving assembly line, which famously brought down the price of automobiles, sewing machine companies were feverishly competing to rationalise production and make their machines more affordable. Today a sewing machine can be purchased from as little as £33 from the likes of John Lewis, Lidl and Hobbycraft.

The popularity of sewing machines ebbed and flowed throughout the course of the 20th century. At first, due to its price, it was a household status symbol. With the rise of steadily cheaper ready-to-wear clothing, it waned in popularity. The world wars gave drive to campaigns like 'make do and mend', reigniting the sewing machine as an essential tool, but by the 1980s onwards, low-cost high street fashion and the steady decline in school needlework lessons saw a big decrease in the popularity of the skill. Since the early 21st century, home sewing has been on the rise, aided by cheaper tools and the rise of blogging and craft fairs, which have made the activity more easily available and accessible. Concerns about climate change and the need to find alternatives to fast fashion have led many to start making their own clothes, while the BBC's *The Great British Sewing Bee* (first aired in 2013) has further fuelled the popularity of the craft. Incidentally, the sixth series of the show returned to popular acclaim on 22 April 2020, one month into the UK's first lockdown.

'Making' is widely recommended as a tool for mindfulness and good mental health, and more than ever people are turning to it as a calming antidote to the stresses of global crises. As a result, the craft sector has flourished. Hobbycraft, the UK's biggest arts and crafts retailer, reported that visits to their website tripled during lockdown and sewing machines more than doubled in sales.

Mindfulness aside, the pandemic boom was also linked to phenomenal grassroots campaigns that saw the sewing machine become an essential tool in combating the virus. The increased turnover of vital personal protective equipment (PPE) and protective clothing created a global scarcity. In response, numerous volunteer groups such as the 'For the Love of Scrubs' Facebook group and local community 'Scrub Hub' groups were set up throughout March and April to bring sewing enthusiasts together and co-ordinate efforts to supply the NHS and other front-line health workers with scrubs during the crisis. Sewers used readily available online templates to craft scrubs from unused or unwanted materials, including curtains, bedding and linen. Organisations such as the Royal Hospital for Neurodisability in Putney specifically asked volunteers to prioritise bright colours and patterns to bring some much needed cheer to the hospital corridors and community.

The voluntary campaign saw thousands of scrubs donated as part of this national effort. It also brought together a diverse network of sewers including local community groups, costume makers at the English National Opera, individual home sewers and fashion designers such as Phoebe English, Holly Fulton and Bethany Williams, who set up the Emergency Designer Network. In contrast, prior to lockdown, policymakers had been keen to trumpet the so-called fourth industrial revolution, where new digital manufacturing hardware such as 3D printers, CNC mills and laser-cutters would herald a new era of flexible and geographically distributed production. Such technologies would, in theory, be invaluable in facing the scarcities and supply chain problems that were highlighted during the pandemic. And while these technologies have been employed, it was the humble sewing machine that emerged as one of the most effective tools when global networks failed.

Text by Becky Knott

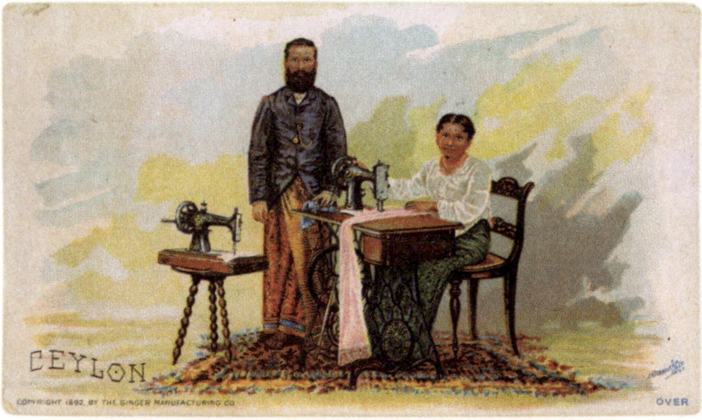

Singer advertisement card, distributed at the World's Columbian Exposition in Chicago, 1893.

MILK

School milk bottle made by
United Dairies, UK, c1950–59.

How the pandemic re-engaged with historical ideas of sourcing food and drink that is local, ethical and waste-free

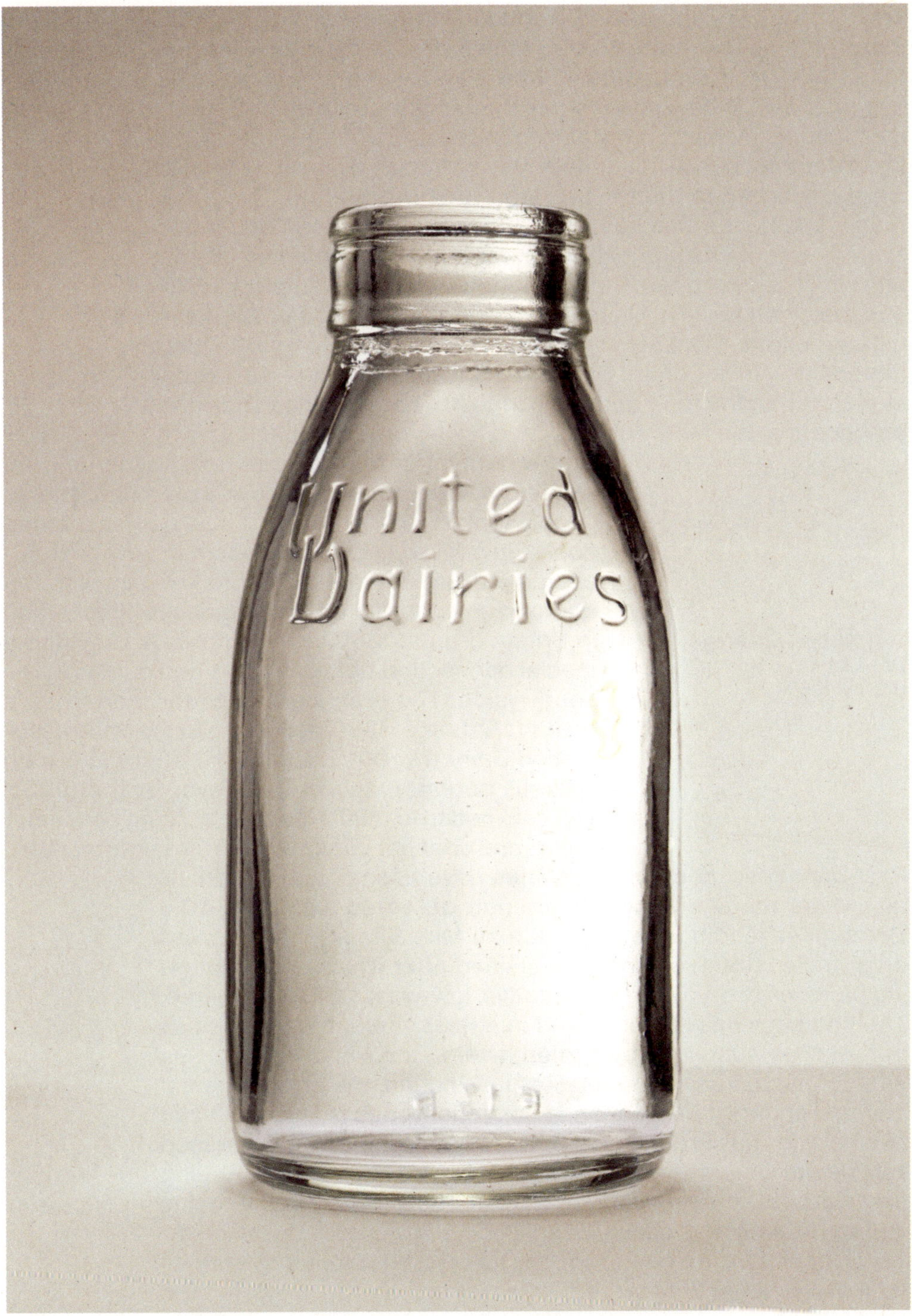

REVIVE

The fragility of industrial food production systems was highlighted during the pandemic. Following the start of the first lockdown in March 2020, huge quantities of fresh milk were thrown away as supply chains were disrupted and demand from cafés and restaurants dropped. Interim data from a Royal Association of British Dairy Farmers survey found that just over one million litres of milk were discarded in the UK between 6–20 April 2020. There are many reasons for this lack of resilience, including an economic system which puts profit above the welfare of people and planet, and which tends towards large monopolies. For example, in 1915, one major wholesaler, United Dairies, controlled half of London's milk supply. In 1918, the government nationalised milk production under a new Milk Control Board, but this soon collapsed. Consolidation within the food and drink industry has continued, leaving producers at the mercy of fewer and fewer large companies.

At the beginning of the pandemic, online delivery slots from supermarkets were at a premium, and so people looked to alternatives. Local dairies offering doorstep delivery reported a boom in new customers, employing additional staff to keep up with the demand. Fresh milk delivery services first began in Britain around 1860, as new railways provided a crucial connection between cities and dairies in the countryside. The practice thrived for more than a century. As late as 1980, according to the trade association Dairy UK, 89% of all milk bought in Britain was still doorstep delivery. However, by the 1990s, this declined to just 30% due to changing consumer habits and cheaper competition from supermarkets.

Toy milk float made by Lines Bros Ltd, Merton, UK, late 1960s.

Post-pandemic, doorstep deliveries have risen again, especially as a wider range of products are now delivered alongside milk. Companies leading the way, such as Milk & More, have thrived on giving customers a more diversified offer while also positioning themselves as a green alternative, low-waste and plastic-free. The company has also invested in a fleet of electric vehicles as part of their sustainable mission, seeing food and transport as interconnected environmental issues. Indeed, the environmental impacts of the intensification of home deliveries is in fact difficult to untangle. This is due to the potential emissions from increased vehicle movements in contrast to a decrease in plastic packaging as glass bottles are reused, a greater focus on local supply chains and so on. What has clearly been a boon, however, is the diversification of options for how food gets to the table, ultimately making for a more robust food system.

Text by Sara Kassam

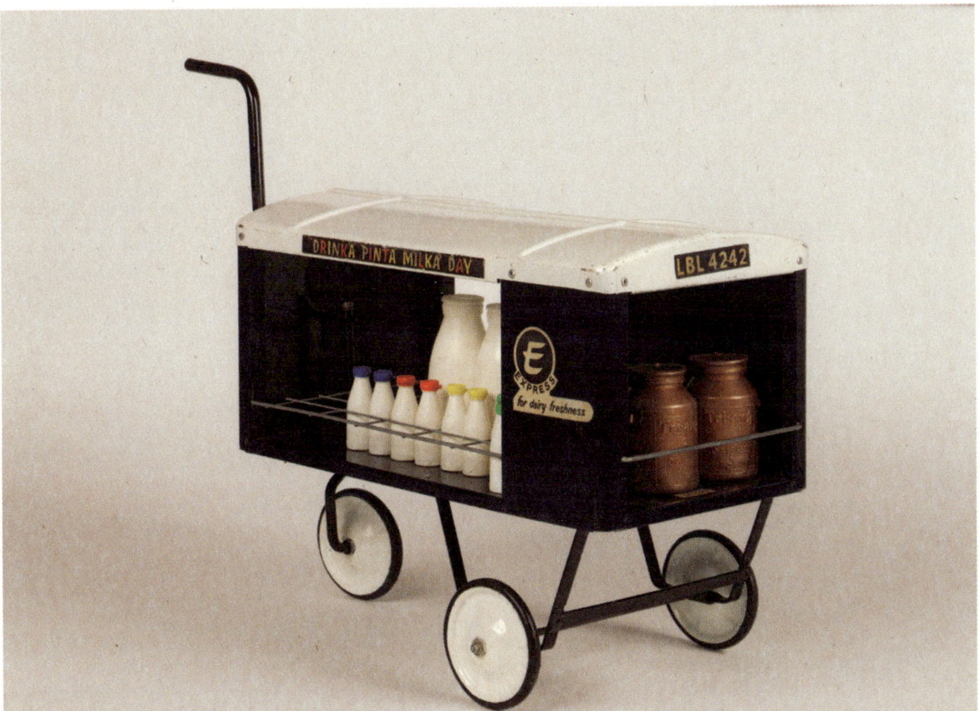

REVIVE

HOPSCOTCH

How spontaneous hopscotch markings recalled the power of play in our streets

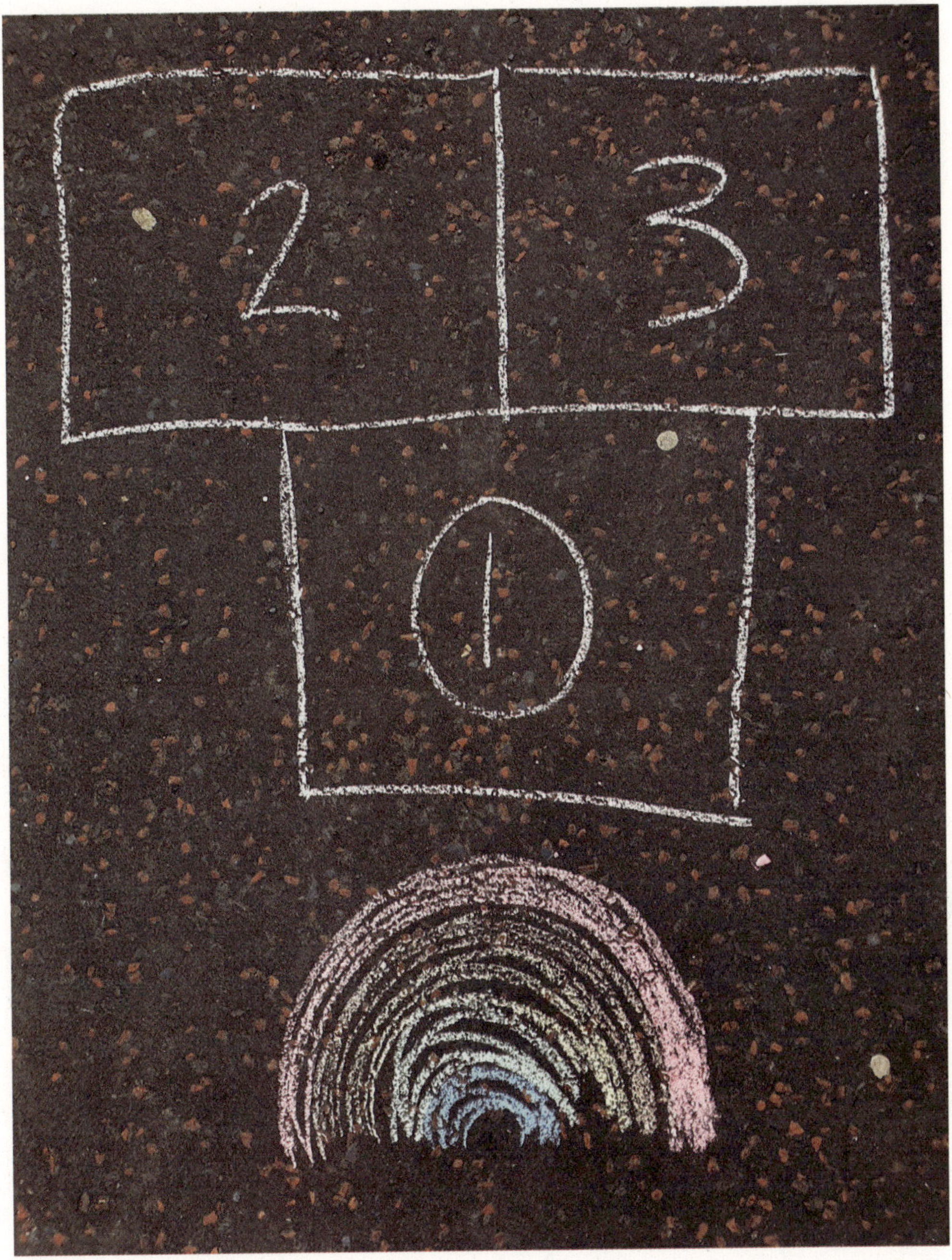

Giant hopscotch initiated and documented
by Jenny Elliott, Edinburgh, 2020.

'How do you bring people together when you can't bring people together?' asked Jenny Elliott, an urban designer and landscape architect based in Edinburgh. Hopscotch, she thought at the beginning of lockdown, might be one way. Elliott drew up a few squares on the pavement outside her home, left a box of chalk and put up a handwritten sign that read: 'Please use the chalk ... for ... HOPSCOTCH!' (see Homemade Signs, p12). This offer also posed a challenge: 'Add some squares to the hopscotch on your walk up the hill, and see if we can make it to the top before it rains.' The weather was dry for the next two weeks and the hopscotch court grew, by a collective effort, into a 400m grid comprising some 1,400 squares. It reached the top of the hill, and even expanded in other directions before being washed away by rainfall. Elliott had to move her sign further up the road several times to keep up with the design, but 'the biggest challenge,' she said, 'was trying to source enough chalk. All the neighbours chipped in, and any chalk at the back of their cupboards came out'.

As the world went into lockdown, many cities saw their pavements and streets slowly transformed by chalk drawings. Hopscotch was a particularly popular motif combining creative chalking with play. A home security camera in Irvine, California caught an Amazon delivery worker hopscotching back to his van after dropping off a parcel; a heartwarming and yet slightly creepy moment due to how the video was captured on the home camera. Clips of refuse collectors and police officers hopscotching down streets while picking up bin bags in Hull, Darlington and Derbyshire circulated on local news websites in March and April 2020. Hopscotch, it seemed, was as popular among the key workers who encountered chalked grids during their shifts as it was among children.

An ancient game, hopscotch is thought to have originated in India; a description is included on the list of games prohibited by the Buddha from the 6th or 5th century BCE, a list which also features dice, ball and board games. In England, it was first recorded by Francis Willughby in the 17th-century *Book of Games*, referred to there as 'scotch-hoppers.' A common hopscotch court consists of a numbered grid of alternating single and double squares through which players hop on either one or both feet, careful not to tread on any lines. Hopscotch teaches co-ordination and counting and, when the pandemic began, was an activity that could be played while observing social distancing rules. As such, it made its way onto new lists – Covid-era ones – that itemised activities parents should encourage their kids to do during lockdown. As *The Scotsman* exclaimed, 'Put the phones and tablets down and grab some coloured chalk for some outdoor fun on your driveway!'

However, unless you have a driveway or a private garden with a paved area, such advice could be deflating, as UK laws restrict such acts. To draw on public streets or pavements, even with chalk, requires permission or a 'play street' permit. While this law has been only loosely enforced over the years, hopscotch has in fact been targeted by law enforcement. In 2013, a 10-year-old girl was threatened with criminal damages by an over-zealous police officer for chalking a hopscotch court outside her home in Kent. During the pandemic a local inspector at a housing estate in Bishopsbriggs, East Dunbartonshire told parents that their children must 'refrain from (playing hopscotch) immediately', arguing that the chalk courts damaged the overall appearance of the property.

Why should it be so transgressive to chalk up a play area in public space? Jenny Elliott, who initiated the Edinburgh hopscotch, thinks the game has an inherent mark-making appeal. 'That's the delight of drawing your own hopscotch as a child,' she says. 'You often draw the grid somewhere that is not normally allowed. But it's alright because it will wash away.' From her perspective as an urban designer, Elliot finds this impulse important as 'it gives you some control over your surroundings as a citizen. I think a lot of people don't feel they have that ability to shape the way their outside environment looks and feels'.

Elliott's hopscotch initiative showed that when given the opportunity, people of all ages can take delight in shaping their immediate surroundings despite restrictive laws. 'We had people personalising their own squares,' she explains. 'When we got to 1,000 squares, somebody did this huge drawing around it.' Participants dedicated squares to NHS staff and other key workers, and wrote birthday messages for local children. The design of the court was also creatively adapted to fit around and respond to urban features along the road. 'There was a small laneway that cuts across the street,' Elliott says, 'so somebody drew a rocket ship to "help" the hopscotch fly over.'

Unfortunately, as lockdown restrictions eased, traffic levels began to return to pre-pandemic levels. While hopscotch courts are normally drawn on pavements, not the road itself, the constant presence of cars made it less likely parents could allow their children to play in an urban environment. After the interlude of the pandemic we were back to the trajectory mapped out in a 2007 report from Play England; it found that while 71% of adults remember playing out on the street as children, only 21% of children in 2007 actually did so.

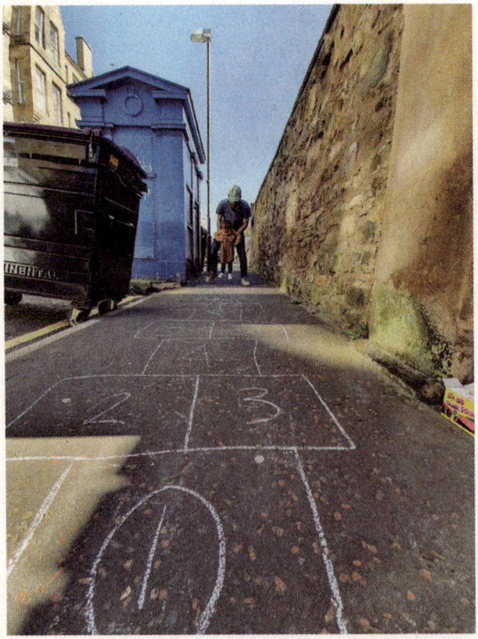

Giant hopscotch initiated and documented by Jenny Elliott, Edinburgh, 2020.

Architects and urban designers have long emphasised the vital importance of spontaneous play in towns and cities. It was no coincidence that, as personal cars became increasingly present on our streets, some of the most powerful design ideas for play emerged during the decades that followed the Second World War. Emerging alongside the so-called 'playground revolution' in the 1960s, Dutch architect Aldo van Eyck envisioned and developed his Amsterdam playground project: hundreds of spaces developed in squares, parks and vacant lots between 1947 and 1978, all featuring minimalist equipment which could be played with creatively (sadly, only 17 of these playgrounds remain). In Britain, civil engineer Colin Buchanan's 1963 *Traffic in Towns* report led to an increased pressure to establish 'home zones' or permanent play streets, where traffic was heavily reduced in favour of pedestrians, cyclists and playing children. Additionally, architects Alison and Peter Smithson championed their concept of 'streets in the sky', traffic-free walkways in housing complexes that could be used communally by residents. Unfortunately, many of these well-intentioned urban visions have disappeared into the rear-view mirror, resulting in an ever-growing presence of cars in our cities. As streets return to pre-pandemic levels of traffic, pollution and congestion have made many cities vow to improve pedestrian spaces to allow for the type of play and urban engagement that the lockdowns briefly provided. As Jenny Elliot points out, it is ultimately a political choice. 'Do we want cars to dominate these spaces? Or do we want to give them over to other uses? Or is there a balance that can be struck?'

Text by Kristina Rapacki

RADIATORS

How the pandemic revived old ideas of collectively heating our homes

PANDEMIC OBJECTS

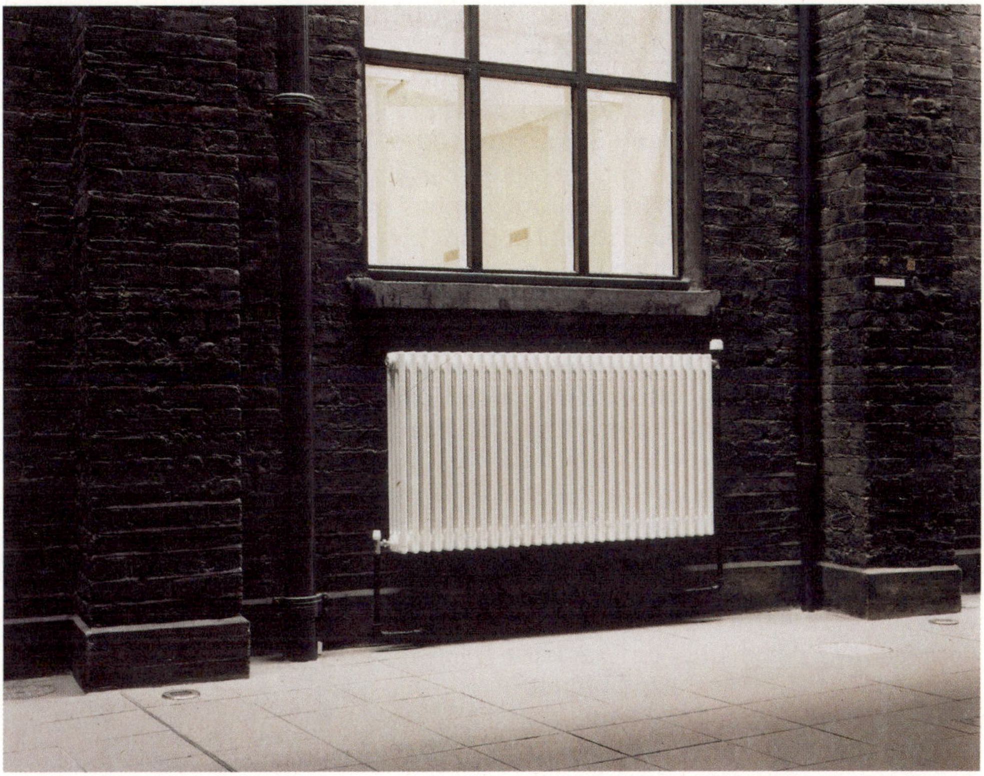

Nigel Shafran, *Untitled (Staff Resturant, Victoria & Albert Museum)*, London, 1999.

The relationship between heating infrastructures and public health – and pandemics in particular – has a long history. Many transformations and innovations in architectural design and city planning introduced in the first half of the 20th century had their origins in an increased understanding of the relationship between living conditions and health. For example, proponents of the early-20th-century 'fresh air movement' in the US referred to unventilated rooms as a 'national poison', promoting access to windows in all habitable spaces as a building standard. Modernism is often understood as a movement focused on germ-free designs, promoting healthy housing for the future. And the 'clean lines' of many iconic modernist homes originated in the tuberculosis epidemic of the early 20th century, informed by a belief in exposure to sun and fresh air as a foundational principle of modernist hygienic ideas.

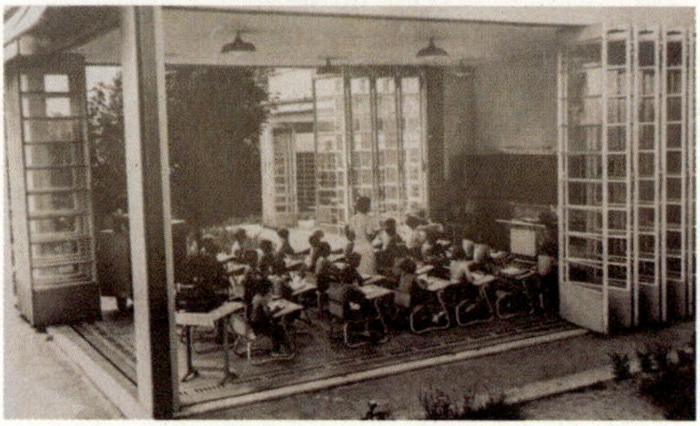

Some of the most significant shifts in thinking about home heating systems and their design date back to the outbreak of the Spanish flu in 1918, which brought with it the radiator as we know it today. While a 'hot box' radiator made of steel, iron or brass that used water or steam to generate heat dates back to the 1850s, our current model of radiator heating came from turn-of-the-century theories of infection control. In the late 19th century, health officials discovered that fresh air could ward off infectious diseases. And while, in the summer, outdoor green spaces offered a viable and popular alternative to staying at home, spending a whole day outdoors proved a less attractive proposition in winter. According to heating expert Dan Holohan, during the Spanish flu epidemic the Board of Health in New York City ordered that windows should remain open to provide ventilation, even in cold weather (a recommendation familiar to anyone who attempted to work in a shared office space during the Covid-19 pandemic). This seemingly contradictory need for fresh air and heat at the same time proved an important factor in the transformation of radiator design. The new radiator still relied on the same steam-powered infrastructure, but was made more effective to keep spaces warm when windows were open during a very cold New York winter. Such robust steam boilers – often operated by local district heating systems, another design innovation of the period – became a standard not only in New York City but also in other cities in the northern United States, such as Chicago, Detroit and Boston.

The effectiveness of the powerful American radiator meant that the design also grew in popularity elsewhere (the American Radiator Company, the leading radiator manufacturer at the time, established factories in France, Italy, Germany and Austria as well as Hull in the UK), fuelling a major transformation on a large scale of the ways in which homes were kept warm.

This thinking about heating provision did not come to an end with the Spanish flu. The realisation that universal access to heating did not only contribute to 'better living' but also helped decrease winter mortality rates was fundamental to radical changes in 20th-century housing policy and modern home design standards. Radiator systems started to gradually replace coal-fired open-hearth heating systems in the first decades of the 20th century and became widespread in the 1960s. In many new housing estates, communal central heating systems, similar to the New York district heating model, were also installed. Thanks to shared boilers controlled by local authorities, these new heating infrastructures supported all the dwellings in their catchment areas at the same time. They made heating and hot water available to their occupants (council and private tenants alike) all year in exchange for a fixed and affordable annual service charge. In many European countries this type of district heating remains an infrastructural standard. In Denmark, for example, more than 70% of all homes are heated through communal neighbourhood heating networks. In the UK, however, where only 2% of homes still rely on them, many of these systems have since been dismantled. They have been replaced by individual household boilers and metered energy systems, moving away from state-managed heat available as a public good and instead favouring provisions of heat as an individual commodity, controlled by private energy suppliers. This approach has ultimately made homes both less affordable and less energy-efficient (a study of Churchill Gardens estate in Pimlico, one of the remaining London estates which still enjoys a publicly-owned heating system, revealed that its CO_2 emissions were 8-10% lower because of its reliance on the communal energy supply than if each individual flat in the estate used its own boiler and energy supplier).

Open air schools were built to combat the spread of tuberculosis in the early 20th century.

Today, while 95% of the UK population reports having access to a heating system, a survey by Ipsos has showed that more than a third of the population describes their homes as cold and damp. Cold homes are a significant cause of winter morbidity and mortality, with a Public Health England report showing that residents of the coldest 25% of homes face a 20% greater risk of death during winter than those in the warmest homes. We also have plenty of evidence that fuel poverty put households at risk of the worst effects of Covid-19. The combination of increased energy use – an inevitable outcome of a much greater reliance on domestic infrastructures during the pandemic – and reduction in income for many, meant that the radiator remained cold at the time of the greatest global health emergency in a century. This crisis has only been exacerbated post-pandemic, with the fuel price hikes driven by inflation, the war in Ukraine's impact on gas supplies into Europe, unsustainable energy policy and the widespread reliance on privatised energy provisions. With the least energy efficient homes in western Europe, the UK has been the most heavily affected by the current energy crisis, as shown by a 2022 International Monetary Fund (IMF) analysis.

It might be time to return to the model of communal heating, as an infrastructure that makes warm and healthy homes accessible to all. As the pandemic made abundantly clear, access to heating that is reliable and affordable should never be considered a privilege but a universal right.

Text by Kaja Marczewska

Churchill Gardens Estate, London, designed by Powell & Moya and photographed by Peter Pitt, 1946.

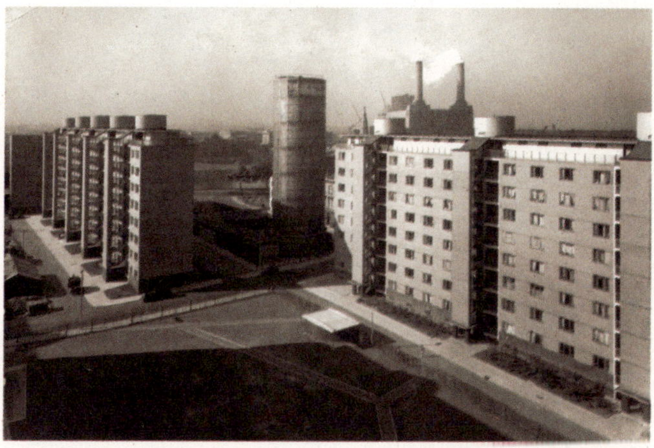

RADIO

How radio's power to connect brought transnational communities together during the pandemic

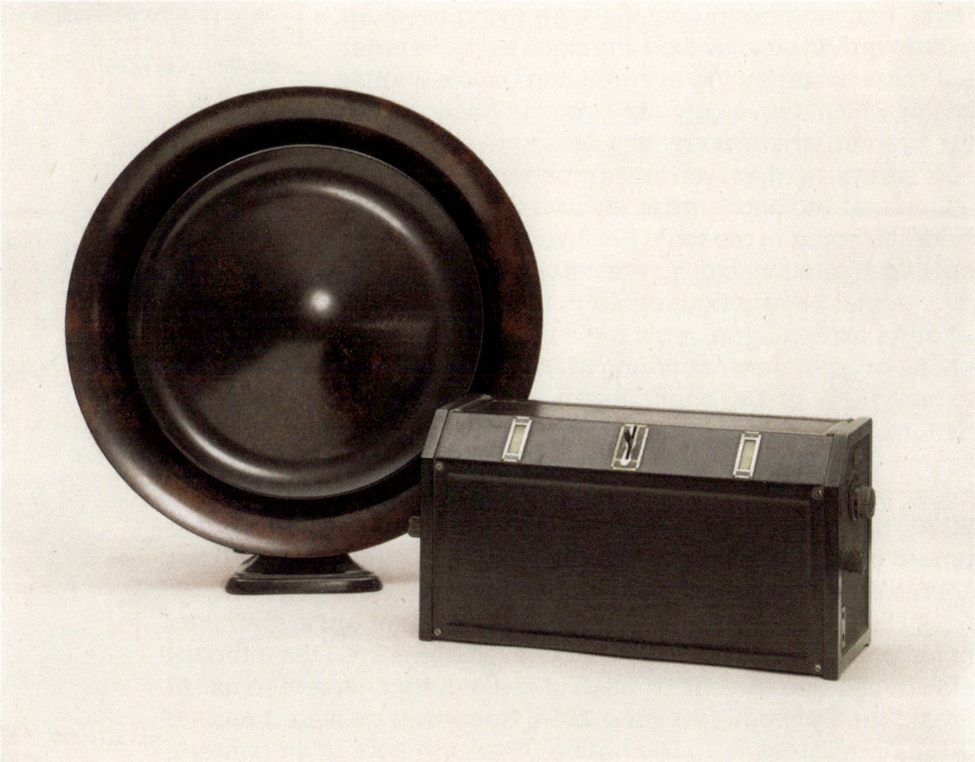

Radio receiver designed by Louis Christiaan Kalff and made by Philips in 1928.

Radio has long been considered a dying medium, overtaken first by television and since by the internet. But there is something evergreen in radio's humble power, which derives perhaps from its relationship to time. Unlike the internet, where everything lives forever, or the podcast – available always, to which you listen independently – radio is essentially ephemeral and anchored to the present. Digital playback services aside, listening to the radio live involves a kind of kinship, however fleeting or subconscious, with others listening elsewhere.

Almost every household in the UK has access to a radio, whether an analogue set, a radio in their car or digital radio on a phone or computer. According to Radio Joint Audience Research, almost 90% of UK adults listen to the radio weekly. All three national lockdowns in the UK saw a marked increase in both listener numbers and listening time, as many were confined to the house or working from home. In the anxious early days of March 2020, news stations saw a particular boost, as many people turned to radio – already a century-old invention – as a trusted source of information, reassurance and company.

Historically, radio has been used to great effect in moments of national urgency. Franklin D Roosevelt harnessed the intimacy of listening and the sheer reach of radio during his tenure as US President. Between 1933 and 1944, Roosevelt delivered around 30 radio addresses to the nation. Although serious in content, his 'Fireside Chats' were characterised by an informal, conversational style, and were designed to make the listener feel as though the president was speaking directly to them. Initially intended to garner support for Roosevelt's New Deal policies, the chats became an important source of hope and security throughout the Great Depression and Second World War. Their nickname conjures images of families gathered around the fireplace, radio on the mantel, listening collectively at the hearth.

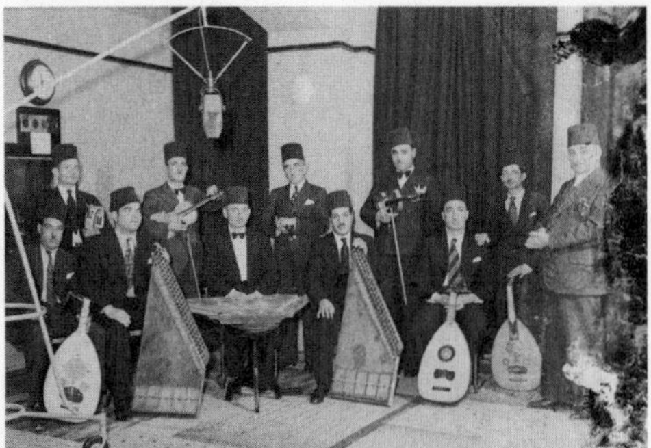

Radio artists from Palestine Broadcasting Service, Jerusalem, c1936–46.

The first radio was patented in 1897 by Guglielmo Marconi, and by the 1920s 'amateur' radio was broadcasting all over the world. The accessibility of radio clashed with desires for national control. A 1933 conference in Lucerne officially assigned frequencies to European countries so that they could manage broadcasts at home and across their colonies in the Middle East and Africa. One such example was the Palestine Broadcasting Service, established in 1936 and modelled after the BBC, which ran until the end of the British Mandate in 1948 and was afterwards taken over by Palestinian broadcasters.

While radio was instrumental for colonialism, it has also been a medium for resisting it. In Algeria, clandestine radio transformed the way independence was understood and imagined in the minds of Algerian listeners. In 1956, the Voice of Algeria began its broadcasts, uniting the Algerian people in solidarity and resistance. Although the French colonial government confiscated radio sets and jammed the Voice's frequencies, its messages got through. As Frantz Fanon writes, 'buying a radio, getting down on one's knees with one's head against the speaker, was no longer just wanting to get the news...it was *hearing* the first words of the nation'.

The pandemic has also been a catalyst for new online radio stations across the Middle East and North Africa. In Palestine, Radio Alhara (the Neighbourhood Radio) began broadcasting on 20 March 2020, run by five friends based between Ramallah, Bethlehem and Amman – architects Elias and Yousef Anastas, graphic designers Saeed Abu Jaber and Mothanna Hussein and artist Yazan Khalili. The station's programming harnesses the reach of the organisers' vast networks, and Radio Alhara quickly became a site for free expression and global communion with others, programmed by its own listeners. Tune in to hear artist Jumana Emil Abboud telling Palestinian folk tales; Raja Khalidi addressing the economy; an hour of 1960s Black nationalist poetry by The Last Poets; and musicians and DJs from all over the world playing sets from their sofas. In July 2020, Radio Alhara organised a three-day protest broadcast, triggered by the proposed annexation of part of the West Bank, which was mirrored on radio platforms from London to Tunis. After the port explosion in Beirut on 4 August 2020, the station ran a 30-hour fundraiser stream to support those affected. In her 'Love letter to radio', written in 2020, Rayya Badran observes, 'These recent communal experiments with radio...are incredibly exciting, not only because they summon us to listen, alone and together, but to harness a transnational collectivity that is otherwise made impossible by harsh and imposed borders'.

While such transnational potential is particularly meaningful in Palestine and across the Middle East, radio is an inherently planetary technology. Radio waves, like light, are a form of electromagnetic radiation, around us all the time, oscillating between the scale of a body and a building. Listening to the radio means tapping into something elemental – to waves bouncing between the ionosphere and earth, to sound sizzling across borders. Radio is pirate and planetary, public and clandestine, reassuring and revolutionary; it resounds during moments of national and global urgency. Radio's power to connect us has rarely felt so precious.

Text by Rachel Dedman

Ayla Hibri performing as part of the Sonic Liberation Front at MMAG Foundation in Amman.

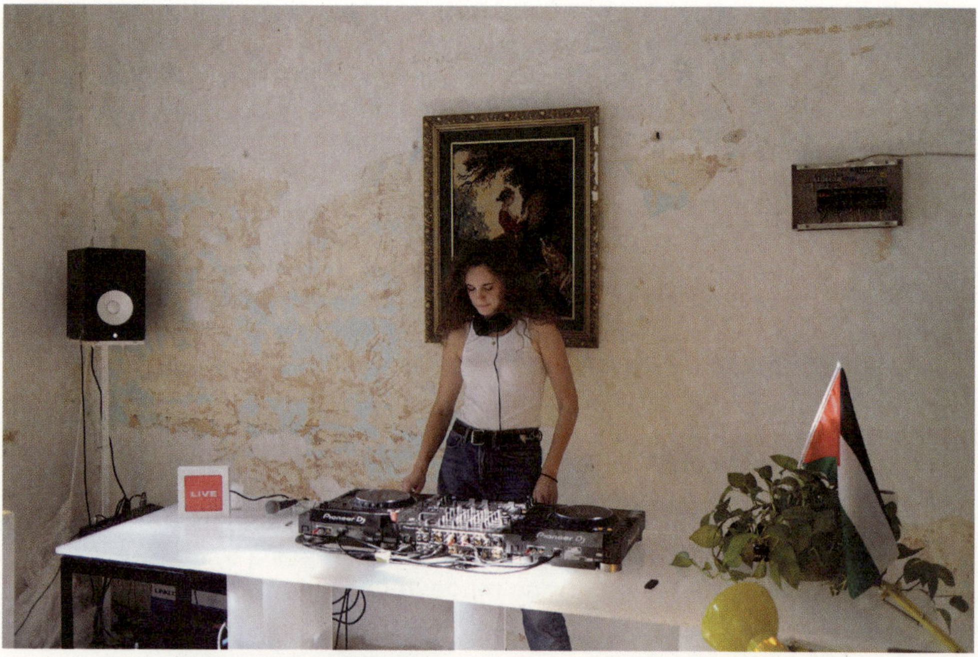

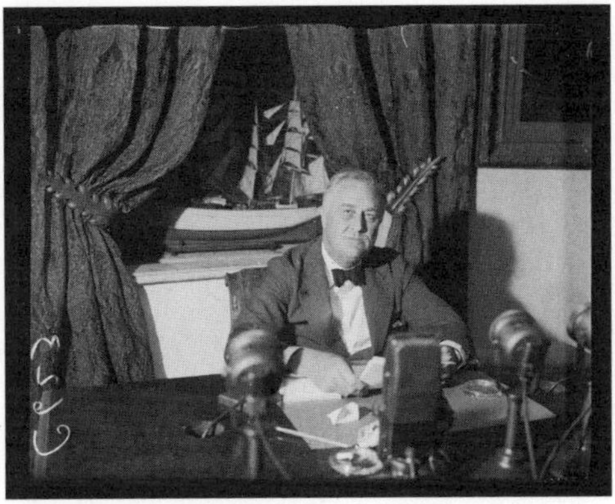

Franklin D Roosevelt's 'Fireside Chats', 6 September 1936.

08

SCALING UP

The most confounding quality of the pandemic was its scale. Reflected in the name – 'pan' meaning everything and everywhere – Covid-19 touched every corner of the world in one way or another. The issue of scale had several knock-on effects for objects. In one sense, the actions of one person were multiplied by millions, made evident where panic buying was visualised in real time with empty supermarket aisles in the early days of the outbreak. But scale also confounded our ability to think of actions and solutions at an international or global level. Designers offering copper and acrylic design hacks – often rightly making these open-source and shareable – failed to think of the material scarcities one would quickly run into, should millions of people adopt their designs. Elsewhere, the pandemic highlighted objects that were crucial to lockdown living, yet still unavailable in millions of households – namely laptops, tablets, phones and a decent Wi-Fi connection. The pandemic offered a shock to the design world, showing how bespoke designs would mean virtually nothing if scale, access and material supply chains weren't considered from the outset.

TOILET ROLL

Greenpeace toilet paper,
UK, c1991.

How the hoarding of toilet roll symbolised societal anxieties about hygiene, and reinforced the effectiveness of advertisement campaigns

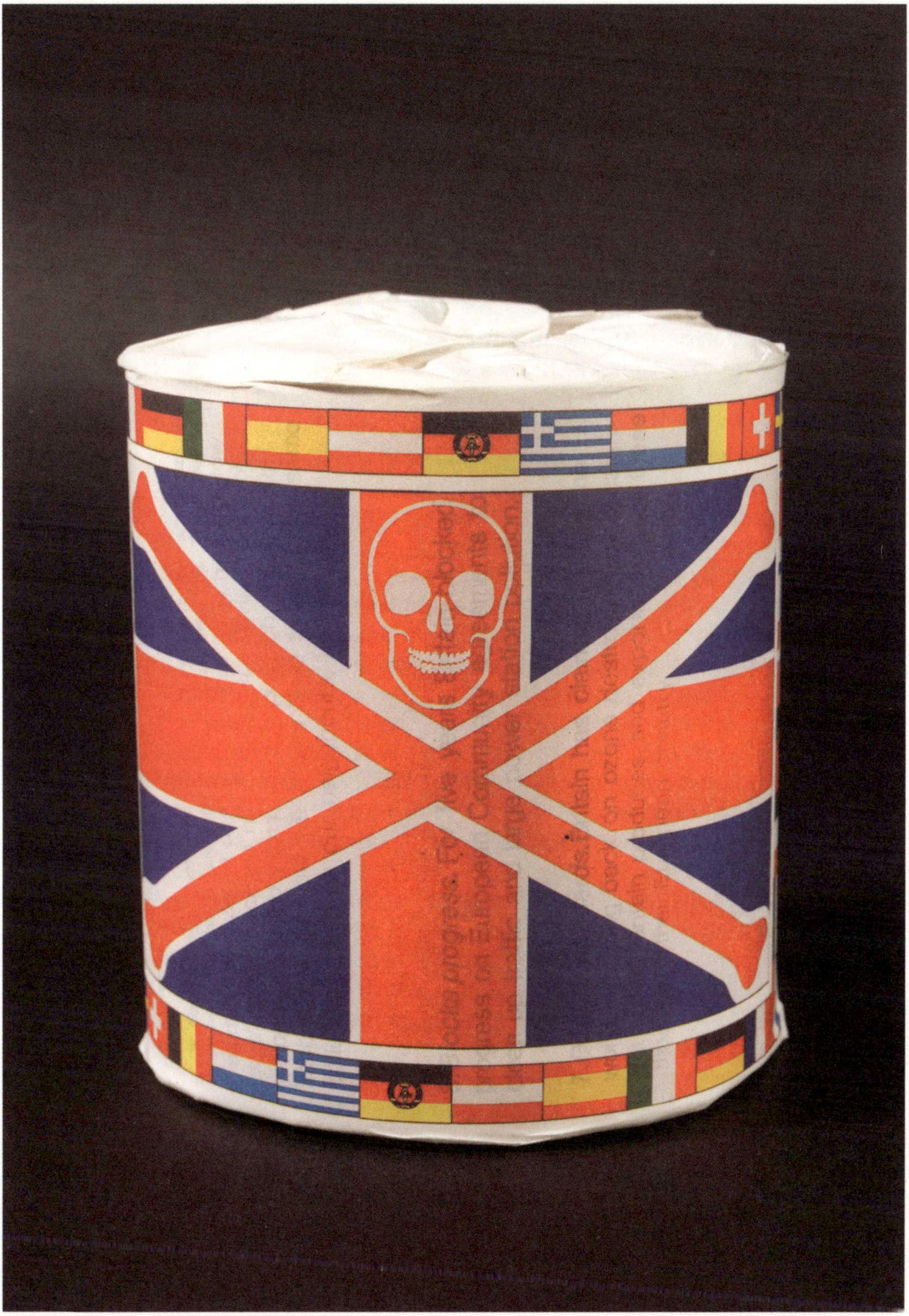

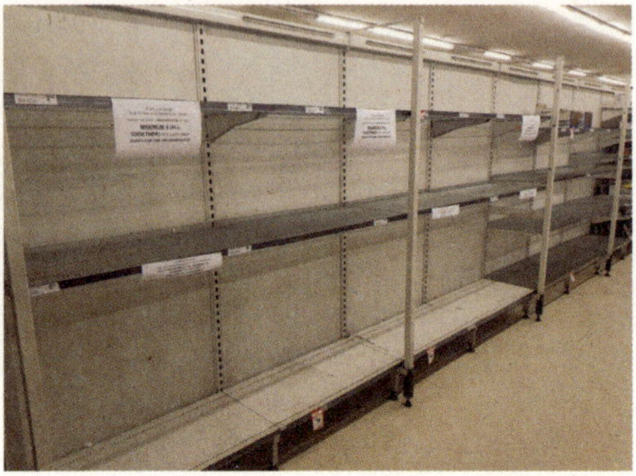

In March 2020, news reports and social media produced a constant stream of photographs showing queues of customers at supermarket check-outs, their trolleys filled with bales of super-saver, multi-ply toilet roll packs. Soon enough, these were replaced by images of long hollow aisles of empty shelves. In Hong Kong, Singapore, Australia, Japan, the US and UK, such images became the signifiers of imminent apocalypse, further driving panic buying in an endless feedback loop. Fights broke out over the precious commodity, and supermarket workers restocking the stripped-bare shelves had to protect themselves from the hordes with hastily constructed barricades. Stockpiling was criticised as an uncivil act, placing unnecessary pressure on supply chains, and rationing was introduced, with customers only allowed to take one pack each.

For about three weeks, as country after country entered lockdown and people prepared themselves for self-isolation, our most private act became a matter of public anxiety and scrutiny. Much of the world prefers a jug of water for their ablutions – but in a crisis, toilet paper, which contributes to massive deforestation, proved the basic necessity that our disposable culture felt it could not live without. The shortage was the subject of analysis by pundits and psychologists, as well as many jokes and memes. Two violinists wearing life jackets went viral with a video in which they played the *Titanic* theme tune in front of supermarket shelves emptied of toilet tissue.

The great toilet paper crisis of 2020 seemed worthy of an epilogue to Charles Mackay's miscellany of folly, *Extraordinary Popular Delusions and the Madness of Crowds* (1841). Mackay's study of 'moral epidemics' such as the South Sea Bubble and 'tulip mania' sought to 'show how easily the masses have been led astray, and how imitative and gregarious men are, even in their infatuations and crimes'. The 2020 frenzy, explained as an example of herd mentality, was not the first time toilet roll was the subject of collective consumer panic. In 1973, at the height of the oil crisis, a throwaway remark made by the TV comedian Johnny Carson warning of looming shortages caused a similar false scare. It was a self-fulfilling prophecy, with panic buying forcing prices up and leading to four months of scarcity.

Shelves in a supermarket in Sydney were emptied on 4 March 2020 from panic buying.

Toilet paper originated in China. In 105 CE, Cai Lun invented a new form of paper made from a mixture of mulberry leaves, fish nets, rags and hemp. Specially perfumed sheets eventually came to be made for use in the Emperor's toilet, and by the early 14th century millions of packets were produced a year. Public conveniences in Britain became popular with the Great Exhibition of 1851, where 827,280 visitors chose to spend a penny to use one of George Jennings' 'monkey closets' in the Crystal Palace Retiring Rooms. However, one Chinese visitor to Britain in the 1860s was appalled to find no purpose-made toilet paper: 'Westerners love to be clean,' he noted in his diary. 'Their bathrooms and toilets are extremely clean, however they use newspapers and books together with other reading materials in the toilet to wipe their filth away. They don't appreciate the value of written works.' Mass manufacture first occurred in the US in 1857, when Joseph Gayetty introduced his brand of 'therapeutic paper', each sheet soaked in disinfecting medicinal oils; it was advertised as 'the greatest discovery of modern time so far as alleviating and preventing human suffering is concerned'. The first perforated toilet paper produced in rolls, as we use it today, was invented in 1879 by British businessman Walter Alcock. The British Perforated Paper Company product, manufactured in Hackney Wick, was not as soft, splinter-free or absorbent as we now expect, but was rough on one side and shiny on the other. The Science Museum in London has in their collection a roll of Bronco, the not-so 'De Luxe Toilet Paper' produced by The British Perforated Paper Company in the 1930s and advertised with the slogan, 'Bronco, for the bigger wipe'.

It also has four rolls of 'Kleenex Quilted' produced in 1997 with a Penrose tiling embossed design. As design critic Alice Twemlow notes in an essay on the marketing of toilet paper in the magazine *Dirty Furniture*, brands with comforting names like Purex, Cushelle and Velvet use images of cupids, fluffy clouds and Labrador puppies in their advertising: 'The hope is that these images will befuddle us sufficiently to prevent us from considering the lack of any real technological innovation in toilet paper over the past 120 years, and to postpone any self-reflection on what we are actually doing with it, which is far from nesting in it, seeking emotional comfort in its embrace, or unfurling it along the corridor'.

It was perhaps this insulating sense of emotional comfort that buyers sought with their recent hoarding and nesting. In *Purity and Danger* (1966), the anthropologist Mary Douglas noted that 'reflection on dirt involves reflection on the relation of order to disorder, being to non-being, life to death'. As we became a nation of germaphobes, when every journey into the dirty public sphere seemed to involve mortal danger, buying toilet roll seemed to offer some kind of defence against the invisible enemy, a reassuring sense that you had prepared for the battle. Sigmund Freud connected the anal phase of a child's development – when they are toilet training – with the learning of control, and hoarding with anal retentiveness. As we all became exiles in our own countries, to cocoon ourselves in toilet paper, in the face of contagion, seemed to offer a final, precarious safety line.

Text by Christopher Turner

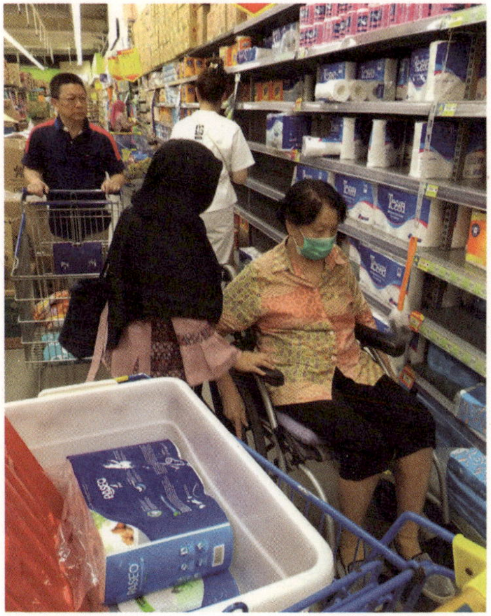

Panic buying in Jakarta
on 14 March 2020.

LAPTOPS

How the pandemic highlighted the ever-growing digital divide through the importance of being able to access a laptop

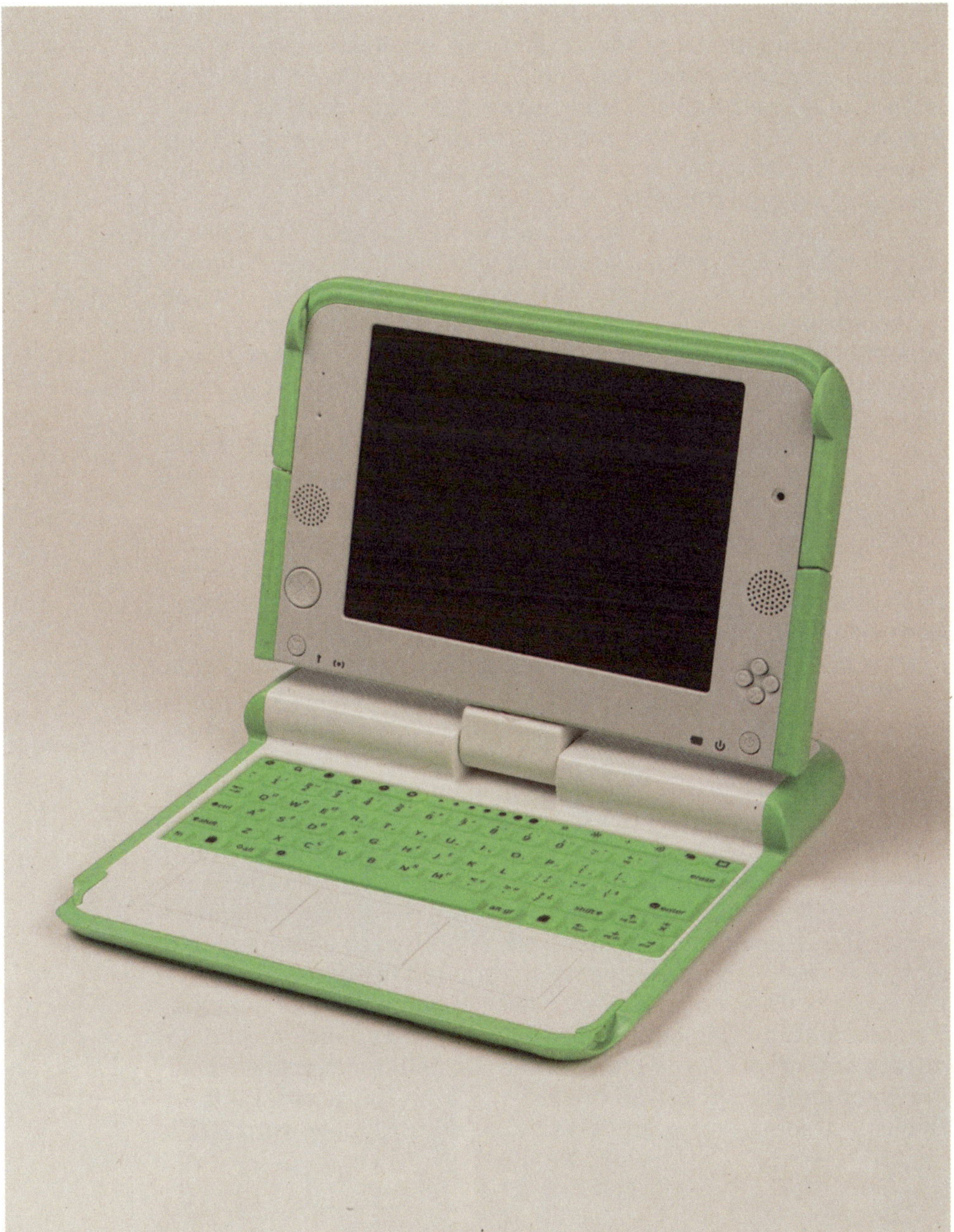

Laptop produced by One Laptop Per Child (OLPC), an initiative to combat digital inequality.

The laptop was an essential object of the pandemic, the vessel that facilitated the forced blending of work and play which resulted in new forms of interaction during lockdown. A society already obsessed with screens was sent into overdrive as people retreated inside domestic spaces, spending their time oscillating between emails, video conferencing, social media and streaming services (p142), all through the laptop.

However, not everyone has access to this essential piece of technology. The pandemic highlighted the drastically different and unequal experiences people had and exacerbated an already widening social division. The digital divide was apparent in every aspect of life under lockdown, from the ability to work from home and socialise with friends, to shopping and entertaining yourself and your family.

The immense scale of digital poverty is astonishing. It has been estimated that 1.9 million families in the UK have no access to the internet at home, with tens of millions more on expensive pay-as-you-go mobile internet tariffs. The poorest and most vulnerable households are the victims of this inadequacy. Prior to the pandemic, the digital divide had long been felt in the education sector. When lockdown was enforced by the UK government in March 2020, many of the solutions that had previously been put in place to address this – such as shared access to computers in schools and public libraries – were suspended, closed or scrapped altogether.

Digital poverty was one of the main factors that caused gaps in how young people were educated during the pandemic. An Institute for Fiscal Studies study from 2020 found that children from families with higher incomes dedicated on average 30% more time to their studies than those from less well-off households. These disadvantaged families often had to share a single laptop, where the time parents were required to access the internet for work often conflicted with their children's online courses. The same study also highlighted a large discrepancy regarding private schools, 79% of which offered their students online learning, in contrast to just 47% of students from the poorest fifth of families attending state-funded schools during lockdown in 2020.

The digital divide is not a new problem. Nearly 20 years ago Nicholas Negroponte, a Massachusetts Institute of Technology professor, started the One Laptop Per Child (OLPC) initiative to help combat digital poverty. The small green and white computer was purposefully designed to resemble a lunchbox, making a connection between how access to a laptop, in an increasingly digital world, is just like food – not a luxury, but a basic right for all children. Expectations for the device, which included a hand crank that could power the laptop in the event that reliable energy sources were not available, were sky high, with headlines forecasting that it would be the 'laptop that would change the world'. Unfortunately, shifts in strategic goals, developments in technology and the complex nature of distribution and educational systems in general, curtailed the initiative, and OLPC has since shifted its focus towards a broader strategy of enabling learning opportunities for children.

However, despite the criticism and setbacks to the OLPC initiative, it is critical to understand that access to a home computer has become a non-negotiable requirement when it comes to the education of children. Throughout the pandemic, schools attempted schemes that involved, for example, loaning laptops to students for them to take home; however, this was predicated on schools having enough or even any laptops to share with the students in need. In the museum sector, several institutions initiated or shifted educational programmes to online platforms. The British Library, Natural History Museum and V&A Dundee all circulated printed educational resources to local food banks. Through its #LetsMakeWednesdays education initiative during lockdown, the V&A drew young people away from their screens by broadcasting art, design and performance learning material through social media channels to encourage them to use everyday objects around the house as educational props.

However, the issue remains: all of these educational programmes are reliant on access to a computer, mobile phone and connection to the internet. The digital divide, which became readily apparent during the Covid-19 pandemic, is alive and well, cutting off large populations of children with a thirst, curiosity and, most importantly, a right to learn. The absence of technological means places all children without access to them at greater risk of isolation and a risk of falling behind; the laptop needs to be seen as an essential tool for the right to an education.

Text by Elizabeth Galvin

School report, London County Council, UK, 1910.

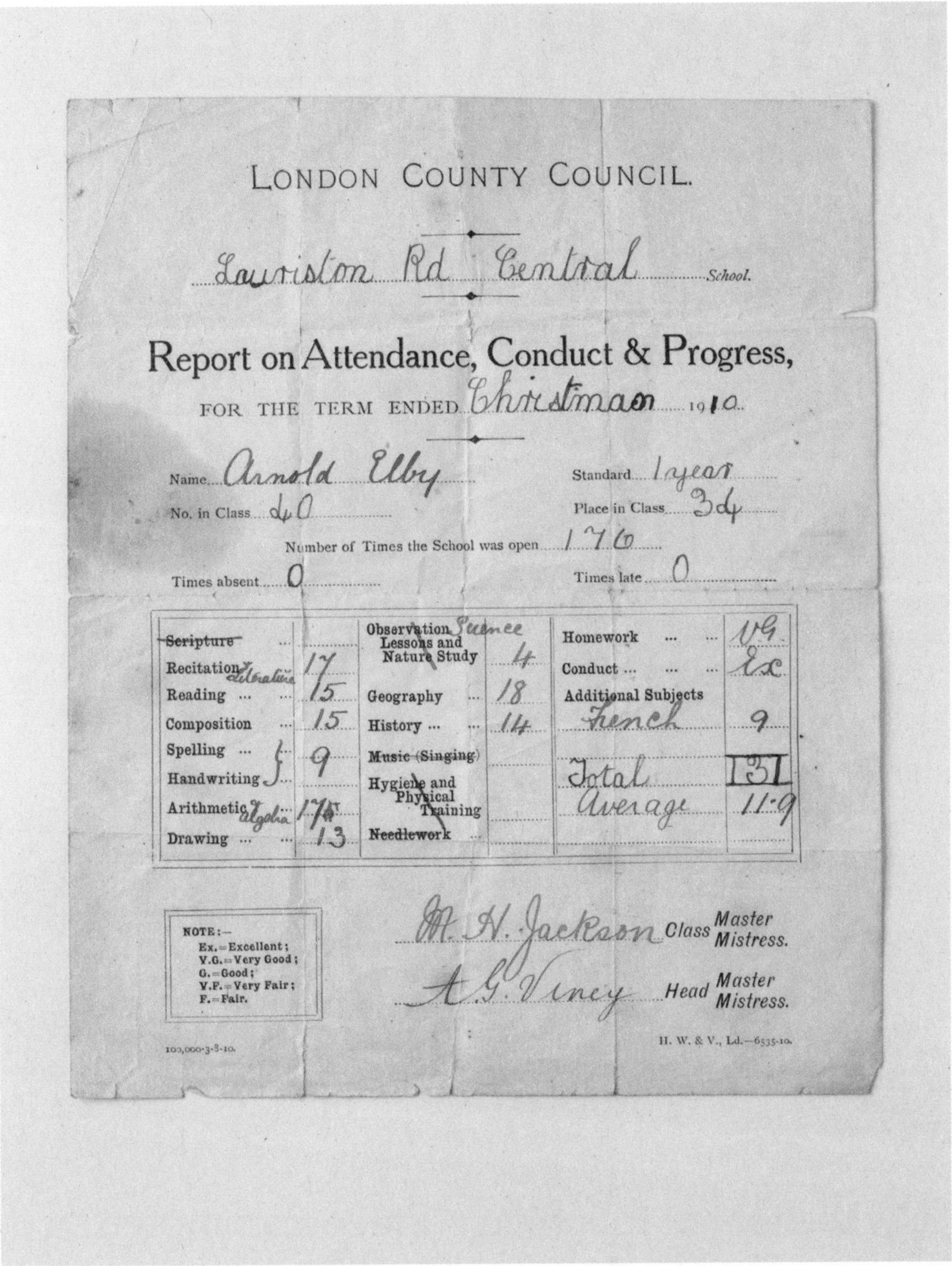

LONDON COUNTY COUNCIL.

Lauriston Rd Central School.

Report on Attendance, Conduct & Progress,

FOR THE TERM ENDED Christmas 1910

Name Arnold Elby | Standard 1 year

No. in Class 40 | Place in Class 34

Number of Times the School was open 176

Times absent 0 | Times late 0

~~Scripture~~ ...		Observation Science Lessons and Nature Study	4	Homework	V.G.
Recitation & Literature	17			Conduct	Ex
Reading	15	Geography ...	18	Additional Subjects	
Composition ...	15	History	14	French	9
Spelling ... }	9	~~Music (Singing)~~			
Handwriting }		~~Hygiene and Physical Training~~		Total	131
Arithmetic & Algebra	17			Average	11·9
Drawing	13	~~Needlework~~ ...			

NOTE:—
Ex. = Excellent;
V.G. = Very Good;
G. = Good;
V.F. = Very Fair;
F. = Fair.

M. H. Jackson Class Master Mistress.

A. G. Viney Head Master Mistress.

100,000-3-8-10.

H. W. & V., Ld.—6535-10.

DOOR HANDLES

How the fear of touching surfaces prompted a flurry of hands-free hacks, while exposing the need for deeper thinking about everyday affordances and accessibility for all

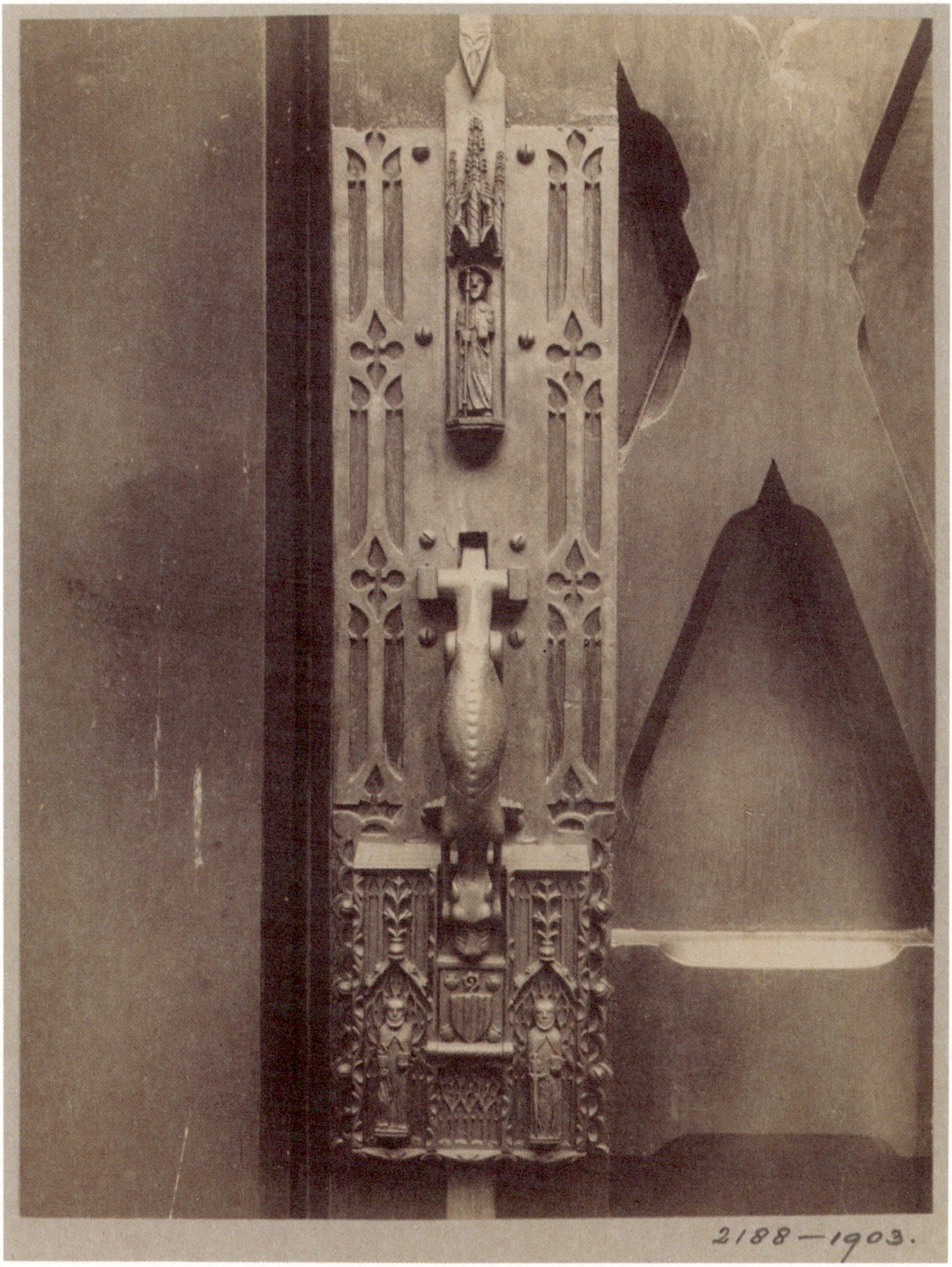

Eugène Atget, *Door Knocker, Hotel de Cluny*, Paris, c1900.

On 17 March 2020, a study published in the *New England Journal of Medicine* revealed that coronavirus can stay on surfaces such as plastic and stainless steel for up to 72 hours. Suddenly some of the most commonly used objects, none more than the door handle, came to be seen as a potential breeding ground and vector for a deadly disease. While transmissibility was still very much in question, the natural response for most was to try to avoid touching things in public, resulting in one common revelation: it is very hard to get around without using your hands.

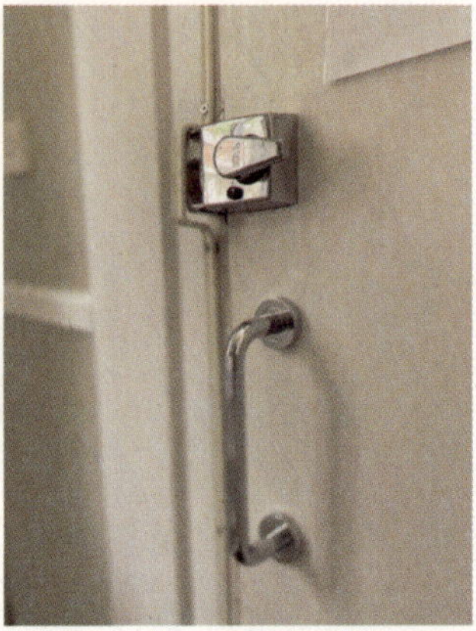

Brendan Cormier's daily dance with danger: the communal door in his building.

3D printing company Materialise quickly produced a suite of 3D-printed door handles that would slot over the top of existing ones, accompanied by the catchy slogan 'Do less harm, use your arm!' According to *Business Insider*, it took the team 24 hours to create and test the door handle before they were able to upload the free open-source designs. If you couldn't print at home, you could order a set for yourself. A pair cost between £29 and £60, depending on the size; the price was entirely driven by the costly 3D printing process, with no profit added.

These designs aimed to reduce harm by stopping people from touching the door with their hands. Instead, you use your forearm to pull the door towards you, or push down to force the lever. Another response from architectural designers Ivo Tedbury and Freddie Hong was more DIY, and didn't need screws – it was held together instead by a pair of cable ties. Such designs served a secondary use beyond the pandemic, as a means to open doors that would otherwise prove challenging for many disabled people. Form, as we know, should follow function, but – with apologies to the design gods of yore – such functions have often been imagined in exclusionary terms, and forms designed without everyone in mind. Your average lever handle, a supposedly 'universal' design, can actually be rather disabling to people with limited dexterity or who don't have a hand, thus becoming an uninviting way to enter someone's home.

Disabled people have been asking for this problem of supposed universality to be addressed for a long time. Now that we have all grappled with the challenge of thinking about new ways to avoid using our hands, this could be an opportunity to invite conversations of adaptation and access for all (and look to where disabled people have been doing it all along), well beyond the pandemic. The design by Materialise, and that by Tedbury and Hong, are yet more considerations for a renewed outlook on the assumptions we make about our most everyday affordances.

Text by Natalie Kane

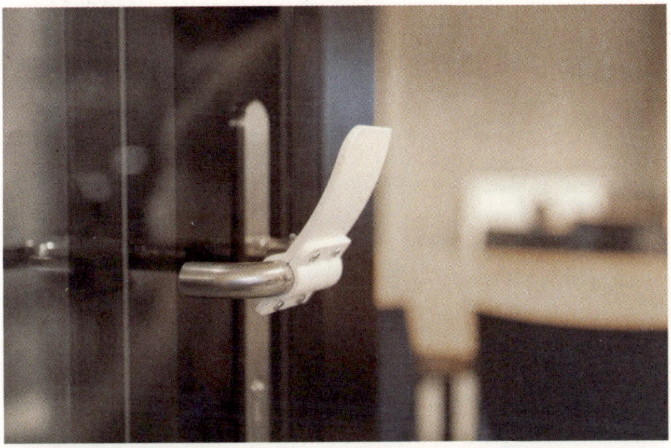

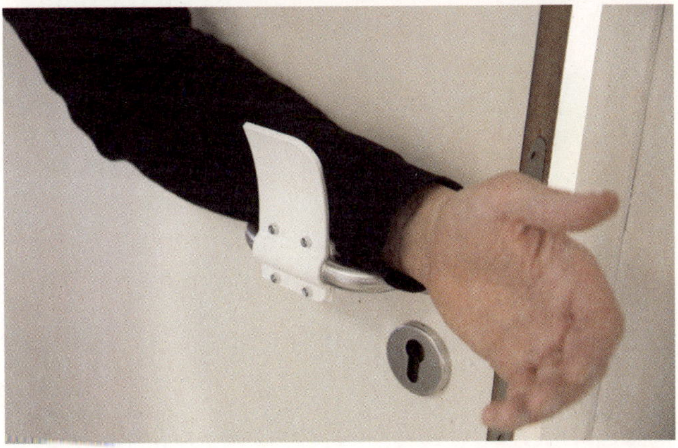

3D printed door handle attachment by Materialise.

COPPER

How copper, due to its antimicrobial properties, became a simplistic go-to for designers seeking solutions to the pandemic, distracting from more effective public measures

PANDEMIC OBJECTS

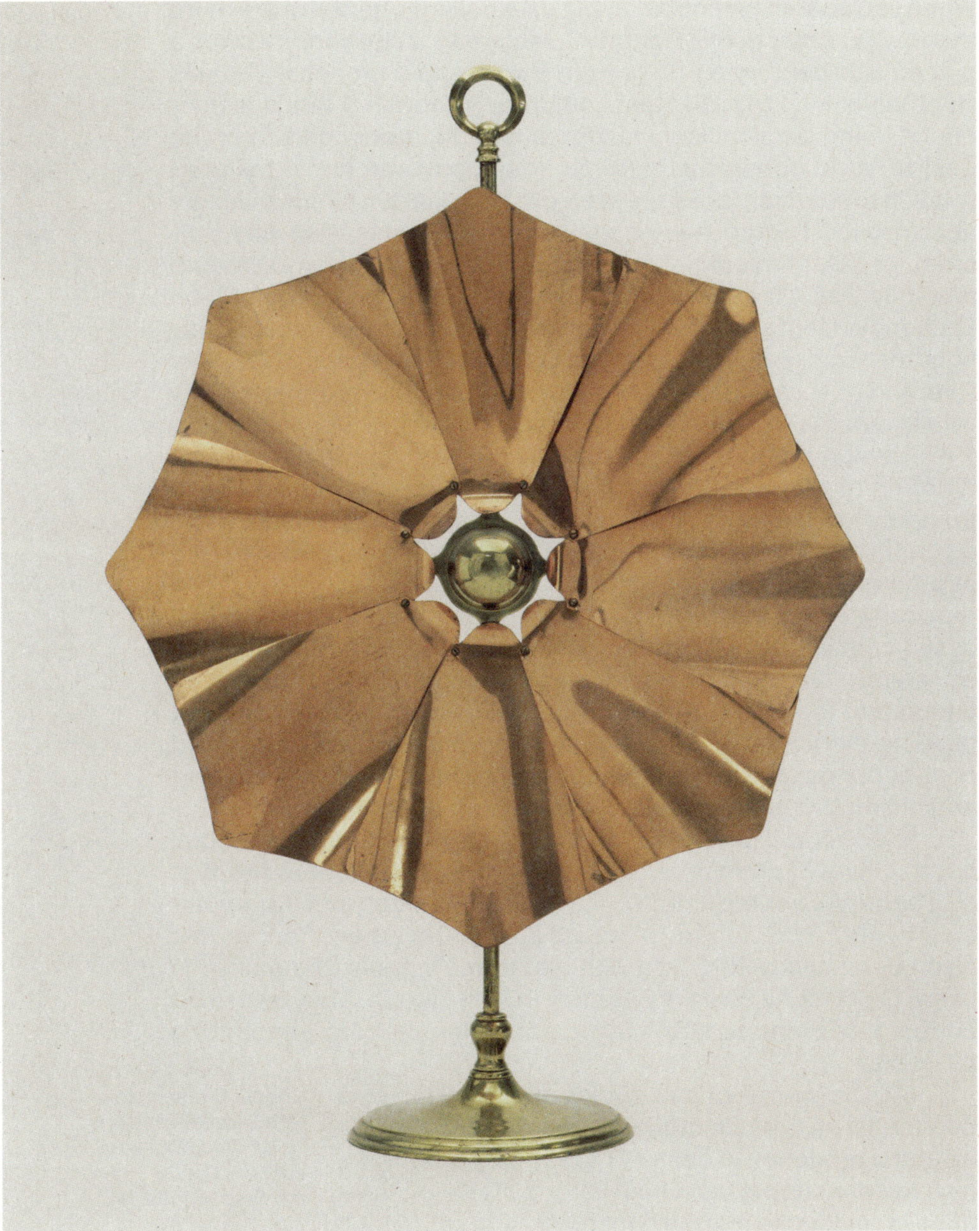

Fire screen made of copper by William Arthur Smith Benson, London, 1884.

When you search for copper in the V&A collections, there are more than 2,000 objects that contain it, including a 7th-century ewer, a pair of 19th-century earrings from Egypt, and a model of Thomas Heatherwick's 2012 Olympic cauldron. Although it has a history of use going back millennia, copper has become a darling of the design world during the past few years, coveted for its textured reddish tone which looks great on everything from lamps to luxury apartments. During the pandemic, copper was also championed for its antimicrobial properties. As a result, between March and July 2020, it had a 40% growth surge on the London Metal Exchange. Central to this was the idea that copper can not only fight the virus, but also look good doing so. How much of this was true, and how have designers in the past balanced copper's utility with its aesthetic allure?

Design and copper have a long history, that mostly places function at the fore. Before the 21st century, copper was used primarily for its mechanical properties. Copper has been used as piping in city infrastructure since at least 2,750 BCE (discovered at a funerary complex in northern Egypt) and many of the pipes that carry water in the UK today are made of copper, which can assist with water purification. Above ground, copper was used as roofing for Grecian temples, as sheet metal for shipbuilding and during the 19th century as a material for interior and exterior building elements. Additionally, printing presses used engraved copper plates to print illustrations and bronze (an alloy of copper and tin) matrices were used for the casting of type metal.

Electronics have also taken advantage of copper's natural conductivity. The material was an essential element in the first true battery, invented in 1800, and in a revolutionary new computer chip by IBM, developed 197 years later. Conversely, copper has also been used to interfere with electronic signals: the buildings of the US National Security Agency in Fort Meade, Maryland used copper sheathing to stop spying radio signals from penetrating the walls.

At the onset of the pandemic, copper was heralded as a miracle material for a different ability: a natural tendency to destroy microbes. This is not a new role for copper, as it has historically been identified in relation to human health, starting with Aulus Cornelius Celsus's 1st-century treatise *De Medicina*, which listed the many ways that copper can be used for medicinal purposes. In 2008, Celsus's ideas were verified by the US Environmental Protection Agency, which confirmed that copper and bronze

Copper printing plate with jewellery designs by Nicolaus Mensma, engraved by CF Frihsch, the Netherlands, 1747.

can kill microbes on contact. This declaration led to a boom in the production of antimicrobial copper objects and surfaces, and was further accelerated by the Covid-19 pandemic, in which a fear of transmission on anything that came into contact with our bodies resulted in designs ranging from touch tools and mobile testing units to 'full metal jackets'.

Is this magical copper-tinted thinking? Copper does have antimicrobial properties, but it takes approximately 45 minutes for pathogens to break down on copper, and not all copper products have the same material integrity. However, for high-contact, stationary objects such as doorknobs, copper remains a great material for reducing microbe transmission. It is for this reason that Bill Keevil, a professor of environmental healthcare at the University of Southampton, has suggested that architects and designers preserve all copper and bronze fixtures in existing buildings and include them in all future design projects.

Though antimicrobial copper does have a capacity to ward off microbes, when planning anti-pathogenic architecture and systems, the emphasis should remain on collective measures such as the design of well-ventilated spaces and new codes that ensure that the correct types of copper are used in new buildings.

Text by Anna Talley

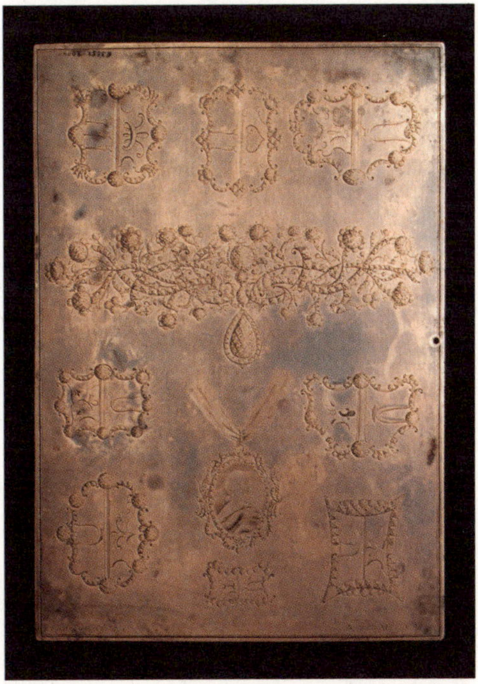

CARDBOARD BOXES

Astronaut helmet made from papier-mâché by Richard Blundel with help from his mother, Maidenhead, 1969.

How a dramatic increase in home deliveries exposed the inherent fragility in a strained global logistics system

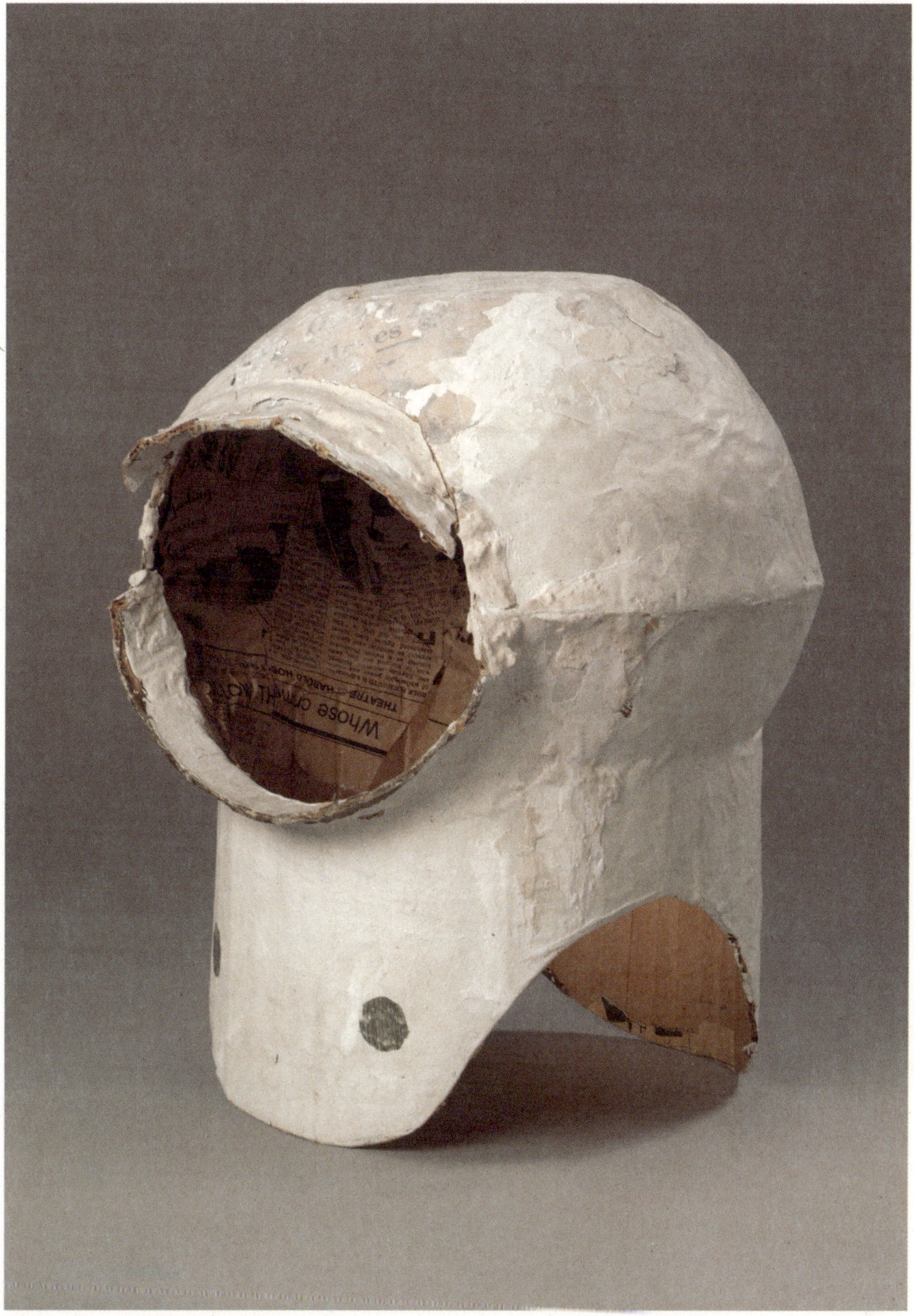

During the Covid-19 pandemic, home deliveries thrived. With the arrival of each package – from a 5kg supply of fruit and vegetables from the wholesaler or a much-needed beard trimmer sold by Amazon, to a long-awaited book enjoyed during another weekend at home – the majority of deliveries often had one thing in common: a cardboard box.

The box itself allowed one to safely shop from the confines of home during the pandemic. Received in a ritual of 'contactless' delivery, it was a portal into a former time when venturing outdoors for shopping was a normality. This desire to have some form of connection with the outside world, through objects delivered in cardboard boxes, was apparent in the surge of home deliveries, with e-commerce giants struggling to fulfil demands (Amazon reportedly recruited more than 100,000 additional staff in March 2020 alone and saw profits double in the first year of the pandemic). On the other hand, the cardboard box represented a new pandemic worry: surfaces that could carry the virus into the safe confines of your sanitised home.

A flurry of articles relayed scientific advice about Covid-19 and its contagious longevity on various surfaces. From the dangers of metal door handles to virus survival rates on plastic buttons on clothes, cardboard was often featured on lists of materials upon which the virus might survive, risking infection (see Door Handles p318, Copper p322 and Tote Bags p252). It thus joined a league of everyday banal objects that suddenly posed a concern and prompted risk management.

US Department of Agriculture's 'Meals to You' program sending supplemental food boxes to children in rural areas during school closures in 2020.

Adding to this double transformation of cardboard is that it also enabled the mass delivery of vitally needed medical equipment for public health services such as personal protective equipment (PPE), testing kits (p332) and ventilation machine supplies. In this sense, cardboard, as a carefully designed packaging system, reached its zenith of functionality – neatly and safely enabling the global distribution of all goods.

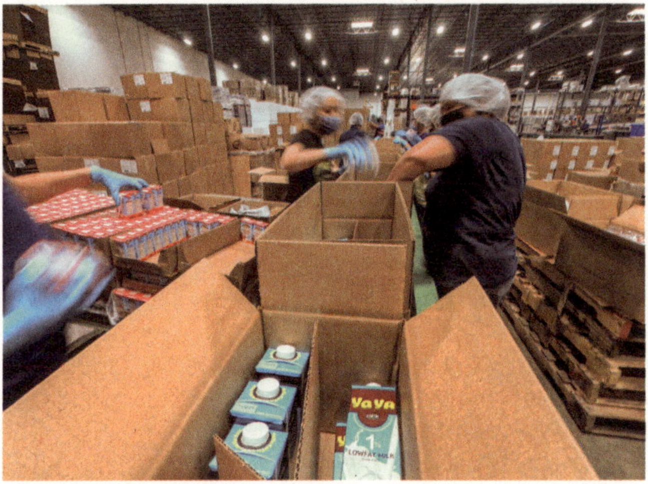

In many ways, this shift in meaning for the cardboard box was seismic. Prior to the pandemic, the cardboard box was so ubiquitous an object, it was almost invisible. It was a mechanism for delivery, but never the main point of interest. The cardboard box has been in use for over a century, used as a shipping material since the 1870s. The invention of one of the first folding cardboard boxes is attributed to paper manufacturer Robert Gair Company of Brooklyn, New York, who dates its creation to a fortuitous machine cutting accident in 1879. Designs for more systematised folding boxes followed with a series of patents in the 1890s, along with many others entering circulation, eclipsing the previously dominant wooden shipping crate. While there have been a few major design innovations in the decades since, such as Tetra Pak food packaging or Amazon's box-finding algorithm, the core look and feel of the corrugated brown cardboard box has barely changed, and has more recently celebrated with its own emoji.

The use of the cardboard box poses another issue – its disposal. A box is typically discarded immediately after receipt, or occasionally repurposed as a raw material – from home DIY projects to works of modern art, such as Pablo Picasso's cardboard guitar and Joseph Beuys' assemblages, and of contemporary design and architecture, such as Frank Gehry's chairs and Shigeru Ban's buildings. The surge in home deliveries and cardboard box shipping triggered by Covid-19 lockdowns, and our continued reliance on the material post-pandemic, has seen this once-mundane object become central to the large-scale disruption of another important system: recycling.

At the end of March 2020, the Recycling Association issued a stark warning on the prospect that the UK would face a cardboard shortage as a result of the pandemic. Increased demand coupled with the challenge of many local councils suspending regular recycling collections during lockdowns posed a threat for an industry that relies on recycled fibre for cardboard manufacture. Moreover, fibre trade is an international market that was strained by border closures. The pandemic provided a stress test for many global systems, and in the case of cardboard, it revealed the fragility of a logistics system that heavily relies on a single material. These recycling challenges also exacerbated the worrying environmental cost of online retail, where packaging waste and over-packaging have long been problems.

Reflecting on the pandemic, it is vital to remember that industries that touch the entire supply chain of delivered goods require more efficiency. Post-pandemic thinking around systems design needs to address packaging more thoughtfully. From optimising material choices to upgrading existing infrastructures for circulating and reusing resources, it is vital to create more resilient systems. Sustainable material practices are more important than ever as we seek to mitigate our environmental impact and safeguard our common future.

Text by Zofia Trafas White

Cosplay of D.Va from Overwatch at the 2016 New York Comic Con.

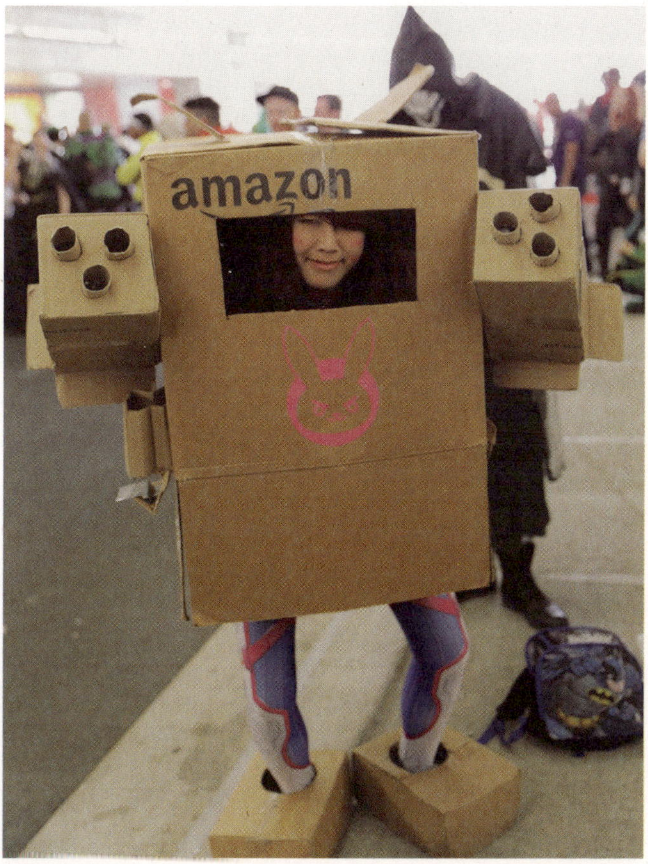

TESTING KITS

How design played an important role in the self-administering of Covid-19 tests and allowed for the spatial navigation of mass testing centres in the UK

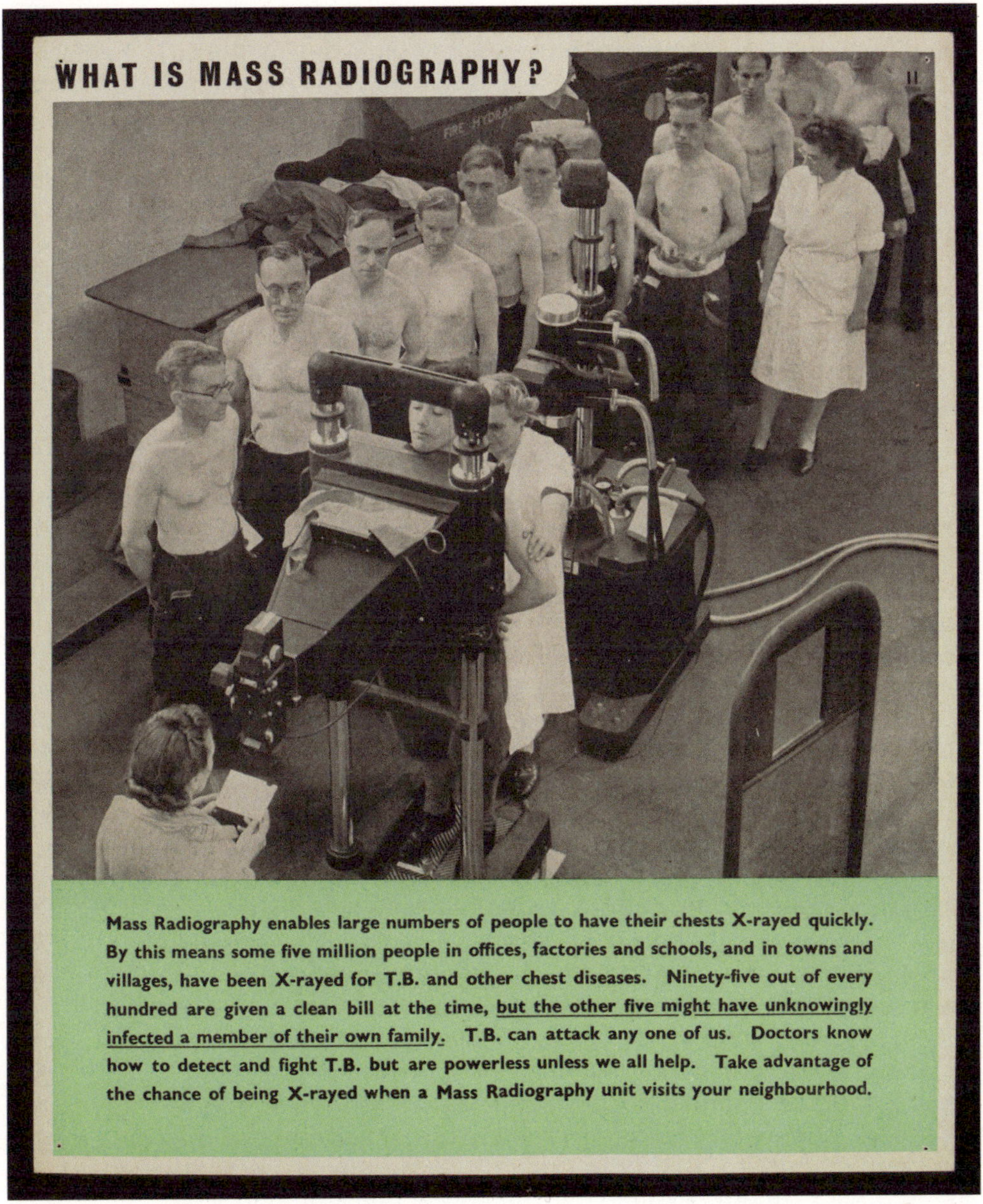

Mass radiography poster commissioned by the Ministry of Health, UK, 1949

'A test is a critical moment, meaningful because it claims to stand for something', argue Noortje Marres and David Stark in 'Put to the test: For a new sociology of testing'. The essay was published in the *British Journal of Sociology* in April 2020, just as the world was closing down to stop the spread of Covid-19. Little did the authors know that the concept of tests and testing would take on such monumental proportions in British society and around the world in the following months.

The idea that tests stand for something was keenly felt throughout the UK in the first year of the pandemic. Low testing capacity at the beginning of the pandemic had devastating consequences for people residing in care homes, while, later on, mass testing in schools led students and parents to question privacy and consent around the data collected during these procedures. In July 2021, the NHS Test and Trace app resulted in a so-called 'pingdemic', where almost 700,000 people in England and Wales were asked to self-isolate during a single week due to potential exposure to someone with a positive Covid-19 test, even if they had not tested positive themselves. At the same time, sceptics took to the streets to protest against Covid-related restrictions, including 'Covid passports', mandatory for most international travel. Despite the mixed reactions, the act of testing was seen by many as something akin to a civic duty and a way to care for fellow citizens. This sentiment was clearly stated in the NHS Test and Trace leaflet which explained that 'around one in three people with Covid-19 do not know they have it', and that to combat this 'with regular self-testing we can slow the spread and help protect the most vulnerable in our families and communities'.

In November 2020, Liverpool pioneered the first attempt at mass testing in the UK for people with no symptoms, with more than 280,000 inhabitants (57% of Liverpool residents) tested in a few months. That December, the government introduced a mass testing programme for all UK schools, which was delayed for two months in favour of another national lockdown. In February 2021, mass testing was implemented in specific postcodes throughout the UK where new and more infectious strains of coronavirus had been diagnosed. And from April 2021, everyone in England and Scotland became eligible for free self-administered Covid-19 tests twice a week. These different testing programmes were accompanied by the development of various visual forms of instruction or communication, designed to provide the public with easy-to-understand information.

Here, design as a means of communication became integral to the access and administering of tests. Rapid Covid-19 tests, or lateral flow tests for self-administration, were issued by the Department of Health and Social Care (DHSC) and manufactured by Xiamen Biotime Biotechnology in China, and came with a 20-page, 20-step instruction manual. These step-by-step instructions were easy to follow, guiding test takers through the process of 'swabbing' with pictograms and simple line drawings. Mostly printed in the sans-serif typeface New Transport (a digital adaption of the Transport lettering designed by Jock Kinneir and Margaret Calvert in the late 1950s to be used for road signage in the UK), the leaflet was a carefully considered piece of interaction design, enhanced by the fact that the cardboard packaging that accompanied the testing kit could also be transformed into an 'extraction tube' holder.

Hundreds of spaces across the UK also suspended their normal use to become test centres. As the need for testing capacity grew, these centres occupied a range of spaces from supermarket car parks, school gymnasiums and community halls to repurposed buses and vans, convention centres (p236) and even racecourses. The selected sites, large in scale and spacious enough to allow for social distancing, needed new signage to communicate direction. Repurposed road signs became familiar sights, both at vaccine and test centres, using the same formats and colours as Kinneir and Calvert's national road signage system. The signs were adapted from a group that was created to alert road users to temporary instructions and diversions, and the all-caps messaging – either in white text against a red background, or black text against a yellow background – is immediate to decipher and insists upon caution. They appeared at the test centres with a medley of eerie pandemic slogans, easily legible at a distance: 'COVID-19 TEST CENTRE'; 'MAINTAIN 2M DISTANCE'; 'DO NOT ENTER IF YOU HAVE SYMPTOMS OF CORONAVIRUS'; 'FACE COVERINGS MUST BE WORN'.

Unlike the quickly executed, hand-drawn paper signs of the early pandemic (see Homemade Signs p12), these signs made of metal composite expressed an air of officiality and reliability. Often held in place by sandbags and accompanied by traffic cones, they provided a sense of bureaucratic familiarity, despite their impromptu nature.

These examples of communication design bring to mind another such effort in the UK following the Second World War. At the conclusion of the 1940s, there was an alarming rise of tuberculosis cases in the general population and a similar initiative to test large groups of British citizens followed as a result. The posters and leaflets designed to promote the mass radiography programme instigated by the Ministry of Health are testament to this effort. Mobile screening units were sent to schools, factories and other local access points to ensure that asymptomatic tuberculosis sufferers were found, isolated and treated before the disease could spread further. The language used in these campaigns is similar to that used in Covid-19 mass testing material and, like the tuberculosis mass-screening posters, the instruction manuals, road signs and other ephemera connected to the UK's effort to mass test the population for Covid-19 form an important material archive of the pandemic. They evidence the role design can play in transforming scenarios that might at first might seem entirely unfamiliar, instead rendering them as commonplace.

Text by Johanna Agerman Ross

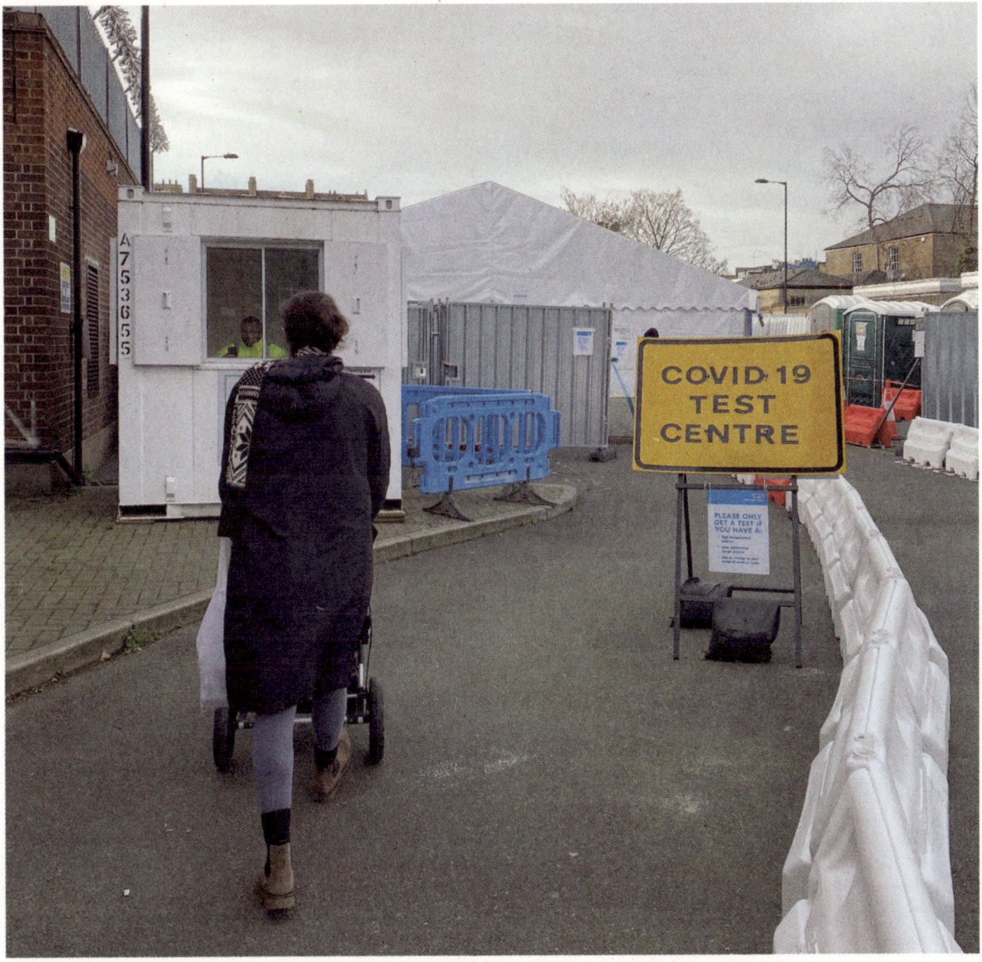
COVID 19
TEST
CENTRE
PLEASE ONLY
GET A TEST IF
YOU HAVE A:

Covid-19 testing centre in a parking lot in Dalston, London.

HANDS

Clapping is not just a gesture of appreciation, but a performance in its own right. Such a performance was especially powerful during the first lockdown in the UK, as across the country every Thursday at 8pm people stood on stoops or leaned from windows to clap in support of the NHS. While the idea had already begun in other European countries, it was proposed in the UK in late March over social media by Annemarie Plas, a Dutch woman living in London. Under the title 'Clap for our Carers', this performance quickly became a national ritual, with politicians and celebrities filming and photographing themselves clapping and sharing said media online, along with millions of others.

For many, the first instance of 'Clap for our Carers' was genuinely moving. Amid so much isolation, hearing your street erupt with noise and knowing that the same thing was happening at the other end of the country was an emotional experience. Criticism was also rightly raised at the perceived hypocrisy of politicians who had mishandled the lockdown and left the NHS ill-prepared for the crisis. After all, clapping wasn't going to save lives, but good governance could. Group fatigue over the ritual gradually set in, and by the end of May, Plas was calling to end the intervention with one last hurrah, which took place on 28 May 2020.

Regardless of its eventual demise, the event was an object lesson in successful group happenings. At the beginning of the pandemic, when hands were vilified as vectors of disease, here they were also a modest way of coming together, at a distance.

Text by Brendan Cormier

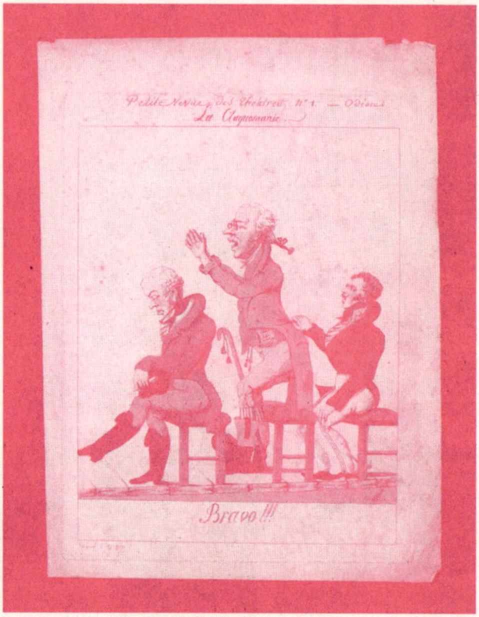

B Julien, *La Claquomanie*, France, 19th century.

STREET TREES

The suspension of everyday rituals during the Covid-19 pandemic led many to focus on their immediate environment, noticing elements that they might otherwise have overlooked. A newfound admiration for street trees became evident, likely prompted in the UK by the permission of a daily constitutional as reason to be outside during the first lockdown. Feeding this surge in enthusiasm were apps such as Tree-Talk London, which helps identify tree species in your neighbourhood, and the grassroots phenomenon of botanists chalking the names of plants growing in the cracks of pavements to show others what is growing where. The realisation that trees bear fruit, and that many wild plants are edible, also sparked a renewed interest in foraging. Such attention to urban nature had a calming effect during the pandemic, but also expressed a simple transformational idea: that more care and mindfulness about the natural infrastructure that makes up cities is the first step to a more ecologically resilient place.

Based on Ella Ravilious's essay
on the *Pandemic Objects* blog

DIGITAL ARCHIVES

In April 2020, Anna Talley and Fleur Elkerton, two postgraduate design historians at London's Royal College of Art and the V&A, set up Design in Quarantine. It was an online database that brought together the various design responses to the Covid-19 pandemic.

Through a simple format consisting of image, title, author and date of appearance, the archive was able to nimbly bring together hundreds of projects from around the world. On the homepage, there is a prompt to submit your own design response, or a design response that you think should be included, adding to the heterogeneity of content. Scanning through the archive today reveals a mixture of the surreal and prosaic: from photographs of vegetables used as ersatz face masks, to packaging for testing kits from Taiwan.

A significant amount of criticism emerged during the pandemic about the way in which certain quickly conceived, undercooked 'design solutions' were being put forward by design firms and disseminated on design websites, more as a way to generate clicks and internet traffic than as earnest proposals. What Design in Quarantine shows, however, is a far richer tapestry of projects conceived during this time and a testament to human creativity during a crisis. While hosting fees and site maintenance requirements mean that little on the internet can promise eternal existence, some precautions have been taken for this archive, which is now permanently stored and viewable on the UK Web Archive.

Text by Brendan Cormier

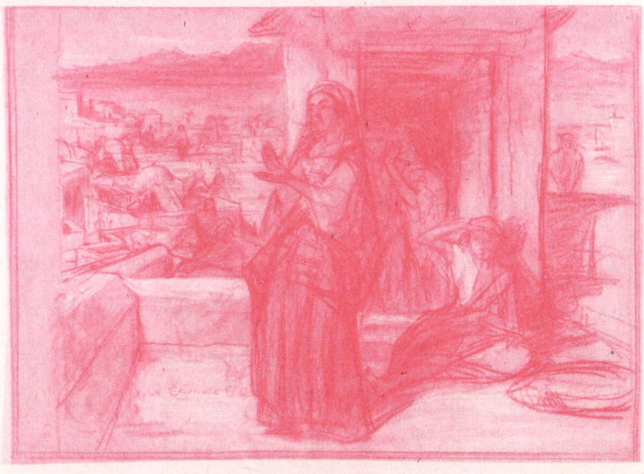

Drawing by Alfred W Elmore, Algeria, 1866–67.

BEARDS

How do we explain the peculiar uptick in men growing beards during the pandemic? Was it an opportunity to experiment with a style otherwise frowned upon in the workplace? Or was it a post-apocalyptic look to match the times? Interpreting the symbolism is a slippery task. Throughout history, the beard has expressed both revolutionary appeal and conservative conformity. Even today, the beard remains a popular symbol of both left-leaning hipsterism and far-right militiamen. Perhaps the real reason for the quarantine beard was something more personal and corporeal: an attempt by many to cast a protective layer between the body and the outside world.

Based on James Robinson's essay
on the *Pandemic Objects* blog

COCKTAIL GLASSES

The 'quarantini' was an aspirational approach to lockdown, an embrace of leisure and online posturing in the absence of being with others. As Richard Godwin wrote in *The Guardian*, 'cocktails have an affinity with strange, uncertain times; celebration and consolation in one hit'. The opulence was reinforced by celebrities drinking cocktails on social media – such as Meryl Streep giving a boozy performance of 'The Ladies Who Lunch' over Zoom, or Stanley Tucci offering up a tutorial for how to make the perfect Negroni – bolstering the comfortable lie that we were all in this together. The cultured affectation of the cocktail glass may have also spurred on a more insidious effect. While drinking rates rose during the pandemic, many did not cut back once the initial crisis settled. Through its nostalgic connotations, the cocktail glass may have been a mask for many partakers, giving them a sense of participation in a collective cultural act rather than a potentially destructive form of self-medication.

Based on Josephine Rout's essay
on the *Pandemic Objects* blog

Barber's bowl, Brislington,
Great Britain, c1710–20.

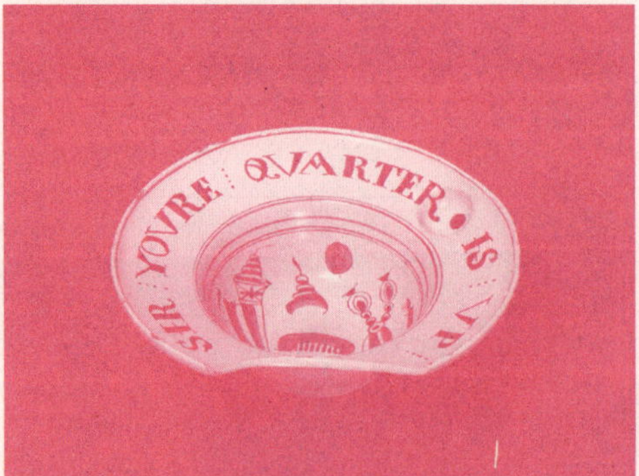

Hagueneau champagne glasses,
designed by René Lalique, France, 1924.

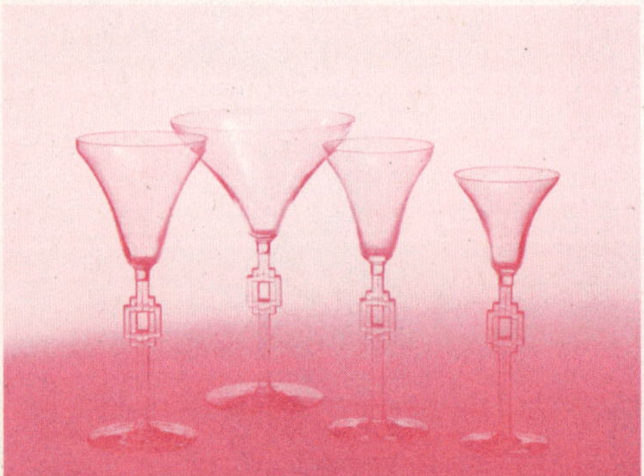

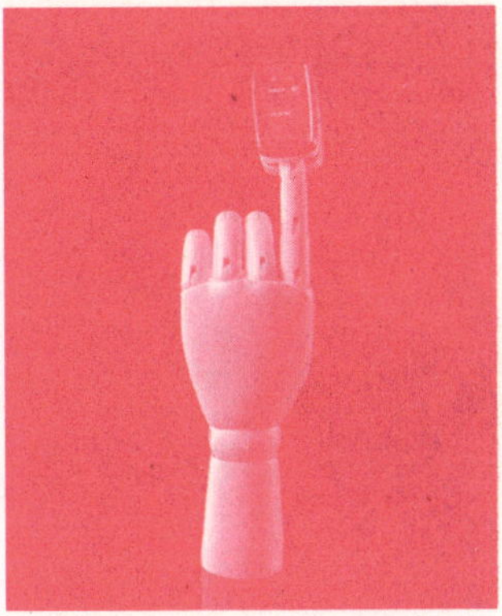

Fingertip pulse oximeter made by ACurio, Shenzhen, 2021.

FINGER OXIMETERS

A small device used to monitor the amount of oxygen carried in the body, the finger oximeter was little considered before the pandemic. One might have encountered them in a hospital or noticed them as a prop in a hospital TV drama, but their function was rarely clear to a broader public. Following the outbreak of Covid-19, with healthcare services in crisis and the need for many infected with the virus to track and manage the progression of their condition at home, many healthcare services, including those in the UK, France and Italy, began recommending that people buy a finger oximeter. The device would warn users if they weren't receiving enough oxygen in their blood, a sign that the disease might be causing them to deteriorate dangerously. In France, amid a shortage of testing kits, many also turned to the oximeter as a way to try and test if they had contracted the virus, although this method was not a reliable indicator. For many, using the oximeter became a daily ritual, recalling superstitious practices from the past that aimed to ward off disease in the absence of a deeper understanding of contagion. More importantly, as hospitals and healthcare spaces remained under strain well after the initial crisis of the early pandemic, the oximeter symbolised the individualisation and decentralisation of healthcare to the domestic environment.

Based on Ana Debenedetti's essay on the *Pandemic Objects* blog

HAND SANITISER

Initially, it was thought that Covid-19 was mainly transmitted by touch, prompting a surge in sales for hand sanitiser. The compulsion to continually sanitise one's hands soon became a ritualistic habit for many, even well after it was determined that the disease was airborne. Hand sanitiser became less a scientifically-proven agent to combat the virus (masks were shown to be far more effective), and more of an emotional and superstitious tic – although regular hand cleaning had many other benefits. Hand sanitiser in the Covid-19 era recalled a long tradition of devices people have held close to their bodies to ward off disease, such as scent-emitting pomanders from the 17th century and masks filled with flowers worn during the Great Plague of 1665 – a talisman for the 21st century.

Based on Antonia Boström's essay on the *Pandemic Objects* blog

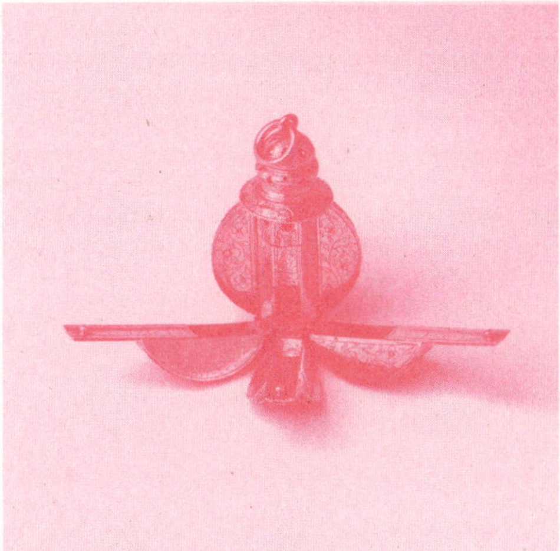

Pomander, England, c1600–10.

MOURNING RINGS

Being able to mourn the loss of loved ones during the pandemic became a particularly acute problem. Traditional spaces for grieving and saying goodbye – the hospital bed, the funeral, the cemetery (p154) – all became relatively inaccessible. Without these venues for collective mourning, grief was often internalised and difficult to resolve. In the absence of funerals, other public ways to acknowledge the loss of life were experimented with, such as newspaper editorials (see Lists p60) and impromptu public memorials.

At the personal level, a common practice from past epidemics was to wear the name or initials of a loved one on the body in the form of jewellery. The tradition of mourning jewellery is a form of rememberance that finds origins as far back as ancient Rome, though it is associated also with the late medieval to Victorian periods. From the 16th century onwards, it became common for written wills to provide instructions and the necessary funds to allow mourners to purchase rings. Mourning rings often name the deceased, sometimes visible to all, sometimes only to the wearer. The mass production of these rings, which could be personalised with inscriptions inside the hoop, began towards the end of the 18th century. Today, this tradition has largely disappeared, but looking back at this piece of jewellery presents both a question and an opportunity: how can objects be used in the long term to retain the personal memory of those we lost in the era of Covid-19?

Based on Catrin Jones' essay
on the *Pandemic Objects* blog

Ring inscribed with the initials of seven children who died within a week, likely of smallpox or cholera, London, 1801.

ICONS

For religious communities, one of the biggest challenges was the closure of places of worship and the consequent need to find new ways of staying spiritually connected during lockdown. In the absence of communal architecture, household objects – such as icons in Orthodox Christianity – helped bridge that gap.

The Orthodox spirituality embodied in the space of the church is a feast for the senses. The visual communication of the holy icons and symbols in the building's decor; the auditory stimulation of the chanting and the rustling of the rich heavy vestments; the sweet scent of the incense burning; the touching of the cross, and the taste of bread and wine form a bridge to the supernatural. With such powerful architecture temporarily unavailable, the icon – which can be found in churches but also in people's homes, offices, shops, boats, cars, motorbikes, even bags and purses – took on renewed importance. Icons are not worshipped as idols but instead are venerated, considered to have the ability to connect Orthodox Christians to the divine. Household and personal icons became a way of making such spiritual connection, recalling the deep power of objects – in their highly decentralised and personalised way – to create bonds with a larger community.

Based on Gina Koutsika's essay
on the *Pandemic Objects* blog

PLAYGROUNDS

One of the most poignant scenes in lockdown was the empty playgrounds. With gates shackled, swings removed or hung high out of reach, red and white barrier tape across the seesaw or looped around the handles of the roundabouts. As vital pieces of civic infrastructure, playgrounds are the result of a long history of advances in developmental psychology and our understanding of early education. From the kindergarten movement, founded by Friedrich Froebel in Germany in 1837, to Donne Buck and others in the 20th century championing play as a fundamental right of children, these spaces are an affirmation that play is a critical foundation for learning. Covid-19 put into stark relief what happens when these spaces are taken away, including damage to young people's learning and emotional wellbeing. Developmental psychologist Alison Gopnik has described children as being the 'R&D department of the human species', where play is a mode of creative experimentation and exploration, a way of developing the 'what ifs' of our imaginative worlds. This chimes with the way designers think and work, exploring the realm of the possible and reifying ideas into material or experiential form. Given how radical a rethink we need to create a world in which everyone can flourish, nurturing and harnessing the potential of play has never been so critical.

Based on Helen Charman's essay
on the *Pandemic Objects* blog

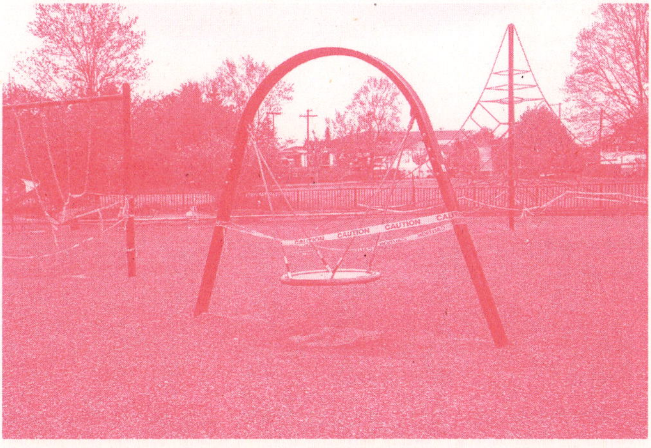

Playground covered in caution tape, Vancouver, 4 May 2020.

SPREADSHEETS

Zoom discos; Houseparty quizzes; WhatsApp groups; Teams meetings: the shutdown amplified and accelerated the use of online apps and software as vital and ersatz interpersonal communication, often bringing with it senses of either vague comfort or deep frustration. Each platform – dependent on the particularities of its pre-shutdown UX design – came with its own constraints. A global pandemic and a series of extended lockdowns were likely never considerations in their initial designs. And so, there we all were, in a situation unanticipated by the software itself, beholden to imperfect platforms to keep relationships alive.

With widespread use, however, came creative takes on how the online world could be hacked for various unanticipated ends (see Google Street View p256). Marie Foulston, a former V&A curator who curated the museum's landmark *Videogames: Design/Play/Disrupt* exhibition in 2018, is an avid explorer of the communicative capacity of different online media. In the first weeks of lockdown, she brought together a virtual field trip through *Black Mesa*, a landscape photography workshop for spacemen in *No Man's Sky* and relocated a keynote talk from Somerset House to an Animal Crossing island (see Animal Crossing p130). Her most unlikely of projects during this period, however, was to turn the online spreadsheet software Google Sheets into a house party.

To do so, Foulston set up a series of tabs, each a different room of the house. On the landing page, she pasted an image of a front door with festive balloons. As people joined the party at a predetermined time, conversations started to appear in the gridded fields of the spreadsheet. People pasted images of snacks, drinks, and other treats they had 'brought along' to the party. The party unfolded in a free-form way: 'The party has grown and evolved,' she recounts. 'A Peep is microwaved in the kitchen. Someone has animated the dance floor. An elaborate backyard has appeared with a perfect lawn, flowers, and a hedge maze. A new sheet is made, it briefly has no purpose. Someone paints every cell blue, it becomes "the blue room". The band Blue appears'.

Prior to the pandemic, Google Sheets had already proved a powerful tool in pooling collective information, most notably to form 'whisper networks' bringing to light sexual misconduct in both the media world as well as the architecture community, in a way that would have been impossible on more public platforms like Twitter.

Explorations such as Foulston's, pushed on by social distancing policies, suggest the potential to yield promising new ways for carving out alternative publics and forums in an increasingly centralised internet ecology. Or at the very least, a new way to have fun online.

Text by Brendan Cormier

BARRIER TAPE

In July 2020, a community of theatre workers in the UK called Scene/Change began staging a nationwide event to draw attention to the plight of theatres in the pandemic. Theatre buildings were wrapped in specially created tape printed with the text 'missing live theatre'. Meanwhile, another initiative organised on behalf of the entire live event industry, called 'Light it in Red', covered stages and venues in red light, drawing attention to the scale and impact of Covid-19 on the workforce behind these now-silent stages (see Music Venues p180).

The site-specific installations created by Scene/Change around UK theatres and performing arts venues were bold and hopeful statements of civic, local and national pride. They were simple scenographic statements, brilliantly executed in individual ways, and inspired and made by a theatre community reaching out and showing solidarity. Sometimes the tape appeared to be exploding from empty buildings, such as the Everyman in Cheltenham or the Swansea Grand Theatre; sometimes it enshrined the theatre like a protective barrier, such as the Theatre Royal Newcastle or the Kiln Theatre in London. Longfield Hall in London turned its building into a kind of maypole, with ribbons streaming from its circular architecture, and many theatres, like Sadler's Wells in London and the Sherman Theatre in Cardiff, used the tape as an inviting enhancement around their entrances.

Introduced during a period of profound uncertainty for live events workers, with drastic redundancies being made by theatres as they struggled to survive lockdown, this clever, bold, playful concept could be shaped and imagined across the profession to suit the architecture and the space, with each transformation part of a clear narrative of support for the struggling industry.

Based on Kate Bailey's essay
on the *Pandemic Objects* blog

Tape, England, c1665–99.

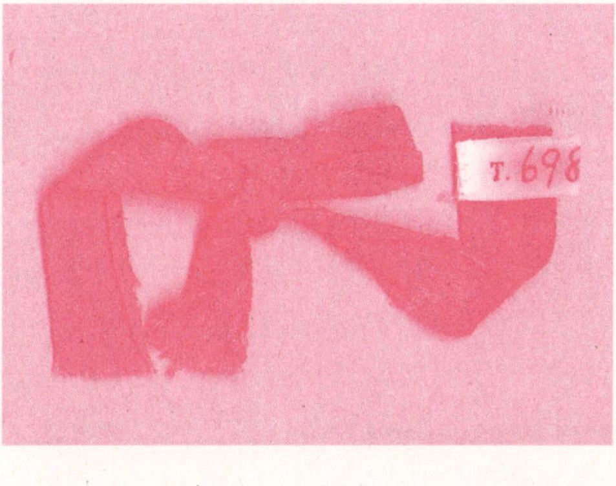

BALCONIES

The balcony became a coveted domestic asset during lockdown. For those who had one, a balcony granted unrestricted access to outdoor space, but also, depending on the location, a way of conversing and being public when most public activities were strictly forbidden. While balconies often ended up under-used as social spaces and overused as storage during non-Covid times, the pandemic was a moment where new social rituals could take place on this de facto stage. An early viral hit was the balcony toasting stick: neighbours in Italy fashioned long bamboo sticks with a glass holder, which could be thrust across balconies to clink glasses with a friend. The balcony also became a scene of serenading and musical performance, and a space to mount banners and signs. The restrictions highlighted the balcony's greatest strength as an in-between space – not quite private, not quite public, but an interface between the two.

Based on Catherine Ince's essay on the *Pandemic Objects* blog

SKIPPING ROPE

With gyms closed during lockdown, people sought out new ways to stay fit. And with so many flats in London too small for at-home workouts, the city's abundant network of parks transformed into outdoor workout zones (see Public Parks p214). Online sales of simple, affordable and portable workout equipment skyrocketed, including skipping rope, resistance bands and medicine balls. And where, prior to the pandemic, working out in parks only seemed acceptable when part of a group, a tipping point occurred during lockdown: the imperative to stay fit outweighed the social anxieties of being seen doing something funny on your own. Suddenly, solo skippers and yogis could be spotted everywhere – a park, after all, presents an infinitely open-ended programme, choreographed by often invisible social codes. The pandemic helped rewrite those codes, with the help of a bit of rope.

Based on Gina Koutsika's essay on the *Pandemic Objects* blog

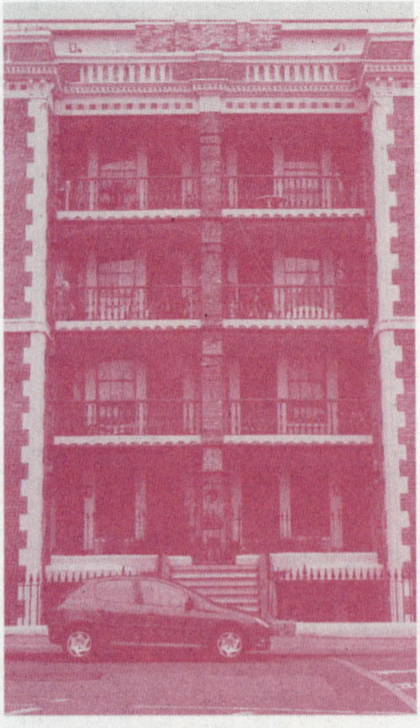

Flats with balconies, Columbia Road, London.

Wallpaper with girls skipping, designed by Walter Crane, Great Britain, 1880.

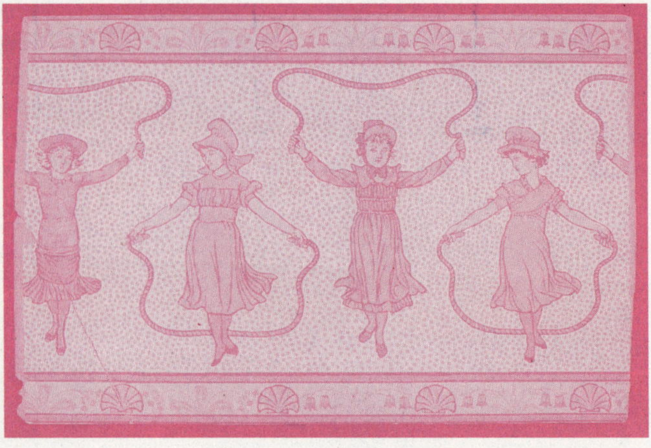

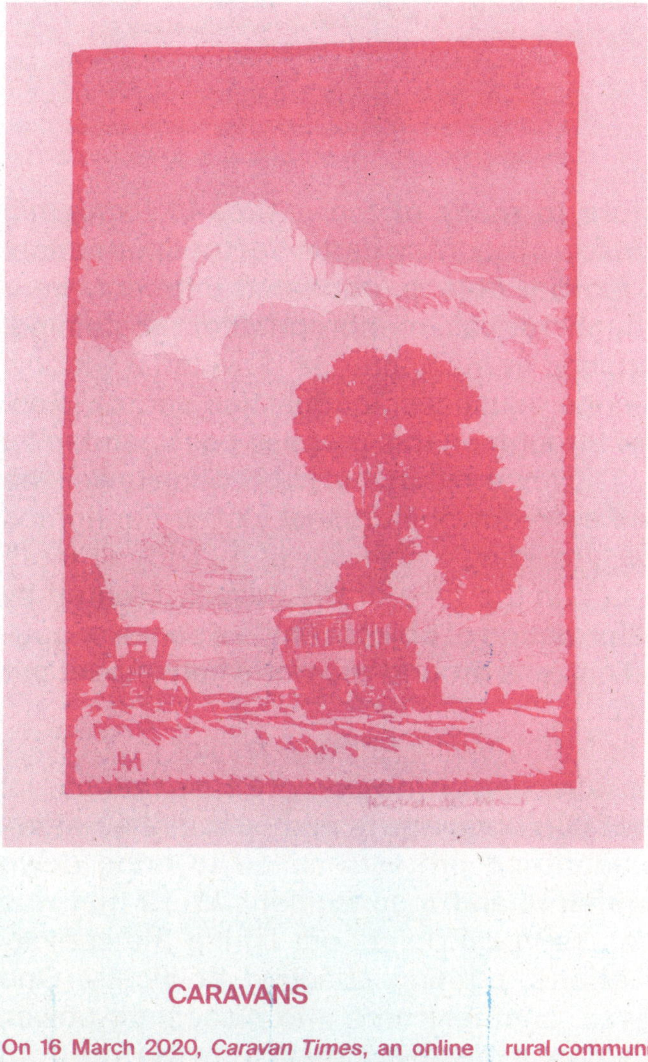

The Caravaners, a linoleum print by Eric Hesketh Hubbard, c1925.

CARAVANS

On 16 March 2020, *Caravan Times*, an online caravanning community, published an article encouraging readers to 'escape the corona hysteria' by taking their caravans to campsites for the duration of the national lockdown. Indeed, national emergencies seem to stoke the appeal for homes on wheels. In May 1939, *The Motor* described the popular caravan model, the Eccles, as an 'emergency retreat' from an 'outbreak of hostilities involving the bombing of our big cities'. The object itself seemed particularly well-suited to a pandemic – as a way, for many, to not only 'escape' to the countryside, but also as a measure of containment for family members who might fall ill. However, for rural communities, the sudden influx of people during the crisis caused pressures on local infrastructures and an understandable fear of potential transmission. Hostile signs directed towards these groups were placed around campsites and in villages. One person's escape was another's burden.

Based on Alice Baddeley's essay on the *Pandemic Objects* blog

Epilogue

Ryan Dillon

There is a cyclical nature to many of the entries in *Pandemic Objects*. Objects often follow a recurring pattern of transformation: the pandemic arrived, familiar objects appeared different, were thus transformed (through revival, reappropriation, abstaining, documenting and so on) and in many entries provided a window into and a call to challenge injustices, inequalities and division. But how might we follow through on this promise post-pandemic, and make real change? The texts within this publication unveil the power possessed by the everyday objects that clutter our homes through an oblique view, providing a new way of thinking or more importantly a spark to act. In the face of the despair created by the pandemic this transformation of objects emits a sense of optimism, and of hope, that citizens around the world can impact our lives from the ground up.

I am reminded of an interview by Enrique Walker in *AA Files* with Paul Virilio, who was reflecting on the journal *Cause Commune*: its response to both the 1968 uprisings in France and their aftermath. In May 1968, student-led protests aimed to bring down capitalist-driven governments and a consumer culture that was eroding society. And yet, as Virilio points out during the conversation, despite these efforts, nothing changed politically. One government was removed, another came into place, into power. Whilst the attempt to dismantle the government from the top, from above, resulted in minimal change for the common citizen, Virilio and those reflecting on these events in *Cause Commune* began to look elsewhere; not from above, but from below. Focused on the 'infra', which means 'below' the writers of *Cause Commune* began to investigate the infraordinary; a call 'to describe the ordinary and habitual aspects of everyday life'. Famously, as part of this aim, the writer Georges Perec asked us to question our teaspoons.

The pandemic provided us the time and the space to look at ordinary objects within our domestic spaces more closely, and to see them afresh with new meanings and uses. *Pandemic Objects* documents this as a particular moment within human history, transforming the book as an object into a time capsule at the scale of a physical archive. Meandering through the collection, you can feel a sense of empowerment, of purpose, of collectiveness, of the good inherent in every one of us to unleash creativity, ingenuity and a sense of freedom to act, for the betterment of each other and for society at large. These pages are full of optimism during a period in which there was every reason to be pessimistic and humour at a time when sadness could have prevailed. The preservation of this moment – to not let it disappear and be rendered meaningless – is to display these transformed artefacts as a reminder that every object we touch daily has an embedded latency capable of being released as long as we are still willing to take the risk to do so.

Acknowledgements

Brendan Cormier

Collaboration underscores all museum life, yet departmental silos still hinder so much of what we do. If anything, *Pandemic Objects* was a radical experiment in breaking down those walls, opening participation to whomever was interested in the project and had something to say. Pre-eminent thanks must be given to all the authors who contributed their time and energy to writing for the blog. I loved the diversity of thoughts, opinions and observations you gave, which all added up, somewhat miraculously, to a coherent whole:

Ella Kilgallon, Kristian Volsing, Catherine Flood, Jessica Eddie, Livia Turnbull, Natalie Kane, Meneesha Kellay, Zofia Trafas White, Becky Knott, Catherine Ince, Christopher Turner, Kristina Rapacki, Gus Casely-Hayford, Samantha Manton, Gina Koutsika, Ella Ravilious, Christopher Wilk, Antonia Boström, Joanna Norman, Jasmine Farram, Caroline McCaffrey-Howarth, Lisa Galvin, Priya Khanchandani, Kathleen Walker-Meikle, Kate Bailey, Harriet Reed, Duncan Forbes, Ana Debenedetti, Melanie Vandenbrouck, Catrin Jones, Helen Charman, Georgia Haseldine, Alice Power, Ruth Hibbard, Josephine Rout, James Robinson, Rachel Dedman, Katy Canales, Alice Baddeley, Kaja Marczewska, Melanie Lenz, Jenna Mason, Hana Kaluznick, Isolde Nicolaysen, Lucia Savi, Esmé Hogeveen, Stephanie Wood, Anna Talley, William Newton, Mariam Rosser-Owen, Gill Saunders, Sara Kassam, Maude Willaerts, Masami Yamada and Johanna Agerman Ross.

I'm especially grateful to Christopher Turner, former Keeper of the design, architecture and digital department, where I worked, for greenlighting the proposal. Tom Windross, Head of Content at the V&A, graciously made accommodations on our blog for the project to happen, lending advice along the way for how to structure it. Keith Hale patiently walked me through the ins and outs of WordPress. Phoebe Moore and Callum Walker in our communications department did incredible work promoting *Pandemic Objects*, resulting in perhaps the most press coverage of a museum blog project in the history of museum blog projects. And a special thanks to the V&A Director and Deputy Director, Tristram Hunt and Tim Reeve, for giving the whole endeavour their institutional backing.

Over at the Architectural Association, I'm permanently indebted to Ryan Dillon, Kristina Rapacki and Maria Shéhérazade Giudici for backing the idea of turning the blog into a book. What seemed like a simple task of taking text from one format to another proved to be, in the end, not an easy task at all, as well as being incredibly time-consuming. I'm very happy we persisted, and that Max Zarzycki could step into the project midway through and lend their fresh eyes to the editorial process, bringing it to the finish line. Thank you to authors who added texts from the AA, Alison Moffett and Anna Lisa Reynolds, to round out the collaboration and bring new perspectives, and to Caspar Bailey for designing the book, and giving it such considered shape and form. Finally, thank you to Ingrid Schroder, for her continued support of the project as she took the helm as Director of the AA.

As this book has thoroughly demonstrated, the pandemic shattered any sense of division between work life, domestic life and social life. My daughter was born six weeks before the first lockdown began, and so almost all of my early work on this project took place in the same 45 square metres where my wife, Azadeh Mashayekhi, and I were learning to be new parents. I'm eternally grateful to her patience and support throughout, and see this book, in part, as a memory to those agonisingly challenging and joyous times.

Credits

Every effort has been made to trace the copyright holders and obtain permission to reproduce the images featured in this publication.

13
Image © Victoria and Albert Museum, accession number PH.230-1982.

16, 17 (top)
Andrew Louis.

17 (bottom)
m-louis / Flickr / CC BY-SA 2.0 DEED.

19
Cloudco. Image © Victoria and Albert Museum, accession number B.1479-1999.

21
Image © Victoria and Albert Museum, accession number 328-1888.

23
Image © Victoria and Albert Museum.

24
Sandra Fauconnier / Wikimedia Commons / CC BY 4.0 DEED.

25
Juliette Lee.

27
Joanne Allnutt. Image © Victoria and Albert Museum, accession number B.2-2018.

28
Image © Victoria and Albert Museum, accession number CIRC.449-1974.

30 (top)
Katy Canales.

30 (bottom)
jimu25702 / Instagram.

33
Christopher Michel / Wikimedia Commons / CC BY 2.0.

35–6
Brendan Cormier.

37
Photograph by Francesco Noferini, courtesy of Caret Studio.

39
Hirbawi. Image © Victoria and Albert Museum, accession number ME.12-2021.

41
Mohammed Musallam. Image © Victoria and Albert Museum, accession number ME.13-2021.

42 (left)
Hirbawi. Image © Victoria and Albert Museum, accession number ME.12-2021.

42 (right)
Mohammed Musallam. Image © Victoria and Albert Museum, accession number ME.13-2021.

43
Hirbawi. Image © Victoria and Albert Museum, accession number ME.12-2021.

45 (top)
Rehgina / Wikimedia Commons / CC BY-SA 4.0 DEED.

45 (bottom)
Dima Srouji.

47
Image © Victoria and Albert Museum, accession number E.13574-1886.

48
Image © Victoria and Albert Museum, accession number E.13841-1886.

50
Image © Victoria and Albert Museum, accession number E.5391-1886.

51
Image © Victoria and Albert Museum, accession number E.13607-1886.

53
Gary Martin. Image © Victoria and Albert Museum, accession number E.516-1993.

57 (top left)
Declan Buckley and Hywel Williams. Image © Victoria and Albert Museum, accession number E.1025-2002.

57 (top right)
Yossi Lemel and G Korisky. Image © Victoria and Albert Museum, accession number E.1229-1995.

57 (bottom)
Gran Fury. Image © Victoria and Albert Museum, accession number E.472-1993.

61
From The New York Times. © 2020 The New York Times Company. All rights reserved. Used under license.

63
Johns Hopkins University.

65
Photo by Victoria Sambunaris, courtesy of Maya Lin Studio.

67
Image © Victoria and Albert Museum, accession number 1872-1899.

69
Seongnam City / Wikimedia Commons.

71
DJI. Image © Victoria and Albert Museum, accession number CD.102-2016.

73
Image © Victoria and Albert Museum, accession number RPS.906-2019.

74–81
Eithne Nightingale.

85–7
Shashank Peshawaria.

89–97
Natasha Durlacher.

99–104
© Simon Roberts. Courtesy of the artist.

109
Catherine Flood.

112
May Rosenthal Sloan.

113
Laura Wilson.

117
Samantha Manton.

121
Image © Victoria and Albert Museum, accession number C.19-1982.

123
Image © Victoria and Albert Museum, accession number 414:253/A-1885.

125
Image © Victoria and Albert Museum, accession number S.133:438-2007.

129
Jill Downs. Image © Victoria and Albert Museum, accession number B.291-2010.

131
Image © Victoria and Albert Museum, accession number 581-1870.

132
Alice Power / Nintendo.

134
Image © Victoria and Albert Museum, accession number P.40-1910.

135
Alice Power / Nintendo.

137
Bill Brandt © Bill Brandt Archive Ltd. Image © Victoria and Albert Museum, accession number PH.28-1978.

141
Cinephonic Music Co. Image © Victoria and Albert Museum, accession number S.600-2014.

143
JVC Ltd. Image © Victoria and Albert Museum, accession number W.661-2001.

145
© Estate of Abram Games.
Image © Victoria and Albert Museum, accession number E.820-2004.

149
Image © Victoria and Albert Museum, accession number E.1479-1991.

151
Anchal Vohra / Voice of America.

152
Wellcome Collection / CC BY 4.0.

153
Max Zarzycki.

155
Image © Victoria and Albert Museum, accession number CIRC.54-1930.

157
Image © Victoria and Albert Museum, accession number 5839-1938.

161
Image © Victoria and Albert Museum, accession number A.2-1964.

164
Image © Victoria and Albert Museum, accession number AL.9254:11.

165 (top)
Hilary Powell. Image © Victoria and Albert Museum, accession number E.3297-2018.

165 (bottom)
Hilary Powell. Image © Victoria and Albert Museum, accession number E.3291-2018.

167
Image © Victoria and Albert Museum, accession number E.219-1987.

171
Cityswift / Flickr / CC BY 2.0 DEED.

173
Image © Victoria and Albert Museum, accession number IS.149-1993.

175
Image © Victoria and Albert Museum, accession number T.331-1982.

177
Image © Victoria and Albert Museum, accession number 02545(IS).

179
Image © Victoria and Albert Museum, accession number PH.1160-1980

181
Image © Victoria and Albert Museum, accession number PH.345-1982.

185
Image © Victoria and Albert Museum, accession number S.1831-2013.

187
Image © Victoria and Albert Museum, accession number W.22-1937.

189
Image © Victoria and Albert Museum, accession number S.2564-2009.

191
Image © Victoria and Albert Museum, accession number E.138-1925.

193
Image © Victoria and Albert Museum, accession number CIRC.427-1971.

194
Brendan Cormier.

195
Oskar Karlin.

199
Image © Victoria and Albert Museum, accession number E.1300-1988.

203
Hinge.

205
Image © Victoria and Albert Museum, accession number E.1904-1934.

207–9
Coltrane McDowell.

211
Image © Victoria and Albert Museum, accession number E.1397-1959.

213
Image © Victoria and Albert Museum, accession number E.208:3911-1994.

215
Brendan Cormier.

219 (top)
Zofia Trafas White.

219 (bottom)
Image © Victoria and Albert Museum, accession number E.4944-1923.

221
James Stirling/Michael Wilford fonds, Canadian Centre for Architecture © CCA.

226
mira66 / Flickr / CC BY 2.0.

227
John Fielding / CC BY 2.0.

229
Image © Victoria and Albert Museum, accession number E.429-1899.

233
Image © Victoria and Albert Museum, accession number PH.1157-1980.

237
Image © Victoria and Albert Museum, accession number E.575-1985.

238
Sludge G / Flickr / CC BY-SA 2.0.

240
BDP.

243
Scope. Image © Victoria and Albert Museum, acccession number E.977-2002.

245
Shakeyjon / Alamy.

249–51
Sports Banger Publishing.

253
Slow and Steady Wins the Race. Image © Victoria and Albert Museum, accession number T.195-2016.

255
Glastonbury Festival.

257
KAC Cresswell. Image © Ashmolean Museum, University of Oxford

259
KAC Cresswell. Image © Ashmolean Museum, University of Oxford

260
Anthony Lobay / Google Street View.

261
O A / Google Street View.

263
Image © Victoria and Albert Museum, accession number FE.1-1971.

265
John Wilson / X.

267
Brendan Cormier.

271
Image © Victoria and Albert Museum, accession number C.740-1924.

272
Image © Victoria and Albert Museum, accession number LOAN:GILBERT.622-2008.

275
Unilever. Image © Victoria and Albert Museum, accession number E.861-1919.

277
Singer Manufacturing Co. Image © Victoria and Albert Museum, accession number T.1600-2017.

281
Singer Manufacturing Co. Image © Library of Congress, Prints and Photographs Division.

283
Image © Victoria and Albert Museum, accession number B.350-2012.

285
Image © Victoria and Albert Museum, accession number B.1-2010.

287–90
Jenny Elliott (CMLI).

293
Nigel Shafran. Image © Victoria and Albert Museum, accession number E.262-1999.

294
Thomas Brenac / Wikimedia Commons / CC BY-SA 4.0.

297
Peter Pitt. Image © RIBA Collections.

299
Philips. Image © Victoria and Albert Museum, accession number W.3&A-1978.

300
Library of Congress, Prints and Photographs Division, LC-DIG-matpc014326.

302
Elias Anastas.

303
Library of Congress, Prints and Photographs Division, photograph by Harris & Ewing, LC-DIG-hec-47251.

307
Greenpeace. Image © Victoria and Albert Museum, accession number E.3167-1991.

308
Maksym Kozlenko / Wikimedia Commons / CC BY-SA 4.0.

311
SquidHomme / Wikimedia Commons / CC BY-SA 4.0.

313
OLPC. Image © Victoria and Albert Museum, accession number W.9-2011.

317
Image © Victoria and Albert Museum, accession number B.284-1999.

319
Image © Victoria and Albert Museum, accession number PH.2188-1903

320
Materialise.

321 (left)
Brendan Cormier.

321 (right)
Materialise.

323
Image © Victoria and Albert Museum, accession number M.37-1972.

325
Image © Victoria and Albert Museum, accession number E.3552-2004.

327
Richard Blundel. Image © Victoria and Albert Museum, accession number B.610-2016.

329
US Department of Agriculture.

331
Richie S / Wikimedia Commons / CC BY 2.0.

333
Image © Victoria and Albert Museum, accession number E.484-2009.

337
Brendan Cormier.

338
Image © Victoria and Albert Museum, accession number S.795-2009.

339
Image © Victoria and Albert Museum, accession number SD.367.

340 (left)
Image © Victoria and Albert Museum, accession number 297-1869.

340 (right)
Image © Victoria and Albert Museum, accession number CIRC.34-1970.

341 (top)
ACurio. Image © Victoria and Albert Museum, accession number CD.2-2022.

341 (right)
Image © Victoria and Albert Museum, accession number LOAN:GILBERT.578-2008.

342
Image © Victoria and Albert Museum, accession number M.18-2004.

343
Rod Raglin / Flickr / CC BY-SA 4.0 DEED.

345
Image © Victoria and Albert Museum, accession number T.698-1997.

346 (left)
Justinc / Wikimedia Commons / CC BY-SA 2.0 DEED.

346 (right)
Image © Victoria and Albert Museum, accession number E.4030-1915.

347
Eric Hesketh Hubbard. Image © Victoria and Albert Museum, accession number CIRC.516-1925.

Pandemic Objects
edited by Brendan Cormier

First published in 2024 by AA Publications
in association with the Victoria and
Albert Museum.

AA Publications are designed, edited and
produced by the Communications Studio
at the Architectural Association School of
Architecture (AA).

DESIGN
Caspar Bailey

EDITORS
Ryan Dillon
Kristina Rapacki
Max Zarzycki

PROOFING
Charlotte Jones

Set in Suisse Int'l
Printed in Belgium by Albe De Coker

ISBN 978-1-919624518

AA Publications
36 Bedford Square
London, WC1B 3ES

For a catalogue of AA Publications visit
www.aaschool.ac.uk/publications or email
publications@aaschool.ac.uk.